$.
#B200CPS
£36.99
616.0754

Clinical Examination

Dedication

June, Daniel, Marc, Morris and Nancy
Harry, George, Josephine, Tom and Ted
Anna, Alastair and Fiona
Anne, John and Joe

Commissioning Editors: Richard Furn, Laurence Hunter
Project Development Manager: Janice Urquhart
Project Manager: Nancy Arnott
Designer: George Ajayi
Illustrator: Marion Tasker, MTG

Clinical Examination

Third edition

Owen Epstein MB BCh FRCP
Consultant Physician and Gastroenterologist,
Royal Free Hospital NHS Trust, London, UK

G. David Perkin BA MB FRCP
Consultant Neurologist, Regional Neurosciences Centre,
Charing Cross Hospital, London, UK

John Cookson MD FRCP
Professor of Medical Education, Hull and York Medical School,
University of York, York, UK

David P. de Bono (deceased)

With contributions from

Neil Solomons MB ChB FRCS
Consultant Surgeon, Otolaryngology – Head and Neck/Facial Plastic Surgery,
Royal Surrey County Hospital, Guildford, UK

Andrew Robins MB MSc MRCP FRCPCH
Consultant Paediatrician,
Whittington Hospital NHS Trust, London, UK

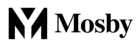 Mosby

EDINBURGH LONDON NEW YORK OXFORD PHILADELPHIA ST LOUIS SYDNEY TORONTO 2003

MOSBY
An imprint of Elsevier Limited

Second edition 1997
Third edition 2003
  Reprinted 2004

ISBN 0 7234 3229 5

British Library Cataloguing in Publication Data
A catalogue record for this book is available from the British Library

Library of Congress Cataloging in Publication Data
A catalog record for this book is available from the Library of Congress

Note
Medical knowledge is constantly changing. Standard safety precautions must be followed, but as new research and clinical experience broaden our knowledge, changes in treatment and drug therapy may becme necessary or appropriate. Readers are advised to check the most current product information provided by the manufacturer of each drug to be administered to verify the recommended dose, the method and duration of administration, and contraindications. It is the responsibility of the practitioner, relying on experience and knowledge of the patient, to determine dosages and the best treatment for each individual patient. Neither the Publisher nor the authors assume any liability for any injury and/or damage to persons or property arising from this publication.   **The Publisher**

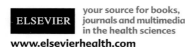

ELSEVIER   your source for books,
           journals and multimedia
           in the health sciences
www.elsevierhealth.com

The
publisher's
policy is to use
**paper manufactured
from sustainable forests**

Printed in Spain

Preface

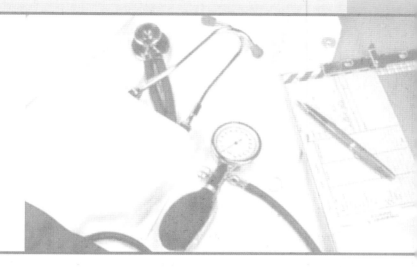

The techniques and skills required for a competent clinical examination can only be mastered by practice at the bedside. However, a thorough and intelligent clinical examination relies heavily on an understanding of normal and abnormal anatomy and physiology as well as 'pattern recognition' of disease. *Clinical Examination* has been written as a companion for medical students and postgraduates acquiring or revising clinical skills. The book guides the user through the anatomy and physiology of each system and builds on this information to describe the normal and abnormal examination

Examining patients draws on the senses of sight (inspection), touch (palpation) and hearing (percussion and auscultation). The detailed text is complemented by almost 1 000 coloured illustrations, clinical photographs, tables and seven distinct types of summary box which are colour coded with icons for easy recognition and quick revision. Although clinical examination of the elderly population differs little from the younger population, the book provides a special reference to those aspects which deserve specific attention in the elderly. At the other end of the spectrum, the paediatric examination differs substantially from the adult and a guide to the examination of the new-born and growing infant and child is also included in the book.

The book is divided into systems and is colour coded to allow easy access to each chapter. The first chapter illustrates the problem orientated approach to case notes and record keeping. The chapter includes a general introduction to history taking with more detailed information available in individual chapters. Chapter 2 deals with the general physical examination and syndrome recognition, and describes those systems which do not fall neatly into the regional examination (endocrine and lymphatic systems). The clinical characterics of most of the common skin, hair and nail disorders are described in chapter 3. This is followed by chapters on regional examination including the ears, nose and throat, cardiovascular system, chest and lungs, abdomen, male and female genitalia, the musculoskeletal system and the nervous system. The final chapter is focused on the examination of the neonate, toddler and growing child, up to and including adolescence. Each chapter is introduced by a description of anatomy and physiology (structure and function), the history and the normal and abnormal examination. Wherever possible, the description of the physical examination is accompanied by artwork and clinical photographs to illustrate the examination technique.

It is well to remember that most medical problems can be solved by careful clinical assessment. This book is a rich resource to help learn and teach these clinical skills.

Acknowledgements

We wish to thank the following individuals and organisations for generously providing illustrative material: Dr Philip Bardsley, Dr Russell Lane, Dr Mike Morgan, Dr P. H. McKee and Dr John Wales; Joan Slack, Dept of Clinical Genetics, Royal Free NHS Trust (Figs 2.3–2.7, 2.9–2.16); Dr Les Berger, Dept of Radiology, Royal Free NHS Trust (Figs 2.36, 2.37, 7.16a); Dr Malcolm Rustin (Figs 3.12, 3.15, 3.23–3.26, 3.30, 3.31, 3.70–3.72); King's College Hospital (Figs 3.13, 3.14, 3.16, 3.37, 3.39–3.43, 3.45–3.47, 3.54, 3.65, 3.73, 3.74) for slides reproduced from Anthony du Vivier: Atlas of Clinical Dermatology (Gower Medical Publishing UK, 1986); Professor Tony Wright (Figs 4.29, 4.31–4.34); Dr James Entwhistle for Figs 5.5–5.10; Dr C. Richards for Fig. 5.13; Dame Margaret Turner-Warwick et al (Figs 5.2, 5.11, 5.12, 5.14, 5.20, 5.29) for slides reproduced from Clinical Atlas of Respiratory Diseases (Gower Medical Publishing UK, 1989); Professor Robert H. Anderson and Dr Sally P. Allwork (Figs 6.4, 6.6, 6.7) for slides reproduced form Cardiac Anatomy (Gower Medical Publishing UK, 1980); Dr James S. Bingham (Figs 8.37, 8.43–8.46, 9.14, 9.15, 9.29) for slides reproduced from Sexually Transmitted Diseases (Gower Medical Publishing UK, 1984); Dr Paul A. Dieppe et al (Figs 10.8, 10.9, 10.38, 10.42, 10.50–10.52, 10.64, 10.66, 10.69, 10.75, 10.77, 10.78, 10.80, 10.81, 10.91) for slides reproduced from Atlas of Clinical Rheumatology (Gower Medical Publishing UK, 1986); Mr David Spalton et al (Figs 11.24–11.28, 11.30–11.39, 11.52, 11.62, 11.64, 11.65) Atlas of Clinical Ophthalmology (Gower Medical Publishing UK, 1984).

The figures listed below were derived with permission from the following sources: Fig. 11.13 from R. B. Strub and F. William Black: The Mental Status Examination in Neurology (F A Davis Co); Figs 11.16, 11.17, 11.19, 11.24–11.26, 11.28–11.41, 11.43–11.45, 11.50, 11.52, 11.62, 11.65) from David Spalton: Atlas of Clinical Ophthalmology (Gower Medical Publishing UK, 1984); Fig. 11.41 (right) from Haymaker, Webb: Bing's Local Diagnosis in Neurological Diseases, 15th edn (St Louis, The C V Mosby Co, 1989); Figs 11.46 and 11.47 from J. S. Glaser: Neuro-ophthalmology (Harper & Row); Figs 11.48 and 11.49 from R. John Leigh and David S. Zee: The Neurology of Eye Movement (F A Davis Co); Fig. 11.110 from Drs J. W. Lance and J. G. McLeod: A Physiological Approach to Clinical Neurology (Butterworths); Fig. 11.107 from Lord Walton of Detchant: Introduction to Clinical Neuroscience, 2nd edn (Baillière Tindall Ltd); Fig. 11.100 from Professor R. S. Snell: Clinical Neuroanatomy for Medical Students, 2nd edn (Little, Brown & Co); Figs 11.108 and 11.109 from Dr V. B. Brooks: Neural Basis of Motor Control (Oxford University Press); Fig. 11.138 from 'Somaesthetic Pathways' Br Med Bull, 33, 113–120, 1977; Fig. 11.146 from Professor Ian A. D. Bouchier CBE and J. S. Morris; Clinical Skills, 2nd edn (W B Saunders); Figs 11.154–11.156 from Dr F. Plum: Diagnosis of Stupor and Coma, 3rd edn (F A Davis Co). Figs 12.1, 12.16–12.27 and 12.29 from Dr Caroline Fertleman, UCL Medical School; Figs 12.3–12.4, 12.30b–12.30k, 12.30m–12.30o, 12.32–12.33, 12.36–12.38 and 12.43 from Dr Heather Mackinnon, Whittington Hospital. Figs 12.5, 12.7 12.10–12.11, 12.44–12.45 and 12.49; Growth charts reproduced with kind permission of Castlemead Publications, Welwyn Garden City; Figs 12.12 and 12.34 with kind permission from Dr T. Lissauer: Illustrated Textbook of Paediatrics (Mosby International); Fig. 12.46 from Professor J. Godfrey.

Contents

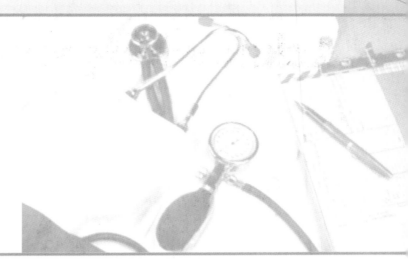

health-related problems. The master problem list is placed at the front of the medical record and each entry is dated (Fig. 1.2). This date refers to the time of the entry, not the date when the patient first noted the problem (this can be indicated in brackets alongside the problem). The dates entered into the problem list not only provide a chronology of the patient's health-related problems but also a 'table of contents' which serves the medical record. Using the entry date as a reference, there should be no difficulty finding the original entry in the notes. In addition to providing a summary and index, the problem list also assists the development of management plans.

Setting up the problem list

Divide the problems into those that are active (or require active management) and those that are inactive (problems that have resolved or require no action but may be important at some stage in the patient's present or future management). An entry of 'Peptic ulcer (1971)' in the 'inactive' column will provide a reminder to someone considering the use of a non-steroidal anti-inflammatory (NSAID) drug in a patient presenting at a later date with arthritis. The problem list is dynamic and the page is designed to allow you to shift problems between the active and inactive columns (Fig. 1.3).

Your entries into the problem list may include established diagnoses (e.g. ulcerative colitis), symptoms (e.g. dyspnoea), physical signs (e.g. ejection systolic murmur), laboratory tests (e.g. anaemia), psychological and social history (e.g. depression, unemployment, parental or marital problems) or special risk factors (e.g. smoking, alcohol or narcotic abuse). The diagnostic level at which you make the entry depends on the information available at a particular moment. Express the problem at the highest possible level but update the list if new findings alter or refine your understanding of the problem. The problem list is designed to accommodate change; consequently, it is not necessary to delete an entry once a higher level of diagnosis (or understanding) is reached. For example, a patient may

---

Problem-related plans

	Problem	Differential diagnosis	Investigation
Dx	jaundice		liver tests, prothrombin time
		acute hepatitis	hepatitis screen (A, B and C)
			auto-antibodies
			(SMA, ANA, AMA)
		alcohol	mean cell volume gamma GT
		drugs	check with family doctor
		obstructive jaundice	ultrasound liver
	anorexia	see jaundice	urea and electrolytes
	weight loss	see jaundice	basal weight
	recurrent rectal bleeding	haemorrhoids	full blood count
		polyp or colon cancer	proctoscopy
			colonoscopy or barium enema
	smoking		chest radiograph

	Problem	Monitor
Mx	jaundice	twice weekly liver tests
	anorexia	monitor diet and caloric intake
	weight loss	twice weekly weight
	recurrent rectal bleeding	haemoglobin weekly

	Problem	Treatment
Rx	jaundice	bed-rest
	anorexia	encourage calorific intake (favourite foods)
	weight loss	special high calorific drink supplements
	recurrent rectal bleeding	treat cause
		(haemorrhoids or tumour) seek surgical opinion
	smoking	encourage relaxation and stress management
	unemployed	arrange meeting with social worker

	Problem	Education
Ed	jaundice	discuss differential diagnosis
	anorexia	explain association with jaundice
	smoking	discuss dangers, techniques for coping
	rectal bleeding	explain need for colonic investigation

Fig. 1.4 Example of a problem-related plan after the creation of a problem list. (Dx, diagnostic tests; Mx, monitoring tests; Rx, treatments; Ed, education)

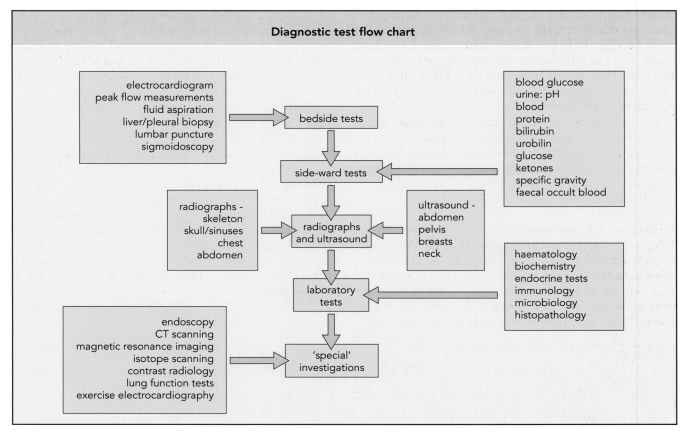

Fig. 1.5   Flow diagram to help plan diagnostic tests.

present with the problems of jaundice, anorexia and weight loss. This information will be entered into the problem list (Fig. 1.2). If, a few days later, serological investigation confirms that the patient was suffering from type A viral hepatitis, this new level of diagnosis can be entered on a new line in the block reserved for active problem 1 (Fig. 1.3). Other problems explained by the diagnosis (anorexia and weight loss) should be amended with an arrow and asterisk to indicate the connection with the solved problem. At this point, viral hepatitis represents the highest level of diagnosis. Once the disease has resolved, an arrow to the opposite 'inactive' column will indicate the point during follow-up that the doctor noted return of the liver tests to normal (Fig. 1.3). Unexpected problems may become evident in the course of investigation (e.g. hypercholesterolaemia) and these are added to the problem list.

The problem list should be under constant review to ensure that the entries are accurate and up to date.

INITIAL PROBLEM-RELATED PLANS

The POMR offers a structured approach to the management of a patient's problems. By constructing the problem list you will have clearly defined problems requiring active management (i.e. investigation and treatment), so it should be reasonably easy to develop a management plan (Fig. 1.4) by considering four headings (see below); all or only some of these headings may be applicable to a particular problem.

Diagnostic tests (Dx)

Write differential next to each problem. Adjacent to each of the possible diagnoses, enter the investigation that may aid the diagnosis. There are a large number of special tests that may be applicable to a particular problem; therefore, it is useful to evolve a general framework for investigation and to adapt this to each problem. You can construct a logical flow of investigations by considering bedside tests, side ward tests, plain radiographs, ultrasound, blood tests and specialised imaging examinations (Fig. 1.5).

Monitoring tests (Mx)

Monitoring information provides evidence of the patient's progress. Consider whether a particular problem can be monitored; if so, document the appropriate tests and the frequency with which they should be performed to provide meaningful information.

Treatment (Rx)

Consider each problem in turn with a view to deciding on a treatment strategy. If drug treatment is indicated, note the drug and dosage. Include a plan for monitoring both side effects and the effectiveness of treatment.

Education (Ed)

An important component of your patient's management is education. Patients are able to cope better with their illness if they understand its nature, its likely course and the effect of treatment. By including this heading in your plans, you will be reminded of the need to talk to your patient about the illness and encouraged to develop an educational plan for your overall management strategy.

PROGRESS NOTES

The POMR provides a disciplined and standardised structure to follow-up notes. These should be succinct and brief, focusing mainly on change. There are four headings to guide you through the progress note (Fig. 1.6).

Subjective (S)

Record any change in the patient's symptoms and, when necessary, comment on compliance with a particular regimen (e.g. stopping smoking) or tolerance of drug treatment.

Objective (O)

Record any change in physical signs and investigations that may influence diagnosis, monitoring or treatment.

Assessment (A)

Comment on whether the subjective and objective information has confirmed or altered your assessment and plans.

Plan (P)

After making the assessment, consider whether any modification of the original plan is needed. Structure

Flow sheet						
Date / Tests	9.1.02	11.1.02	13.1.02	14.1.02	7.2.02	14.2.02
Bilirubin (<17)	233	190	130		28	10
AST (<40)	1140	830	500		52	23
ALT (<45)	1600	650	491		61	31
Albumin (35–45)	41	40	41		42	43
Pro-time (s)	14/12	14/12	13/12	discharged	13/12	12/12
Haemoglobin (11.5–16.2)	12.1	12.3	12.1		12.2	12.6
Blood urea (3.5–6.5)	3.1	4.2	4.8		6.0	6.2
Blood glucose (3.5–6.5)	5.5	6.8	5.0		5.6	6,0
Hepatitis screen			IgM Hep A +ve			
Cholesterol (3.5–6.8)			8.1			8.4

Fig. 1.7 Example of a flow sheet.

Progress notes
date
11/1/02   S – nauseated, fatigued

O – less jaundiced
            liver less tender
            taking adequate calories and fluid
            ultrasound liver/biliary tract: normal
         A – seems to be improving
            no obstruction
         P – check liver tests tomorrow
            phone laboratory for hepatitis markers

13/1/02   S – feels considerably better, appetite improving
         O – transaminase levels and bilirubin falling
            IgM antibody to hepatitis A positive
            sigmoidoscopy: bleeding haemorrhoids
            hypercholesterolaemia
         A – resolving hepatitis A
            rectal bleeding in young patient likely
            to be haemorrhoids
         P – reassess patient, explain hepatitis A
            consider discharge if next set of liver tests
            show sustained improvement; ask surgeon
            to consider treating haemorrhoids
            recheck cholesterol in 3 months

Fig. 1.6 Example of follow-up notes.

this section according to the headings listed earlier (Dx, Mx, Rx and Ed).

If there is no subjective or objective change from one visit to the next, simply record 'No change in assessment or plans'.

FLOW CHARTS

Clinical investigations and measurements are often repeated to monitor the course of acute or chronic illness. For example, patients presenting with diabetic ketoacidosis require frequent checks of blood sugar, urea, electrolytes, blood pH, urine output and central venous pressure. In chronic renal failure, the course of the disease and its treatment is monitored by repeated measurements of blood urea and electrolytes, creatinine, creatinine clearance, haemoglobin and body weight. A flow sheet is convenient for recording these data in a format that, at a glance, provides a summary of trends and progress (Fig. 1.7). Graphs may be equally revealing (Fig. 1.8).

ADVANTAGES OF THE POMR

The POMR encourages all the members of the healthcare team to standardise their approach to record-keeping. This, in turn, enhances communication and

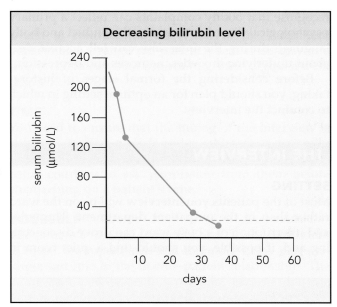

Decreasing bilirubin level

Fig. 1.8 Example of the use of a graph to illustrate changes in bilirubin levels following acute type A hepatitis.

guarantees that everybody involved in the patient's care can contribute to the medical biography. Furthermore, careful structuring of the problem list, care plans and follow-up notes encourages logical, disciplined thinking and ensures that the record is comprehensive and accurate. The POMR approach to record-keeping counteracts the tendency for the 'weight' of a single problem to overwhelm and to distract from other subsidiary but potentially important problems.

Peer review and medical audit have become an integral part of quality assurance and continuing medical education. The structure of the POMR exposes the clinician's thoughts and decision-making processes. This, in itself, is educational for both the clinician and anyone else reading the notes and makes the system particularly suited to the process of audit. The pressure to record meticulous and detailed information is also of intrinsic value to research workers embarking on retrospective or prospective clinical studies. Perhaps most importantly, the POMR helps to maintain a perspective of the 'whole' patient, thereby providing an overview of physical, psychological and social problems and their interaction in health and disease.

CONFIDENTIALITY

Clinical notes contain confidential information and it is important that you protect this confidentiality. Ensure that there is control over access to the medical record and that only individuals directly involved in the patient's care should read or write in the notes. In certain circumstances special security may be necessary. Patients with HIV infection and AIDS and individuals attending sexually transmitted or psychiatric

clinics may have a separate set of clinical notes that are maintained distinct from the general medical records. Access to these classified records is usually restricted to doctors working in that department and the notes never leave the area of the specialist unit.

INTERVIEWING TECHNIQUES AND HISTORY-TAKING

Studies indicate that over 80% of diagnoses in general medical clinics are based on the interview. It is clear that the way in which the interview is conducted and the type of questions asked determine the amount of diagnostically useful information the patient reveals.

For many patients, particularly those seen in the outpatient clinic, the process of history-taking is liable to take longer than the physical examination. Your first step should be to read the referral letter. Sometimes the information provided is inadequate and barely legible (Fig. 1.9) but often you will find a wealth of clinical detail (Fig. 1.10) relating to the patient's history that the patient has either forgotten or chosen not to reveal. During the interview, you will use a combination of open-ended and closed questions. The former deal in generalisations.

 Questions to ask
Open-ended questions

- What's troubling you?
- What brought you to see the doctor?
- What brought you to the hospital?
- What are your symptoms?
- The referral letter tells me something of your symptoms but can you describe them to me?

Other questions require a more specific response: 'Do you experience chest pain when you exercise?' A history confined to closed questions takes the form of an interrogation; taken to its extreme, the patient would simply need to answer 'yes' and 'no' to a succession of questions. Open-ended questions allow the patient freedom to respond, but therein lies the danger. The successful interview allows the patient to set the course but the interviewer keeps a steady hand on the tiller and makes adjustments whenever the course seems to veer. As you learn to structure history-taking, a balance between these two types of question will emerge. Generally start with open-ended questions, then gradually introduce closed ones if certain aspects of the history remain unclear.

Both students and doctors often overlook the psychodynamic components of a physical illness or fail to

of the symptom, its mode of onset, its progression or regression and aggravating or relieving factors.

For each symptom, explore the three items listed in the summary box below:

> **Symptoms and signs**
> **Symptoms helping distinguish different sources of chest pain**
>
> - Myocardial ischaemia – pressure, crushing, pressing retrosternal pain
> - Pleuritic and chest wall pain – localised, sharp, distinct exacerbation with deep inspiration
> - Gastro-oesophageal reflux pain – burning retrosternal discomfort (heartburn) arising from behind the sternum

For the assessment of pain, use the framework shown in the box. The quality of the pain is important in determining the organ of origin. Patients often find it difficult to describe the quality of their symptom, so assist them by providing a list of possible descriptions: colicky, crampy, griping, gripping, dull, throbbing, tight, knife- or vice-like. Ask whether medication has been necessary to alleviate the pain and whether the pain interferes with work or other activities. It is difficult to assess pain severity. Offering the patient a numerical score for pain, from '0' for no pain to '10' for excruciating pain, may provide a quantitative assessment of the symptom. For each presenting complaint, grade the severity by determining its effect on lifestyle. For example, if the patient has intermittent claudication, ask how far the patient can walk before pain forces a rest. If breathlessness is a problem, ascertain whether the symptom occurs on the flat, climbing stairs, doing chores in the home or at rest.

Social history

Enquire about schooling, employment (past and present), social skills, friends and relationships with partners and families. This is a convenient section in which to ask about past and present drug therapy as well as the use of tobacco and alcohol.

Education

Enquire about the age at which the patient left school and whether he or she attained any form of higher education or vocational skill. This may provide useful background information and, in particular, provide a baseline for assessing any deterioration in intellect.

Employment history

Enquire about working conditions as this may be of critical importance if there is suspicion of exposure to an occupational hazard.

Patients may attribute symptoms to work conditions, for example, a headache from working in front of a com-

> **Symptoms and signs**
> **Pain assessment**
>
> - Type
> - Site
> - Spread
> - Periodicity or constancy
> - Relieving factors
> - Exacerbating factors
> - Associated symptoms

> **Differential diagnosis**
> **Occupational disease**
>
> - Asbestos workers, builders: asbestosis, mesothelioma
> - Coal miners: coal worker's pneumoconiosis
> - Gold, copper and tin miners: silicosis
> - Farmers, vets, abbatoir workers: brucellosis
> - Aniline dye workers: bladder cancer
> - Healthcare professionals: hepatitis B

puter screen. Depression, chronic fatigue syndrome and general malaise may be blamed on poor working conditions (the 'sick building' syndrome). Although many such associations are prejudicial or coincidental, avoid dismissing them too readily. Frequent job changes or chronic unemployment may reflect both socioeconomic circumstances and the patient's personality. It is useful to enquire about specific stress in the workplace or threats of unemployment.

Drug history

Many patients do not know the names of their medication and it is useful to ask for the labelled bottles or a written medicines list. Remember to ask about non-prescription medicines: NSAIDs commonly cause dyspepsia, codeine-containing analgesics cause constipation and antihistamines may cause drowsiness. Ask about the duration of medication. Remember that iatrogenic disease is very common and always consider drug-related side effects in the differential diagnosis. Ask women of reproductive age about their choice of contraceptive, and postmenopausal women about hormone replacement therapy. Ask about and list any drug allergies.

Now ask the patient about the use of illicit drugs. Your enquiry needs to be sensitively phrased and will be influenced by the patient's age and background, few 80 year olds smoke pot or eat magic mushrooms! Ask first about marijuana, LSD and amphetamine derivatives. If the response suggests exposure, enquire about the use of the harder drugs such as cocaine and heroin.

Tobacco consumption

Patients usually give a fairly accurate account of their smoking. Ask what form of tobacco they consume and

Symptoms and signs
Units of alcohol equivalents

1 unit is equal to
- 1/2 a pint of beer
- 1 glass of sherry
- 1 glass of wine
- 1 standard measure of spirits

for how long they have been smoking. If they previously smoked, when did they stop and for how long did they abstain?

Alcohol consumption

Unlike smoking, alcohol history is often inaccurate and the tendency is to underestimate intake. Many patients consider beer and wine to be less problematic than spirits. Establish the type of alcohol the patient consumes as this makes estimating consumption more straightforward. Calculate the amount in units. If the patient is vague, ask them how long a bottle of sherry or spirits lasts. Alcohol-dependent patients often erect a firm defence when questioned about alcohol consumption and a third party history from friends and family is often revealing and helpful. Certain questions may reveal dependency without asking the patient to specify consumption. Ask about early morning nausea, vomiting and tremulousness, which are typical features of dependency. Ask whether they ever drink alone or during the course of the day as well as the evenings. Do they have days without alcohol?

Foreign travel

Ask the patient if they have been abroad recently. If so, determine the countries visited and the levels of hygiene maintained. If the patient has returned from an area where malaria is endemic, ask about adequate prophylaxis for the appropriate period.

Home circumstances

At this stage, ascertain how the patient was coping in the community before the illness. The issue is particularly relevant for elderly patients and individuals with poor domestic and social support networks. Do they live on their own, have they any support systems provided by either the community or their family? If the patient's condition has been present for some time, determine how effectively the patient is coping. For example, in a patient with motor neuron disease, is work still possible? Can the patient climb stairs? If not, what provisions are required for the patient to remain at home? Can the patient attend to personal needs such as bathing, shaving and cooking? What assistance may be on hand during the day or at night? What effects will the patient's illness have on the financial status of the family?

Risk factors
Travel-related risks

Viral diseases
- hepatitis A, B and E
- yellow fever
- rabies
- polio

Bacterial diseases
- salmonella
- shigella
- enteropathogenic *Escherichia coli*
- cholera
- meningitis
- tetanus
- Lyme disease

Parasite and protozoan diseases
- malaria
- schistosomiasis
- trypanosomiasis
- amoebiasis

MEDICAL HISTORY

Patients recall their medical history with varying degrees of detail and accuracy. Some will provide a meticulously typed sheet, others need reminding of major events. You can jog a patient's memory by asking if he or she has ever been admitted to hospital or undergone a surgical procedure. Include caesarean sections in your enquiry. If the patient mentions specific illnesses or diagnoses, explore them in detail rather than accepting them verbatim. If a patient mentions migraine, ask for a full description of the attacks so that you can decide whether or not the assumed diagnosis is correct.

FAMILY HISTORY

Although enquiry into the family history may primarily reveal evidence of an inherited disorder, information about the immediate family may have considerable bearing on the patient's symptoms. Start by asking if the patient is married or has a regular partner. If so, determine if that individual is well or whether he or she has had a recent or more chronic illness. If the patient has children, determine their ages and state of health. Find out if any offspring died in childhood and from what cause? Then move on to the patient's siblings and parents. Did any family members die at a relatively young age and, if so, from what cause. When there is suspicion of a familial disorder (e.g. Huntington's disease), it is helpful to construct a family tree (Fig. 1.14). Ages can be added to the tree or listed separately. If the pattern of inheritance suggests a recessive trait, ask whether the parents were related, in particular whether they were first cousins.

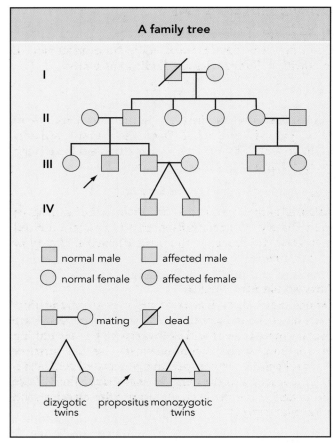

A family tree

I

II

III

IV

☐ normal male ☐ affected male

○ normal female ○ affected female

☐—○ mating ⬛ dead

dizygotic twins   propositus   monozygotic twins

Fig. 1.14   A standard family tree

Dx   Differential diagnosis
Common disorders expressed in families

- Hyperlipidaemia (ischaemic heart disease)
- Diabetes mellitus
- Hypertension
- Myopia
- Alcoholism
- Depression
- Osteoporosis
- Cancer (bowel, ovarian, breast)

SYSTEMS REVIEW

Before focusing on individual systems ask some general questions about the patient's health. Is the patient sleeping well? If not, is there a problem getting to sleep or a tendency to wake in the middle of the night or in the early hours of the morning? Has there been weight loss, fevers, rashes or night sweats? This leads in to the systems enquiry. The questions surrounding the presenting complaint will often have completed the systematic enquiry for that organ and there is no need to repeat questions already asked: simply to indicate 'see above'. Develop a routine that helps to avoid missing out a particular system.

CARDIOVASCULAR SYSTEM

Chest pain

Determine the location of any chest pain, its quality and its periodicity. Find out if there are specific triggering factors. Does the pain radiate? If the patient describes an exercise-induced pain, remember that angina can be confined to the throat, jaw or left arm rather than centring on the chest.

Dyspnoea

Ask if the patient is readily short of breath and quantify the problem: does it occur after climbing one flight of stairs, after walking on the flat for 100 m and so on? Does the patient become short of breath on lying flat (orthopnoea) or does the patient wake up breathless in the middle of the night (paroxysmal nocturnal dyspnoea)?

Ankle swelling

Has the patient noticed any ankle swelling? Is it confined to one leg, or does it affect both? Is the swelling persistent or only noticeable towards the end of the day.

Palpitations

Few patients record their pulse but most will register an abnormal heart rhythm, particularly one that is rapid or irregular. Try to establish whether the abnormal rhythm is regular or irregular and for how long it lasts. Can the patient give you an idea of the frequency by beating out the rhythm with a hand? Do any other symptoms appear (e.g. dizziness, fainting or loss of consciousness) while the heart is beating abnormally?

RESPIRATORY SYSTEM

Cough

Cough is difficult to quantify, particularly if dry. Does the cough wake the patient from sleep? If productive, work out the amount, an eggcupful a day perhaps? Is the sputum mucoid (white or grey) or purulent (yellow or green)?

Haemoptysis

If the patient has coughed up blood, ask whether this is bloodstaining of the sputum or more conspicuous frank bleeding. Is it a recent event, or has it happened periodically over several years? Did it follow a particularly violent bout of coughing? Was it associated with pleuritic chest pain or breathlessness?

Wheezing

Is the wheezing constant or intermittent, and are there trigger factors? Is the wheeze triggered by exercise? If the patient is using bronchodilators, determine the dosage and the frequency of use.

Pain

If the patient complains of localised chest pain, ask whether the pain is aggravated by or tender to the touch (chest wall pain).

GASTROINTESTINAL SYSTEM

Change in weight
Ask the patient if there has been any recent weight loss or gain. If there is uncertainty about weight change, ask the patient whether any alteration in the fit of clothes or belts has been noticed.

Abdominal pain
Ask about abdominal pain. Determine its site, quality and relationship to food. Does it appear soon after a meal, or 3–4 h later? Is it then relieved by adopting a certain posture? Can the pain disappear for weeks or months or is it more persistent? Does the pain cause night waking?

Vomiting
Ask the patient about nausea and vomiting. Is the vomiting violent (projectile) or does it represent effortless passive regurgitation of stomach contents? Is the vomiting lightly bloodstained or does it look like coffee-grounds, suggesting partly altered blood? Are items of food eaten some hours before still recognisable? Is there recognisable (green) bile in the vomit?

Flatulence and heart burn
Does the patient complain of flatulence or burping? Is there heart burn, particularly in certain postures? Does the mouth suddenly fill with regurgitated fluid (waterbrash)?

Dysphagia
Has there been difficulty in swallowing? Does this affect solids more than liquids or the reverse? Is the difficulty swallowing progressive or fluctuant and unpredictable? Can the patient identify a site where they believe the obstruction occurs (this correlates poorly with the site of the relevant pathology).

Bowel habit
Many patients believe they are constipated simply because they do not have a daily bowel action. If the patient has always emptied the bowels three times a week and there is no change, there is little likelihood of pathology. A change in bowel habit is what is significant, whether in terms of frequency or consistency of stool. Has the appearance of the stool altered? Are they black or pale or are they difficult to flush away? If there has been a change in bowel habit, ask the patient what drugs they are taking. A common cause of constipation is the use of codeine-containing analgesics. Has there been rectal bleeding or mucous discharge? Finally, ask about incontinence or soiling of underwear. Although this is not uncommon and particularly in parous women, few patients volunteer this symptom.

GENITOURINARY SYSTEM

Frequency
Determine the daytime and night-time frequency of micturition. Summarise the findings as a ratio:

$$\frac{D}{N} = \frac{6\text{–}8}{0\text{–}1}$$

Has there been an increase in the actual volume of urine passed (polyuria)? Does the patient wake at night to void urine? This is usually associated with increased thirst and fluid intake.

Pain
Ask the patient if there is any pain either during or immediately after micturition. Has the patient noticed a urethral discharge? Is the urine offensive, cloudy or bloodstained?

Altered bladder control
Determine if there has been urgency of micturition, with or without incontinence. Does the patient have urinary incontinence without warning? Does coughing or sneering cause incompetence? Has the urinary stream become slower, perhaps associated with difficulty in starting or stopping (terminal dribbling)? Does the patient have the desire to empty the bladder soon after micturition?

Menstruation
Ask about menstrual rhythm. Use a ratio to summarise the duration of menstruation and the number of days between each period (e.g. 7/28). Are the periods heavy (menorrhagia) or painful (dysmenorrhoea)? Have they changed in quality or quantity? Are they predictable?

Sexual activity
Although sexual dysfunction is common, few patients volunteer this information. Ask whether they have a sleeping partner and whether they are able to achieve a satisfactory physical relationship. Ask whether the partner is male or female. Does the patient practise 'safe sex'? Has the patient ever had a sexually transmitted disease? In addition, ask whether intercourse is painful or whether the patient is concerned about a lack of sexual activity, whether due to loss of libido or to actual impotence. This introduction might prompt the patient to volunteer information on libido, potency and pain.

NERVOUS SYSTEM

Headache
Many individuals have experienced headache. Follow the enquiry you use for other forms of pain but, in addition, ask if the pain is affected by head movement, coughing or sneezing. If the patient mentions migraine, find out what the individual means by the term. One of the most important questions to ask about headache is whether it is a recent problem or whether longstanding over months or years.

Loss of consciousness

Has the patient lost consciousness? Avoid terms like blackouts even if the patient tries to use them. Find out if there are any warning symptoms before attacks, whether they have been witnessed and whether they have led to incontinence, injury or a bitten tongue. Do the episodes occur only in certain environments or can they be triggered by certain activities (e.g. standing suddenly)? How does the patient feel after the attack? Most patients recover quickly from a simple faint but, after an epileptic seizure, patients often complain of headache and then sleep deeply for several hours. If the patient mentions epilepsy, get him or her to specify the exact nature of the attacks. There may be specific symptoms accompanying the attack that assist in making a diagnosis. Is there first pallor followed by facial flushing or is there a clear-cut warning with faintness, sweating and nausea?

Dizziness and vertigo

Dizziness (or giddiness) is a common complaint, describing an ill-defined sense of dysequilibrium usually without any objective evidence of imbalance. Some patients describe a continuous feeling of dizziness but most refer to attacks. If the symptom is paroxysmal, does it occur in particular environments or with particular actions? For instance, hyperventilation attacks, where dizziness is often an associated symptom, tend to occur in crowded places, whereas patients with postural hypotension will notice dizziness triggered by standing suddenly. Only use the term vertigo if the patient describes a sense of rotation, either of the body or of the environment. Again, detail any triggering factors. In benign positional vertigo, the symptom is induced by lying down in bed at night on one particular side.

Speech and related functions

Ask about the patient's speech. Is there simply a problem of articulation, or does the patient use wrong words, with or without a reduction in total speech output? Carefully note the patient's handedness, which should include questions about the limb used for a variety of skilled tasks, rather than just writing. Does the patient have difficulty understanding speech? Has there been any change in reading or writing skill? For the latter, ask not just about the quality of the script but also the content.

Memory

The patient may not complain of memory disturbance but, if he or she does, determine whether this applies to recent events, to events further back in the patient's youth or to both. Is the memory problem persistent or does the patient have 'good and bad days'? Many individuals mention difficulties with memory, although further enquiry often suggests that the problem is influenced by the patient's psychological state.

CRANIAL NERVE SYMPTOMS

Vision

Ask about any visual disturbances. Do these take the form of negative symptoms (i.e. visual loss) or positive symptoms such as scintillations or shimmerings? Most patients assume that the right eye is concerned with vision to the right and the left eye with vision to the left. Consequently, few will cover-test during attacks of visual disturbance to determine whether the problem is monocular or binocular. Ensure you ask whether the patient has cover-tested before accepting his or her account of the distribution of the symptoms. Is the visual disturbance intermittent or continuous? Is it accompanied or followed by headache?

Diplopia

If the patient has or has had diplopia (double vision), determine whether the images were separated horizontally or in an oblique fashion. Can the patient tell you in which direction of gaze the diplopia is most evident? Is it relieved by covering one eye or the other?

Facial numbness

Can the patient outline the distribution of any facial sensory loss? Does the involvement include the tongue, the gums and the buccal mucosae?

Deafness

Has the patient become aware of deafness? Is it bilateral or unilateral? Was there a history of chronic exposure to noise or a family history of deafness? Is the hearing particularly troublesome when there is an increased level of background noise? Is the hearing problem accompanied by tinnitus?

Oropharyngeal dysphagia

Has the patient problems with swallowing? Does this principally affect fluids or solids? Is there spluttering and coughing associated with swallowing?

Limb motor or sensory symptoms

Is the problem confined to one limb or to the limbs on one side of the body, to the lower limbs alone or to all four limbs? Does the patient describe loss of sensation or some distortion of sensation (e.g. a feeling of tightness round the limb)? If the patient complains of weakness, find out whether it is intermittent or continuous and, if the latter, whether it is progressing. Does the weakness mainly affect the proximal or the distal part of the limb? Has the patient noticed muscle wasting or any twitching of limb muscles?

Loss of coordination

Few patients with a cerebellar syndrome will describe their problem in terms of loss of coordination. Some will complain of clumsiness, others will simply refer to the problem as weakness. When assessing the loss of limb coordination, it is useful to ask the patient about everyday activities (e.g. writing and eating). Ask the patient about the sense of balance. Does the patient tend to deviate to a particular side or in either direction? Has the patient had falls as a consequence?

ENDOCRINE HISTORY

The history may give clues to endocrine disease. Diabetes mellitus is characterised by weight loss, excessive thirst (polydipsia) and large volume urine production with night waking (polyuria). An overactive thyroid is suggested by recent onset heat intolerance, weight loss, irritability, palpitations and increased appetite. An underactive thyroid is suggested by constipation, weight gain, altered skin texture, poor cold tolerance and depression.

MUSCULOSKELETAL SYSTEM

Has the patient had bone or joint pain? If the latter, has it been accompanied by swelling, tenderness or redness? Is the problem confined to a single joint or is it more diffuse? Does the pain predominate on waking or does it appear as the relevant joint is used (e.g. in walking)? Is there a history of trauma to a joint now painful or is there a family history of joint disease?

SKIN

Has the patient noticed any rashes? What was their distribution? Were or are they accompanied by itching? Is the patient's occupation a possible guide to the cause of the rash? Find out about chemicals or cosmetics which might have been in contact with the skin. Have metal bracelets or necklaces caused the rash (nickel allergy)? Does the patient wear protective gloves when washing up in the kitchen?

PARTICULAR PROBLEMS

The patient with depression or dementia

There is some logic in coupling these clinical problems. In both cases the patient can appear withdrawn and uncommunicative. Patients with depression may well dwell on their vegetative symptoms (e.g. insomnia and loss of appetite) and be reluctant to discuss their mood change. Determine whether or not there has been any suicidal intent. Patients with dementia initially retain some insight and in particular may have reasonable grasp of distant events. However, their recent recall, orientation for person, place and time' and logical thought patterns may be obviously disabled. A characteristic feature of Alzheimer's dementia is loss of insight and failure to recognise memory loss. This contrasts with senile dementias in which the patient is often concerned at their memory loss. When depression or dementia interferes with history-taking, it is crucial to involve family, friends and carers in the assessment. In addition, the history may only be complete with a visit to the patient's home.

The hostile patient

If a patient is hostile to your attempts to take a history, back off with dignity but use the experience to try and analyse the reasons for the reaction. There is often much information to be gained from patient's actions. The reaction may reflect anger at being ill, separated from family and work, and the doctor or student provides an easy focus for the emotion. You may wish to conclude the interview, although you may feel it reasonable to question the patient gently about their anger and use the encounter to recreate trust and confidence, allowing you to explore the history more formally. If the hostility persists, terminate the interview and discuss the problem with another member of the medical or nursing staff.

History-taking in the presence of students

Usually, when eliciting the history, you will be seeing the patient on a one-to-one basis. At other times you will observe the process in the outpatient department. Occasionally patients find the presence of a group of students intimidating or an infringement of confidentiality. Although most often an explanation of their presence will satisfy the patient, rarely it is appropriate to leave the consultation and allow the patient the right of privacy (Fig. 1.15).

PRESENTING YOUR FINDINGS

All the information from the interview will be recorded in the medical record, the structure of which is outlined earlier in this chapter. Consider history-taking as a stage-set with appropriate props and a dialogue where you, like any good actor, have command over the script but develop the plot with the help of your patient. Most importantly, know your lines and the sequence in which you are going to use them (Fig 1.16).

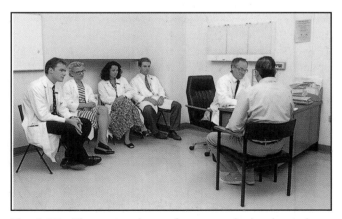

Fig. 1.15   The patient has to face not only the doctor but a number of students. Some patients will have difficulty coping with a 'mass' audience.

Patient history

Mrs G. W. 76 years old female
Date of birth: 11/1/31 Retired shop assistant

Date: 1/6/02

Presenting complaint(s): (1) Constipation
           (2) Stomach pain

History of presenting complaint:
(1) Constipation: Started on 7/4/02. Normally bowels open once a day, but didn't go for 6 days. Subsequently has been going once every 2–4 days.
(2) Stomach pain: Pain started at the same time. Site of pain is in the left iliac fossa. Patient thought it was due to 'straining'. Episodes of pain are of sudden onset and are a 'sagging dull ache'. They last 1 hour and occur anything between 2–3 times a day to once every 3 days. There are no alleviating or exacerbating factors. Pain unrelated to eating or defecation and there are no preceding events. Pain appears not to fluctuate.
  Patient went to visit GP after 6 days constipation. GP felt a mass on abdominal palpation which on bimanual examination was thought to be of ovarian origin. Patient referred to the gynaecological outpatient department.

Social history:
Retired at age of 60 as shop assistant. Married. Husband is a retired bus driver. Alive and well. Live together in own terraced house. Self-sufficient. No pets.

Smoking:
Ex-smoker, 4–5 a day for 5 years as a teenager.

Alcohol:
Only on Christmas Day and birthdays.

Past obstetric history:
Menarche – 12   Menopause – 50 Gravidity 3 Parity 3

(1) Female 41   Spontaneous vaginal delivery full term
             (7 lb)
(2) Female 38   Spontaneous vaginal delivery full term
             (8 lb 4 oz)
(3) Female 35   Spontaneous vaginal delivery
             39 weeks (6 lb 8 oz)

Past medical history:
Hypertension for last 6 years treated by GP with atenolol.
No previous operations.

Drug history: Atenolol

Allergies: None known

Travel abroad: Never

Family History

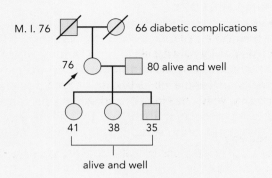

M. I. 76 ☐   ◯ 66 diabetic complications

76 ◯   ☐ 80 alive and well

41 ◯   38 ◯   35 ☐

alive and well

No family history of TB.

Systems review

General:
No weight change, appetite normal, no fevers, night sweats, fatigue or itch.

Cardiovascular system:
No chest pain, palpitations, exertional dyspnoea, paroxysmal nocturnal dyspnoea, orthopnoea or or ankle oedema.

Respiratory system:
No cough, wheeze, sputum or haemoptysis

Gastrointestinal system:
No abdominal swelling noticed by patient, no nausea or vomiting, no haematemesis. Bowels open once every 2–3 days. Stool normally formed. No blood or slime. No melaena.

Genitourinary system:
No dysuria, haematuria. Frequency $\dfrac{D}{N} = \dfrac{2-3}{1}$
No vaginal discharge. Not sexually active.

Nervous system:
No fits, faints or funny turns. No headache, paraesthesiae, weakness or poor balance.

Musculoskeletal system:
No pain or swelling of joints. Slight stiffness in morning.

Summary:
A 76-year-old hypertensive woman, referred to gynaecological outpatients with a short history of constipation and stomach pain. She has no other previous medical history.

Fig. 1.16   A specimen case history taken from a student's notes. Note the brief summary at the end, the writing of which gives useful practice in the art of condensing a substantial volume of information.

Examination of elderly people
History-taking

There are special problems when recording a history from elderly patients. Consider the following.

Hearing loss
- Common in the elderly
- May be helped by hearing aid
- Important to speak clearly and slowly
- Face the patient and avoid extraneous sound
- If necessary, write questions in bold letters

Visual handicap
- Cataracts, glaucoma and macular degeneration are common in the elderly
- Ensure the room is well lit
- Engage an assistant or carer to help patients move in and out of the consulting room and examination area

Dementia
- Often occurs in patients who appear physically fit
- Forgetfulness, repetition and inappropriate answers characterise responses
- Family members, friends and carers often note the development of dementia

Important aspects of a history from elderly patients include:

- State of the domestic environment and general living conditions
- Provision of community and social services
- Family support structures
- Economic status and pension provision
- Mobility (at home and in the local environment)
- Detailed drug history and compliance
- Provision of laundry services
- Legal will

Review
The history

- Welcome
- Note the patient's body language
- Begin with an open-ended question
- Take a history of the presenting complaint(s); use closed-questions to answer the following:
  - which organ system?
  - likely cause?
  - predisposing factors?
  - complications?
- Social history
- Medical history
- Education
- Employment
- Medicines, drugs and tobacco
- Alcohol consumption
- Foreign travel
- Home circumstances
- Family history
- Systems review
  - cardiovascular
  - respiratory
  - gastrointestinal
  - genitourinary
  - nervous
  - endocrine
  - musculoskeletal
  - skin and hair

2.
The General Examination

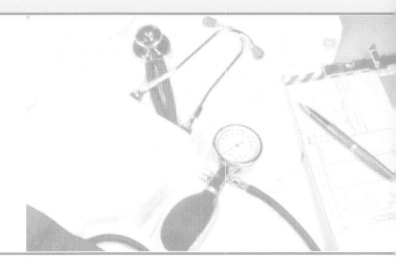

The dividing line between the history and examination is artificial. The examination really begins from the moment you set eyes on the patient. During the course of the history you will examine the patient's intellect, personality, family and genetic background, as well as gather information on the presenting complaint and medical history. In addition, you will have the opportunity to assess speech, orientation for person, place and time, and mood (affect). Throughout the history and examination you should sense information from the patient's unspoken body language. These physical signs are rarely taught, although the patient's body language may provide many useful signs. The patient's facial expression and tone of voice often impart more information than verbal communication. Hunched shoulders, a slow gait and poor eye contact may convey a reluctant patient, unable or unwilling to confront or expose anxieties or fears. Facial expression, tone of voice and body attitude may signal depression, even if the patient does not complain of feeling depressed. Try to look, listen and then write, this will give you the opportunity to see, as well as listen to, the patient's complaints.

The formal physical examination follows on from the history and calls on your major senses of sight, touch and hearing. Inspection, palpation, percussion and auscultation form the foundation of the physical examination and this formula is repeated each time you examine an organ system. The otoscope and ophthalmoscope extend your vision into the ear and eye, respectively, whereas the stethoscope provides an amplification system to help you listen to the heart, lung and bowel sounds. With the help of technology, we are now able to extend our vision deep into the body: radiographs (including computerised axial tomography scanning), ultrasound, magnetic resonance imaging and fibreoptics greatly broaden our powers of observation.

The physical examination begins with a general examination and is followed by examination of the skin, head and neck, heart and lungs, abdominal organs, musculoskeletal and neurological systems.

With practice it is possible to perform the 'routine' examination in 10–15 min, although if you discover an abnormality, considerably more time will be spent refining the findings. From the outset you should aim to choreograph an economical, aesthetic and complete examination.

GENERAL EXAMINATION

The general examination permits you to obtain an overview of the general state of health and provides an opportunity to examine systems that do not fall neatly into a regional examination. For the patient, the general examination is also a gentle introduction to the more intense systems examination to follow.

FIRST IMPRESSIONS
The examination commences as the patient walks into the consulting room or as you sit down at the bedside to take a history. At this first encounter, even before you initiate the history, decide whether the patient looks well or not and whether there is any striking physical abnormality. You will also gain an immediate impression of dress, grooming and personal hygiene.

As the patient approaches you in the consulting or examination room, observe the posture, gait and character of the stride. Diseases of nerves, muscles, bones and joints are associated with abnormal gaits and postures. You should quickly recognise the slow shuffling gait and 'pill rolling' tremor of Parkinson's disease or the unsteady broad-based gait of the ataxic patient. Patients with proximal muscle weakness may have difficulty rising from the waiting room chair and their gait may have a waddling appearance. Patients with osteoporosis lose height as the vertebrae progressively collapse: you may be struck by the typically stooped (kyphotic) appearance and 'round shoulders' of these patients. Take note if the patient walks with a stick or some form of additional physical support. A white stick indicates partial or complete blindness. The gait also conveys body language: the patient may have a spring in the step, make rapid eye contact and immediately offer a firm handshake. This contrasts with the patient with drooping shoulders and a slow (but otherwise normal) step who avoids eye contact.

When making your initial acquaintance with the patient, a warm handshake serves a number of functions (Fig. 2.1). The touching of hands may reassure the patient and serve as a gentle and symbolic introduction to the more intimate physical contact of the examination that follows the history. Before shaking hands, glance momentarily at the hand to ensure that you will not be grabbing a prosthesis or deformed hand. A well-made prosthesis may cause considerable embarrassment as you suddenly realise that the hand you are shaking is hard and lifeless. You may also note other abnormalities such as a potentially painful rheumatoid hand or missing fingers. The grip of the handshake usually provides some useful information. A normal grip conveys different information from a weak, lethargic handshake, which may imply distal muscle weakness, general ill-health or depression. The handshake is a useful physical sign in patients with myotonia dystrophica, a rare autosomal dominant inherited disease of muscle. A feature of this disease is the abnormally slow relaxation of the grip on completion of the handshake. The syndrome is also characterised by premature frontal balding, testicular atrophy and cataracts.

On first contact with the patient, you may be struck by an unusual physical stature. Unusually short stature may reflect constitutional shortness, a distinct genetic syndrome or the consequence of intrauterine, childhood or adolescent growth retardation. Unusually tall stature is most often constitutional, although hypothalamic tumours in childhood or adolescence may cause excessive growth hormone release, resulting in abnormally rapid linear growth and gigantism. If excess growth hormone release occurs after the bony epiphyses have fused, body shape changes (acromegaly). Severe malnutrition and obesity are readily recognised on the first encounter with a patient.

In hospitalised patients, posture may provide helpful information. Patients with acute pancreatitis find some relief lying with knees drawn towards the chest. Patients with peritonitis lie motionless, as any abdominal wall movement causes intense pain. The pain of acute pyelonephritis or perinephric abscess might be partly relieved by lateral flexion to the side of the pathology. In acute pericarditis, the patient finds modest relief by sitting forward; and in left ventricular failure, patients breath more easily when lying propped up on 3 or 4 pillows (orthopnoea).

FORMAL EXAMINATION

On completion of the history, prepare the patient for the formal examination. Always remain sensitive to the apprehension most patients feel when laid out naked on the examination couch or bed. Imagine yourself in that position, confronted by a near stranger who is about to inspect, palpate, percuss and auscultate your body, a daunting thought. The history should provide you with the opportunity to build a confident professional relationship with the patient. It is cultural and established fact that it is quite acceptable for a doctor to undertake a comprehensive physical examination, although remain sensitive to some cultural norms where same-sex examinations might be preferable. This acceptance usually extends to medical students who can be reassured that most patients welcome students and recognise their need to learn the examination technique. Explain the necessity of undertaking a full physical examination. The examination adds information to the clinical database and a thorough examination provides considerable reassurance to the patient.

 Differential diagnosis
Growth failure

Genetic
- Achondroplasia
- Turner's syndrome
- Down's syndrome

Constitutional
- Family members who have short stature

Endocrine
- Hypopituitarism
- Hypothyroidism

Systemic disease
- Crohn's disease
- Ulcerative colitis
- Renal failure

Malnutrition
- Intrauterine growth retardation
- Marasmus
- Kwashiorkor
- Starvation

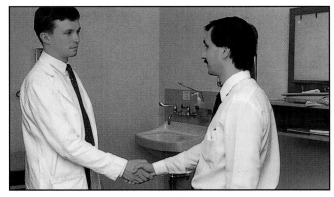

Fig. 2.1 The handshake serves as a gentle introduction to the physical contact that will occur during the formal physical examination.

The examination requires full exposure: men and women should be asked to remove superficial clothing and vests or undershirts. For a chest examination, women should be asked to remove their bra. Ensure a clean and presentable examination grown is available in the examination room for the patient to don before you enter the room. When a patient of the opposite sex is to be examined, always ask the chaperone to check whether the patient is ready.

SETTING

A separate examination room or adequate screening should be provided to ensure privacy while the patient is undressing and being examined. The room should be comfortably warm. Ensure that there are fresh sheets (either linen or disposable) and a clean blanket for cover. The examination couch should be positioned to allow you to examine from the patient's right side and there must be good general illumination. You should be fully equipped to undertake the examination without disruption. Ensure you have a working penlight torch and stethoscope. Close at hand there must be a sphygmomanometer, ophthalmoscope, otoscope, tongue depressors and disposable gloves (for genital and rectal examination). Basic equipment for the neurological examination should be available. This includes a patellar hammer, tuning fork, cotton wool buds, sterile disposable needles for testing pin-prick responses, test tubes to fill with hot and cold water for temperature testing and hat pins with red and white tops to assess visual fields. A cupful of drinking water should also be available, as you may ask the patient to swallow a mouthful to check for a thyroid goitre or other neck swelling.

As you approach the patient, re-establish both verbal and eye contact. You may ask the patient whether they feel comfortable and are prepared for the examination. Start the examination with the patient supine and the head and shoulders raised to approximately 45° above the horizontal. Most modern examination couches and hospital beds are designed to allow easy adjustment of the upper body. Most of the examination takes place with the patient comfortably resting in this position (Fig. 2.2). Three further adjust-

ments will be made in the course of the examination. When auscultating the mitral area of the heart it is helpful to roll the patient towards the left lateral position as this brings the apex closer to the stethosope. To examine the neck, posterior chest, back and spine you will ask the patient to sit forward. For assessing the abdomen, reposition the patient to lie flat, as this provides optimal access for the abdominal examination. Plan the examination to ensure the most economical movements for both you and the patient.

Following the history, reflect on which physical signs may help you to confirm or refine your initial assessment. Anticipation of physical signs will help you to direct and focus the examination. For example, if a patient complains of breathlessness, you may anticipate anaemia or respiratory or cardiac disease, therefore, you should gear the examination towards determining which of these possibilities is responsible for the symptoms.

Begin with an inspection of overall appearance.

> **Symptoms and signs**
> **Observation of general appearance**
>
> - Does the patient look comfortable or distressed?
> - Is the patient well or ill?
> - Is there a recognisable syndrome?
> - Is the patient well nourished?
> - Is the patient well hydrated?

RECOGNISABLE SYNDROMES AND FACIES

When inspecting the face, you might be struck by a single sign such as a red eye or the characteristic facies associated with discrete syndromes.

THE EYE

The history might be helpful in distinguishing possible causes of the red eye. Ask about duration, previous attacks, pain (and its character), photophobia and possible direct causes of traumatic damage. It is useful to

> **Symptoms and signs**
> **Down's syndrome (trisomy 21)**
>
> - Facies – oblique orbital fissures, epicanthic folds, small ears, flat nasal bridge, protruding tongue, Brushfield's spots on iris
> - Short stature
> - Hands – single palmar crease, curved little finger, short hands
> - Heart disease (endocardial cushion defects)
> - Gap between first and second toes
> - Educationally subnormal

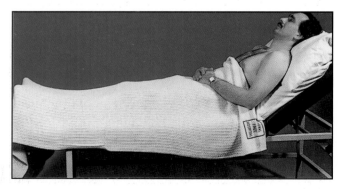

Fig. 2.2 The position of the patient at the start of the examination.

Questions to ask
Red eyes

- Is vision affected? Can the patient read ordinary print with the affected eye/s?
- Is there foreign body sensation?
- Is there photophobia?
- Is there a pus discharge?
- Was there trauma?
- Are you a contact lens wearer?

Differential diagnosis
Main causes of red eye

- Conjunctivitis (infective, allergic, toxic)
- Keratitis (infective, foreign body, sicca syndrome)
- Acute closed angle glaucoma
- Iritis
- Reiter's syndrome

distinguish the sensation of a foreign body from less specific symptoms such as 'grittiness' and 'itching'. A foreign body sensation feels as if there is something in the eye and is associated with some difficulty opening the eye. This symptom is characteristic of an active corneal process causing the red eye.

Begin the examination by inspecting the eyes. In lid and conjunctival disorders, there is no foreign body sensation or photophobia and the patient sits in a brightly lit room without discomfort. In bacterial conjunctivitis the patient complains of pussy discharge (especially in the morning on waking) and this might be seen on inspection. A foreign body sensation (rather than gritty or itchy sensation) is typical of active corneal disease. In infectious keratitis the patient has difficulty keeping the affected eye open, and a similar sign occurs with contact lens abrasion. Patients with iritis may present with difficulty keeping the eye open and some photophobia but without the complaint of a foreign body sensation. In acute angle closure glaucoma the patient often clutches the affected eye and complains of associated headache and malaise. Visual acuity may be affected in red eye and should be assessed. The pinhole test helps distinguish refractive errors from other cause of visual loss. In refractive visual disturbances (e.g. myopia), vision is improved when peering through a small hole. In nonrefractive disorders, improvement does not occur.

Next, use a penlight to inspect the pupils and anterior segment. In angle closure glaucoma the pupil may be fixed in mid-dilation and may not respond to light. In corneal abrasion, acute keratitis and iritis, the pupil might be pinpoint. A purulent discharge suggests bacterial conjunctivitis or keratitis. The pattern of redness might be helpful. Diffuse injection of both the palpebral and bulbar conjunctivae suggests primary conjunctival disorders (bacterial, viral, allergic, toxic or associated with dry eyes). In contrast, more serious disorders such as keratitis, iritis and angle closure glaucoma present with a 'ciliary flush' with injection most marked at the limbus (the sclerocorneal junction). A white spot or opacity on the cornea indicates keratitis and further slit-lamp examination with fluorescein is required to delineate the lesion. Hypopyon is seen as a layer of pus in the anterior chamber and is associated with infectious keratitis, acute iritis and endophthalmitis and is an ophthalmic emergency. Hyphaema refers to the presence of a layer of blood in the anterior compartment and is usually caused by injury.

Symptoms and signs
Quick testing of visual acuity

- Assess ability of each eye to read newspaper print
- Pinhole test
- Snellen chart

Symptoms and signs
Penlight inspection of the red eye

- Does the pupil react to light?
- Is the pupil smaller than expected or pinpoint?
- Is there a purulent discharge?
- What is the pattern of the redness?
- Is there a corneal 'white spot'?
- Is there hypopyon or hyphema?

FACIES AND SYNDROMES

Certain diseases are readily identified by a distinctive combination of physical characteristics. There are a large number of recognisable congenital syndromes that were probably diagnosed during childhood and should not present as an undiagnosed problem to physicians caring for teenagers or adults. In addition, only a proportion survive into adulthood. There are several recognisable genetic or chromosomal syndromes that may present to clinicians caring for adults; examples include Down's syndrome (Fig. 2.3),

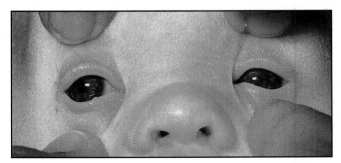

Fig. 2.3 Down's syndrome: epicanthic folds, Brushfield's spots and hypertelorism (increased interorbital distance).

Turner's syndrome (Fig. 2.4), Marfan's syndrome (Fig. 2.5), tuberous sclerosis (Figs 2.6, 2.7), albinism (Fig. 2.8), the fragile X chromosome (a common genetic cause of mental subnormality in which affected males have unusually large testes), Peutz–Jeghers syndrome (Figs 2.9–2.11), Waardenburg's syndrome (Fig. 2.12), familial hypercholesterolaemia (Figs 2.13–2.17) and neurofibromatosis. Other readily recognisable syndromes include the endocrine disorders and major organ failure (liver, heart, lungs and kidneys).

Symptoms and signs
Turner's syndrome (XO karyotype)

- Failure of sexual development
- Short stature
- Facies – micrognathia (small chin), low-set ears, fish-like mouth, epicanthic folds
- Short, webbed neck with low hairline; widely spaced nipples (shield-shaped chest)
- Heart disease (coarctation)
- Short fourth metacarpal or metatarsal
- Abnormally wide carrying angle of the elbow

Symptoms and signs
Marfan's syndrome

- Arm span greater than height
- Above average crown to heel height
- Long slender fingers
- Hyperextensible joints
- Kyphoscoliosis and anterior chest wall deformity
- High-arched palate
- Aortic incompetence and dissecting aortic aneurysms
- Subluxation or dislocation of the lens

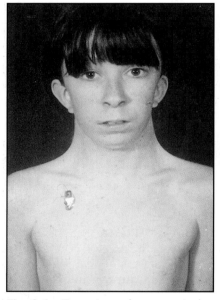

Fig. 2.4 Turner's syndrome: typical facial appearance, webbed neck and widely spaced nipples.

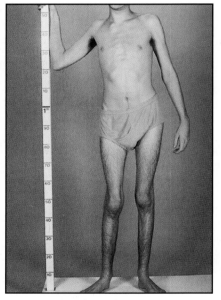

Fig. 2.5 Marfan's syndrome.

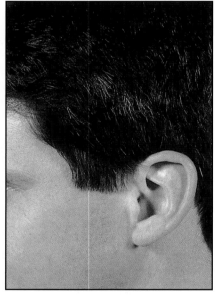

Fig. 2.6 Tuberous sclerosis: flecks of white hair.

Symptoms and signs
Tuberous sclerosis (Bourneville's disease, autosomal dominant choromosome 9)

- Epilepsy
- Mental deficiency (in 67%)
- Skin lesions (facial adenoma sebaceum, shagreen patch, fibromas near toenails and eyebrows)
- Flecks of white hair
- Retinal haemorrhages

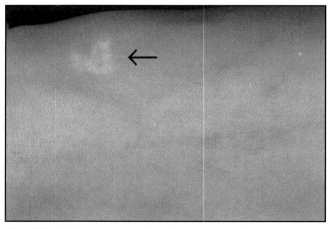

Fig. 2.7 Tuberous sclerosis: shagreen patch.

Symptoms and signs
Oculocutaneous albinism (autosomal recessive)

- Hypomelanosis or amelanosis of skin
- White hair
- Photophobia, nystagmus
- Hypopigmented fundus and translucent iris

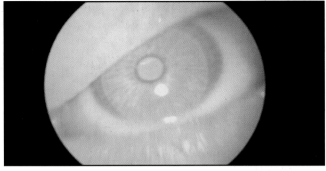

Fig. 2.8   Albinism: typical translucent iris.

 Symptoms and signs
Peutz–Jeghers syndrome (autosomal dominant)

- Pigmented macules (1–5 mm in diameter)
- Occur in profusion on lips, buccal mucosa and fingers
- Gastric, small intestinal and colonic hamartomatous polyps that sometimes give rise to abdominal pain, bleeding and intussusception

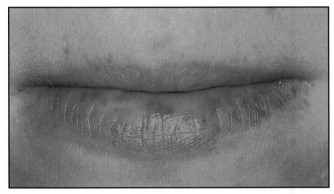

Fig. 2.9   Peutz–Jeghers syndrome: freckles on lips.

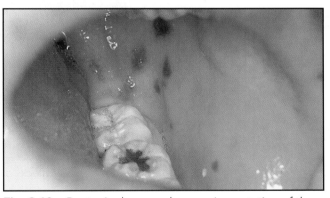

Fig. 2.10   Peutz–Jeghers syndrome: pigmentation of the buccal mucosa.

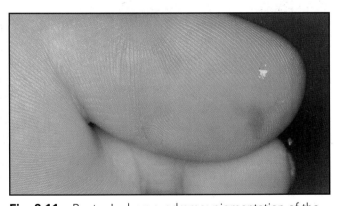

Fig. 2.11   Peutz–Jeghers syndrome: pigmentation of the big toe.

 Symptoms and signs
Waardenberg's syndrome (autosomal dominant)

- Cochlear deafness
- Frontal white lock of hair
- Wide-set eyes
- Different coloured irises
- White eyelashes
- Piebaldism

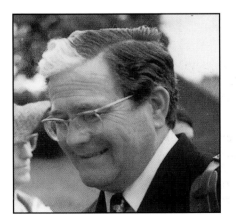

Fig. 2.12
Waardenberg's syndrome: typical white forelock.

Symptoms and signs
Familial hypercholesterolaemia (autosomal dominant)

- Xanthelasmas, skin xanthomas
- Tendon xanthomas
- Arcus senilis
- Marked artherosclerosis
- Ischaemic heart disease, peripheral vascular disease

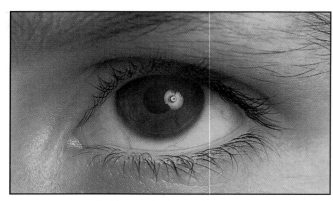

Fig. 2.13 Familial hypercholesterolaemia: cornea (arcus senilis)

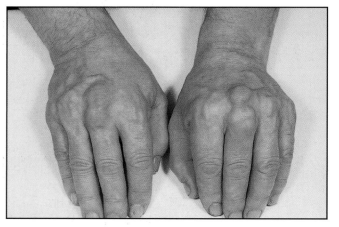

Fig. 2.14 Familial hypercholesterolaemia: tendon xanthomas.

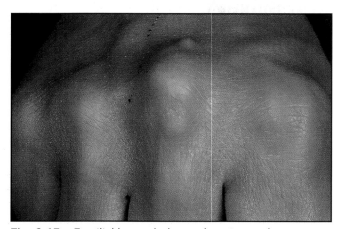

Fig. 2.15 Familial hypercholesterolaemia: tendon xanthomas.

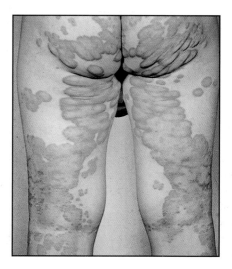

Fig. 2.16 Familial hypercholesterolaemia skin xanthomas.

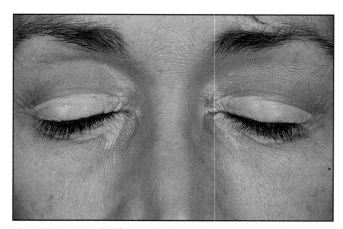

Fig. 2.17 Familial hypercholesterolaemia: xanthelasmata around the eyelids.

ENDOCRINE SYNDROMES

The endocrine glands are scattered throughout the body (Fig. 2.18). It is practical to consider the examination of the endocrine glands in the context of the overall general examination. Both over- and under-activity of the endocrine glands can be suspected from the patient's facies, body build and skin colour; endocrinopathies are often readily recognised in the course of the general examination.

Distinct clinical syndromes occur in diseases of the thyroid, parathyroid, adrenal and pituitary glands. An overview of the structure and function of each of these organs will help your clinical assessment and syndrome recognition.

STRUCTURE AND FUNCTION OF THE THYROID GLAND

The thyroid gland develops from a ventral pouch of the fetal pharynx. This pouch evolves into the thyroid gland by migrating caudally to a resting place in front of the trachea. The migration may leave thyroid remnants along the embryonic tract which extends from the back of the tongue (where a residual lingual thyroid 'rest' may occur). A midline thyroglossal cyst may develop if the migration tract fails to obliterate.

The thyroid gland consists of two lateral lobes joined by an isthmus. The gland lies in front of the larynx and trachea with the isthmus overlying the second to fourth tracheal rings (Fig. 2.19). The lateral lobes extend from the side of the thyroid cartilage to the sixth tracheal ring. Two nerves lie in close proximity to the thyroid gland: the recurrent laryngeal nerve runs in the groove between the trachea and the thyroid; and the external branch of the superior laryngeal nerve lies deep to the upper poles. In thyroid cancer, these nerves may be invaded and damage may occur in the course of thyroid surgery.

THYROXINE SYNTHESIS AND SECRETION

The anterior pituitary hormone, thyroid stimulating hormone (TSH), stimulates the synthesis of thyroxine (T_4) (Fig. 2.20). The functioning unit of the thyroid is the follicle, which consists of epithelial cells lining a central colloid space. The epithelial cells concentrate iodide, which is oxidised to iodine and incorporated with tyrosine to form mono-iodotyrosine and di-iodotyrosine. These two iodinated tyrosines are combined in the colloid to form either tri-iodothyronine (T_3) or tetra-iodothyronine (T_4). The two active hormones, T_3 and T_4, are stored in the colloid and bound to a specific binding protein (thyroglobulin). The protein-bound hormones are taken back up into the follicle epithelium by endocytosis. In the cells, the

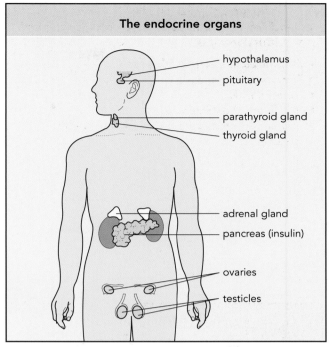

Fig. 2.18 The positions of the main endocrine organs.

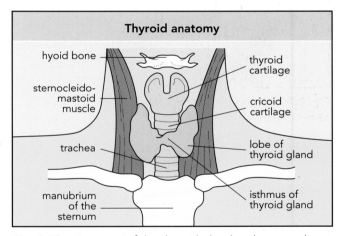

Fig. 2.19 Anatomy of the thyroid gland and surrounding structures.

colloid droplets are disrupted by proteolytic enzymes, allowing the release of T_3 and T_4 into the circulation where most circulate bound to thyroid binding globulin (TBG). Free hormone levels dictate the metabolic effects of T_4. T_4 is synthesised only in the thyroid but T_3 can also be produced from conversion of circulating T_4 in the liver, the kidney and other tissues. The hepatic conversion of T_4 results in two species of T_3: an active T_3 and an inactive reverse T_3.

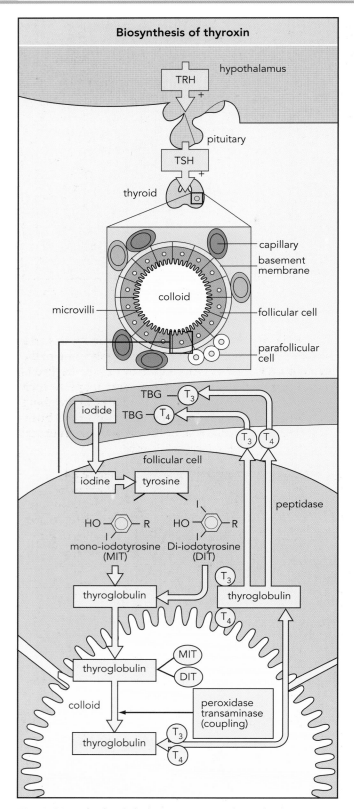

Biosynthesis of thyroxin

Fig. 2.20 The hypothalamus secretes thyroid releasing hormone (TRH) which stimulates the anterior pituitary to produce thyroid stimulating hormone (TSH). This stimulates the synthesis of thyroxine (T_4) in the follicles. Iodide taken up into the follicular cell is oxidised to iodine and then incorporated into tyrosine to form mono-iodotyrosine (MIT) and di-iodotyrosine (DIT), which binds with thyroglobulin

CLINICAL EXAMINATION OF THE THYROID GLAND AND FUNCTION

Although considered part of the general examination, the thyroid gland is usually examined when examining the head and neck (see Ch. 4).

Like any other organ, the thyroid examination relies on inspection, palpation, percussion and auscultation. Examine the thyroid gland with the patient sitting forward in bed or seated in a chair.

Ensure complete exposure of the neck and upper chest. Inspect the thyroid from the front of the neck. The normal thyroid gland is neither visible nor palpable. An enlarged thyroid (known as a goitre) is seen as a fullness on either side of the trachea below the cricoid cartilage, or as a distinct, enlarged, nodular organ with one or both lobes easily visible (Figs. 2.21–2.23). If the lobes are visible, determine whether they look symmetrical or irregular. Ask the patient to sip a little water and hold it in the mouth. When you give the instruction to swallow, watch for the characteristic upward movement of the goitre as the pharyngeal muscles contract. This test helps distinguish a thyroid mass from other neck masses (e.g. enlarged lymph nodes, which hardly move with swallowing). The midline remnant of the thyroid (thyroglossal cysts or thyroid remnants) also moves with swallowing.

Next, explain to the patient that you wish to feel the front of the neck for the thyroid gland. Position yourself to the right and slightly behind the patient. Feel for the left and right lobes with the finger pulps of both

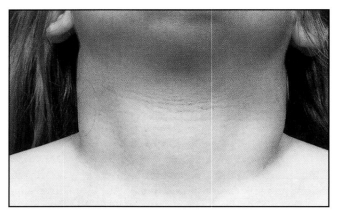

Fig. 2.21 Smooth goitre appearing as fullness in the anterior neck.

and is secreted into the colloid where T_3 and T_4 are synthesised. These are taken back into the follicular cells taken up by endocytosis where the T_3 and T_4 are split from thyroglobulin and released into the circulation, where they are bound to T_4 binding globulin (TBG).

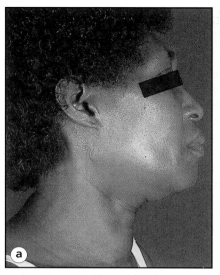
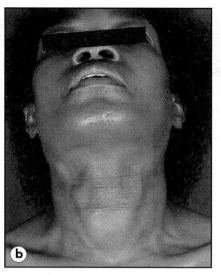
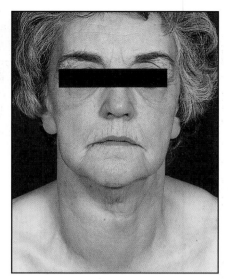

Fig. 2.22 Readily visible multinodular thyroid goitre.

Fig. 2.23 Asymmetrical multinodular goitre.

hands (Fig. 2.24). Ensure a gentle examination, as your hands are positioned in a throttling posture; reassure the patient by standing to the side rather than at the rear so that you remain in the patient's peripheral field of vision. Assess the texture (hard or soft, single or multiple nodules), symmetry and extent of the goitre. A soft, smooth goitre may be more easily seen than felt. It is unusual for the goitre to be tender unless the enlargement is caused by acute inflammatory thyroiditis. In the course of thyroid palpation, again ask the patient to take a sip of water and to swallow when you indicate. As the patient gulps, you should feel the goitre move beneath your fingers. Complete the palpation by feeling for the carotids, which may be encased by a malignant thyroid gland. Thyroid carcinoma may spread to local neck lymph nodes, so it is important to conclude the palpation by checking for palpable regional lymph nodes.

The thyroid gland may also enlarge in a downward direction behind the manubrium sterni. This retrosternal goitre may extend deeply into the superior mediastinum and may even cause compression symptoms (i.e. breathlessness and dysphagia). Retrosternal extension can be assessed by percussing over the manu-

brium and upper sternum (Fig. 2.25). Normally, this area resonates, yet when there is retrosternal enlargement the percussion note is dull. Auscultate the gland for bruits by applying the diaphragm of the stethoscope to each lobe in turn (Fig. 2.26). Ask the patient to stop breathing for a moment while you listen on either side for a bruit. A soft bruit is characteristic of the smooth symmetrical hyperthyroid goitre of Graves' disease.

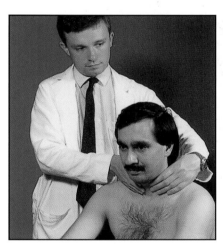

Fig. 2.24 Position for palpation of the lateral lobes and isthmus of the thyroid.

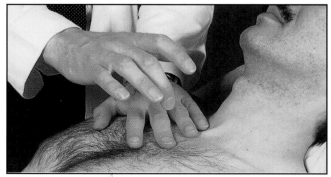

Fig. 2.25 A retrosternal goitre is suggested by dullness to percussion over the manubrium sterni.

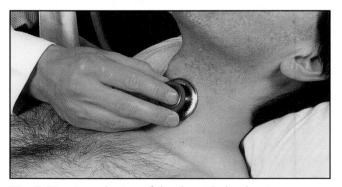

Fig. 2.26 Auscultation of the thyroid gland.

CLINICAL ASSESSMENT OF THYROID FUNCTION

T_4 has a number of important metabolic effects and over- or underactivity results in characteristic clinical syndromes that may readily be recognised. Diagnosis of hyperthyroidism is confirmed by measuring the serum levels of T_4 and T_3, whereas in hypothyroidism the serum TSH level is elevated and T_4 is subnormal.

HYPERTHYROIDISM

Hyperthyroidism occurs most commonly in young women with smooth diffuse goitres (Graves' disease). However, in elderly people, hyperthyroidism may be caused by an autonomous 'toxic' adenoma and, rarely, a functioning carcinoma. Rarely factitious hyperthyroidism caused by excessive T_4 intake masquerades as classical hypothyroidism. In both young and older thyrotoxic patients, you may be alerted to the diagnosis by a history of weight loss, recent intolerance to hot weather, sweating, palpitations, abnormal irritability and nervousness and increased bowel frequency. Most hyperthyroid patients feel warm and sweaty, have a

Questions to ask
Hyperthyroidism

- Have you lost weight recently?
- Has your appetite changed (e.g. increased)?
- Have you noticed a change in bowel habit (e.g. increased)?
- Have you noticed a recent change in heat tolerance?
- Do you suffer from excessive sweating?
- Does your heart race or palpitate?
- Have you noticed a change in mood?

tachycardia, staring eyes (caused by lid retraction) and abnormally brisk tendon reflexes. A fine peripheral tremor is common in thyrotoxicosis. This can be demonstrated by placing a sheet of paper on the back of the outstretched hand and watching the tremor, which is amplified by the sheet of paper 'trembling' (Fig. 2.27). Although similar signs of hyperthyroidism may occur in the young and old, Graves' disease is

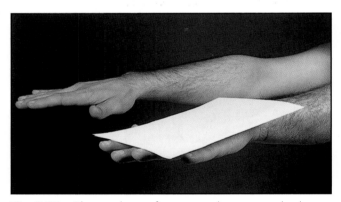

Fig. 2.27 Place a sheet of paper on the outstretched fingers to demonstrate the fine tremor of hyperthyroidism.

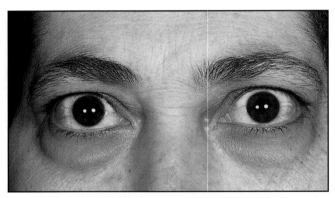

Fig. 2.28 Bilateral lid retraction in a patient with Graves' disease. Note that the upper lid is positioned well above the pupil and the palpebral fissure is widened.

Symptoms and signs
Hyperthyroidism

- Weight loss, increased appetite
- Recent onset of heat intolerance
- Agitation, nervousness
- Hot, sweaty palms
- Fine peripheral tremor
- Bounding peripheral pulses
- Tachycardia, atrial fibrillation
- Lid retraction and lid lag
- Goitre, with or without overlying bruit
- Brisk tendon reflexes

Symptoms and signs
Hyperthyroidism in Graves' disease and toxic nodular goitre

	Graves' disease	Nodular goitre
Sex	female >> men	female = men
Eye signs	very common, exophthalmos	less severe
Goitre	diffuse, overlying bruit	may be multinodular
Heart	tachycardia, atrial fibrillation	also angina, congestive heart failure
Weight	may lose weight	often profound

more readily recognisable from the characteristic facial appearance and associated physical signs.

GRAVES' DISEASE

The facies in Graves' disease is dominated by a staring appearance caused by retraction of the upper eyelid. Normally, during a relaxed forward gaze, the upper lid protects the eye by lying in a horizontal position which crosses the eye in a plane just above the upper pole of the pupil. In Graves' disease, autonomic overactivity causes increased tone and spasm of levator palpebrae superioris. This causes retraction of the upper lid, which exposes most, if not all, of the iris, exposing sclera above the iris and creating the typical staring appearance (Fig. 2.28). Spasm of the muscles supplying the upper lid also results in an abnormal following reflex. Normally, if you ask a patient to follow the movement of an object (e.g. your fingertip) (Fig. 2.29) from a point above eye level to a vertical point below eye level, you will note that as the eye moves, the

upper lid follows the upper margin of the pupil in a fully synchronised downward movement. In hyperthyroidism, this coordination is lost and the movement of the upper lid lags well behind the pupil (this is termed 'lid lag') (Fig. 2.30).

In progressive Graves' disease, abnormal connective tissue is deposited in the orbit and external ocular muscles. The globes are pushed forward, resulting first in proptosis and in the more severe form, exophthalmos (>18 mm protrusion). To examine for exophthalmos, seat the patient in a chair and inspect the globes from above by looking over the forehead or from the side of the profile (Fig. 2.31). A Hertel exophthalmometer can be used to make an accurate baseline measurement of the degree of exophthalmos and this measurement is used to monitor progression and regression. Other eye signs of Graves' disease include ophthalmoplegia caused by weakness and infiltration of the external ophthalmic muscles. These patients complain of double vision (diplopia) and on examina-

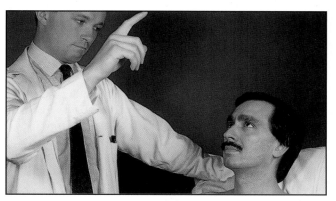

Fig. 2.29   Lid lag. With the patient sitting, position yourself on the patient's right side. Watch how the lid moves with the downward movement of the eye as the patient follows your finger moving from a point approximately 45° above the horizontal to a point below this plane. Normally, there is perfect coordination as the lid follows the downward movement of the eye.

 Symptoms and signs
Graves' disease (autoimmune hyperthyroidism)

- Diffuse goitre with audible bruit
- Pretibial myxoedema, finger clubbing
- Onycholysis (Plummer's nails)
- Lid retraction, lid lag
- Proptosis, exophthalmos
- Conjunctival oedema (chemosis)

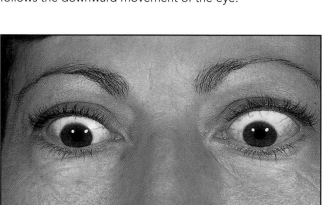

Fig. 2.30   In hyperthyroidism, the downward movement of the lid lags behind the movement of the bulb as it follows your finger through an arc.

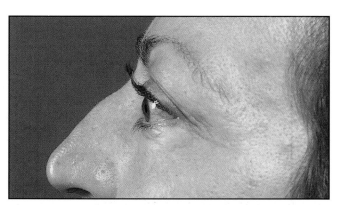

Fig. 2.31   Graves' disease: proptosis of the eye.

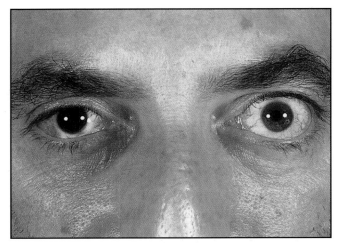

Fig. 2.32 Graves' disease: unilateral eye condition.

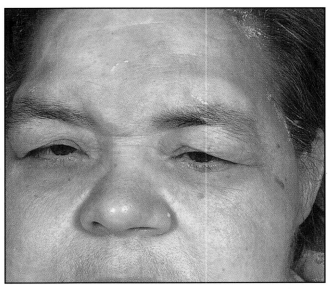

Fig. 2.33 Myxoedema.

tion there is a loss of gaze symmetry. Conjunctival oedema (chemosis) may also occur. The eye signs can be either bilateral or unilateral (Fig. 2.32), although, in the latter, always consider a space-occupying lesion of the orbit. Other features of Graves' disease include finger clubbing, onycholysis (separation of the nail from its bed), pretibial myxoedema (brawny swelling of lower legs), and periostitis (inflammation of the periosteum).

A rare complication of hyperthyroism is thyroid storm. This is an exaggerated manifestation of hyperthyroidism and is life threatening. Always consider this disorder in hyperthyroid patients who develop severe acute disease. While thyroid storm can develop in patients with longstanding untreated hyperthyroidism, it is more often precipitated by an acute event such as thyroid or nonthyroid surgery, trauma, infection or an acute iodine load.

HYPOTHYROIDISM

Hypothyroidism presents insidiously; the diagnosis may be readily apparent on general examination. Suspect hypothyroidism in patients complaining of unexplained lethargy, weight gain, newly noted cold intolerance, constipation, generalised hair loss and

pain in the hand suggestive of a carpal tunnel syndrome. Poor memory and general intellectual deterioration may also be presenting features. While taking the history you might have noticed on unusually hoarse voice. The disorder may occur at any age, although it is most common in elderly individuals. There are a number of possible causes to consider. On first sight you may notice the characteristic puffy facial appearance, the pale 'waxy' skin and diffuse hair loss from the scalp and eyebrows. Look for other signs to confirm your clinical suspicion of myxoedema (Fig. 2.33). The delayed relaxation phase of the Achilles tendon jerk is especially helpful (Fig. 2.34).

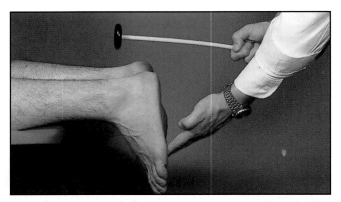

Fig. 2.34 The ankle jerk in hypothyroidism. Although all the reflexes show a distinct slowing of the relaxation phase of the tendon reflex, this sign is best observed and felt with the Achilles tendon jerk. Ask the patient to kneel on a chair or examination couch with the feet hanging over the edge. Expose the Achilles tendon and percuss with a patellar hammer while gently resting one hand on the sole of the foot. Watch and feel for the unusually delayed return of the foot to its resting position after the reflex contraction that follows the tendon tap.

 Emergency
Assessment of thyroid storm

- Thermoregulation – monitor temperature for hyperpyrexia
- Cardiovascular dysfunction – monitor heart rate and development of high output failure
- CNS – monitor for agitation, delirium, psychosis, extreme lethargy, seizure and coma
- Gastrointesinal dysfunction – abdominal pain, nausea and vomiting, diarrhoea, unexplained jaundice
- Assess precipitating event

Questions to ask
Hypothyroidism

- Has your weight changed?
- Has your bowel habit changed (e.g. constipation)?
- Is your hair falling out?
- Have you noticed a change in weather preference (e.g. cold intolerance)?
- Has there been a change in your voice (e.g. hoarse)?
- Do you suffer from pain in your hands (e.g. carpal tunnel syndrome)?

Symptoms and signs
Hypothyroidism

- Constipation, weight gain
- Hair loss
- Angina pectoris
- Hoarse, croaky voice
- Dry flaky skin
- Balding and loss of eyebrows (beginning laterally)
- Bradycardia
- Xanthelasmas (hyperlipidaemia)
- Goitre (especially with iodine deficiency)
- Effusions (pericardial or pleural)
- Delayed relaxation phase of tendon reflexes
- Carpal tunnel syndrome

Differential diagnosis
Hypothyroidism

Congenital
- Congenital absence
- Inborn errors of thyroxine metabolism

Acquired
- Iodine deficiency (endemic goitre)
- Autoimmune thyroiditis (Hashimoto's disease)
- Postradiotherapy for hyperthyroidism
- Postsurgical thyroidectomy
- Antithyroid drugs (e.g. carbimazole)
- Pituitary tumours and granulomas

STRUCTURE AND FUNCTION OF THE PARATHYROID GLANDS

There are usually four parathyroid glands (two superior and two inferior). Ninety per cent of parathyroid glands lie in intimate contact with the thyroid gland, although in 10% of patients the inferior glands lie in an aberrant position. These pea-sized glands usually lie embedded in the posterior aspect of the upper and lower poles of the thyroid or superficially on the surface of the thyroid.

PARATHYROID HORMONE

Parathyroid hormone (PTH) is synthesised in a precursor form known as pre-pro-PTH, which is first cleaved to pro-PTH and then cleaved again to the 84 amino acid polypeptide, PTH (Fig. 2.35). PTH secretion is regulated by the level of calcium in the blood; hypocalcaemia stimulates its release. In the circulation, the 84 amino acid PTH is cleaved to smaller fragments, most of which are inactive; the only active fragment is that containing the first 32 amino acids. The hormone's prime effect is on the renal tubule, where it stimulates calcium resorption from the tubular fluid and phosphate excretion in the urine. PTH also stimulates calcium resorption from bone.

HYPERPARATHYROIDISM

Hyperparathyroidism is usually detected by finding an abnormally high serum calcium level on routine blood testing or in patients presenting with renal colic caused by stones. Hyperparathyroidism may be caused by hyperplasia or one or more autonomous adenomas (often associated with the multiple endocrine neoplasia syndromes). In chronic renal failure, longstanding stimulation may result in loss of feedback and an autonomous secretion of PTH leading to hypercalcaemia (this is known as tertiary hyper-

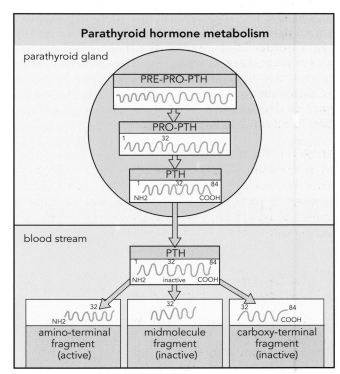

Fig. 2.35 Parathyroid hormone (PTH) metabolism: a large precursor molecule (PRE-PRO-PTH) is cleaved to form an 84 amino acid molecule PTH which is secreted into the blood stream. The molecule, which has an amino and a carboxy terminal, is cleaved to smaller fragments. Only fragments with the first 32 amino terminal amino acids are metabolically active.

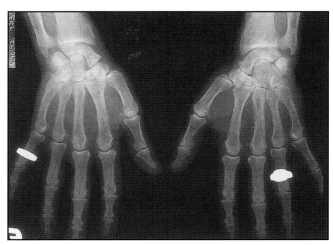

Fig. 2.36 Hyperparathyroidism: a radiograph of the phalanges may show subperiosteal erosions and bone cysts.

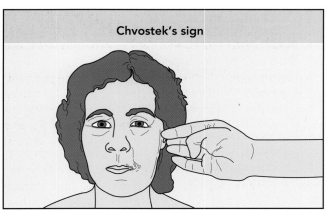

Fig. 2.38 Chvostek's sign. Tap over the facial nerve in front of the ear, this causes a momentary twitch of the corner of the mouth on the same side as the irritable facial muscles contract.

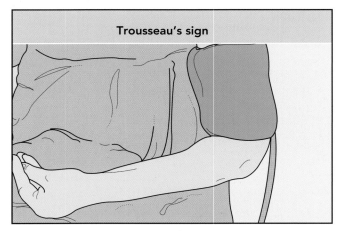

Fig. 2.39 Trousseau's sign. Inflate a sphygmomanometer cuff to above systolic pressure. Within approximately 4 min, there is characteristic 'carpopedal' spasm of the hand. There is opposition of the thumb, extension of the interphalangeal joints and flexion of the metacarpophalangeal joints. This posture reverses spontaneously when the cuff is deflated.

parathyroidism). The clinical syndrome may be difficult to recognise, because the symptoms ('moans') dominate the signs ('stones and bones'). The patient complains of tiredness and lethargy, excessive thirst (polydipsia), and symptoms of increased urine output (nocturia and frequency). There may be profound changes in the mental state and, in severe cases, drowsiness and even coma may occur. The patient may complain of gastro-intestinal symptoms, including nausea and constipation. Renal stones are common and the patient may present with severe acute unilateral abdominal pain radiating towards the groin. On examination, there may be proximal muscle weakness (due to a myopathy), a thin opaque ring around the limbus of the cornea, and bone pain or radiological evidence of hyperparathyroidism (Figs 2.36, 2.37).

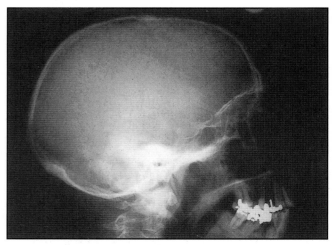

Fig. 2.37 Hyperparathyroidism: skull radiograph shows thinning of the cortex and small osteolytic areas, known as 'pepper pot' skull.

HYPOPARATHYROIDISM

Surgical damage or removal of three or four parathyroid glands during neck surgery (usually thyroidectomy) is the most common cause of hypoparathyroidism. Rarely, autoimmune destruction may cause hypoparathyroidism. The serum calcium level is low (in the presence of a normal serum albumin). The major symptoms of acute hypoparathyroidism are paraesthesiae around the mouth, fingers and toes. Abnormal nerve and muscle irritability can be elicited with Chvostek's (Fig. 2.38) and Trousseau's signs (Fig. 2.39). In chronic hypoparathyroidism, the physical effects develop slowly. The symptoms include tiredness, fatigue, muscle cramps and epilepsy. Premature cataracts should also alert you to the possibility of underlying chronic hypoparathyroidism.

STRUCTURE AND FUNCTION OF THE ADRENAL GLANDS

The high fat content of the adrenal glands (suprarenal) gives the organ a distinctive yellow colour. The adrenals lie on the upper poles of the kidneys abutting the diaphragm. Each gland weighs approximately 4 g and has a rich arterial blood supply from vessels derived from the aorta and renal and phrenic arteries. A single adrenal vein drains from the hila of the glands to the inferior vena cava on the right and to the renal vein on the left. The gland has an outer cortex derived from mesoderm and central medulla, which is derived from neuroectoderm.

The cortex comprises 90% of the gland and consists of three distinct layers: the subcapsular zona glomerulosa, the middle zona fasciculata and the zona reticularis, which lies adjacent to the medulla (Fig. 2.40).

HORMONE REGULATION

The adrenal cortex synthesises three steroid hormones: the mineralocorticoids, glucocorticoids and androgens. Aldosterone is produced in the cells of the zona glomerulosa. Aldosterone secretion is primarily regulated by the renin–angiotensin system, which in turn is influenced by the intravascular volume (Fig. 2.41). In contrast to the glucocorticoids, mineralocorticoid metabolism is not influenced by adrenocorticotrophic hormone (ACTH). When adrenal failure is secondary to pituitary failure, mineralocorticoid function is preserved, whereas glucocorticoid function may be seriously impaired. Aldosterone promotes the entry of sodium into cells and the secretion of potassium from cells; consequently, the overall effect of aldosterone is to cause sodium retention and potassium loss. This effect on renal tubular cells plays a central role in the regulation of sodium and potassium and water balance. Aldosterone-producing tumours of the adrenal cortex cause Conn's syndrome, which is characterised by hypertension, oedema (due to sodium and water retention) and hypokalaemia.

The cells of the zona fasciculata and reticularis synthesise cortisol and adrenal androgens. Glucocorticoid

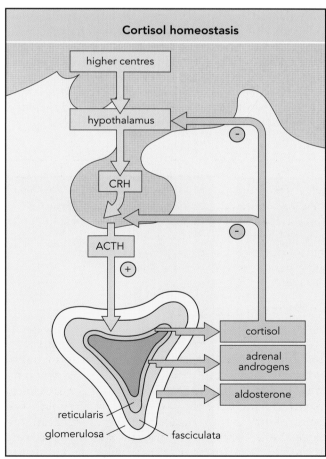

Fig. 2.40 Secretion of cortisol is stimulated by adrenocorticotrophin (ACTH) secretion, which is under the influence of hypothalamic cortisol releasing hormone (CRH). Both ACTH and CRH are under negative feedback control by circulating cortisol. Aldosterone is secreted from the zona glomerulosa by the stimulatory effect of angiotensin II.

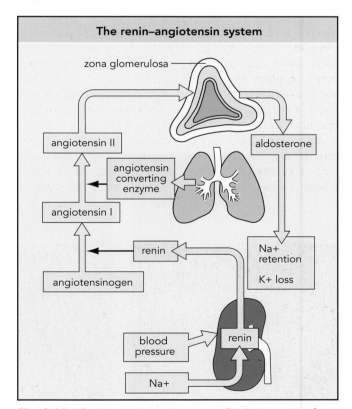

Fig. 2.41 Renin–angiotensin system. Renin is secreted from the juxtaglomerular apparatus of the kidney in response to reduced serum sodium or reduced renal blood pressure. Renin converts angiotensinogen to angiotensin I, which in turn is converted to angiotensin II by angiotensin converting enzyme (ACE) from the lung. The angiotensin II stimulates aldosterone release from the zona glomerulosa cells of the adrenal gland.

synthesis and secretion is under the direct control of ACTH secreted by the anterior pituitary. The secretion of ACTH is itself regulated by the release of hypothalamic corticotrophin releasing hormone (CRH). There is a feedback loop between the hypothalamus and pituitary on one side of the axis and the adrenal on the other. Although ACTH stimulates glucocorticoid and adrenal androgen synthesis and secretion, cortisol (and exogenous corticosteroids as well) inhibits ACTH secretion by impairing the release of CRH and directly inhibiting ACTH release from the anterior pituitary.

The hormones of the adrenal cortex have a circadian rhythm: blood levels of cortisol and aldosterone are highest on waking and lowest at and around midnight. Glucocorticoids promote the conversion of protein to glucose (gluconeogenesis) and inhibit the peripheral use of glucose. The corticoids increase blood pressure and support kidney function by increasing the glomerular filtration rate. Diagnosis of adrenal disease is based on measurement of ACTH, blood cortisol and the adrenal response to ACTH stimulation.

HYPERADRENALISM (CUSHING'S SYNDROME)

Excessive glucocorticoids (either endogenous or exogenous) cause a significant change in body appearance which can be readily recognised as Cushing's syndrome. A cushingoid appearance is most commonly caused by treatment with exogenous steroids. The most characteristic feature is the rounded, 'moon-shaped' face (Fig. 2.42), an obese body (Fig. 2.43) and thin limbs (Fig. 2.44). A typical cushingoid appearance may also occur in chronic alcoholism and, in this setting, it is called pseudo-Cushing's syndrome. The diagnosis is suspected if the physical appearance of Cushing's syndrome occurs against a background of excessive alcohol consumption. The physical and biochemical abnormalities of pseudo-Cushing's syndrome regress when alcohol is discontinued.

HYPOADRENALISM AND ADDISON'S DISEASE

In acute adrenal failure, the clinical features may be nonspecific and puzzling. The patient usually presents with malaise, weakness, nausea, vomiting and abdominal pain with an acute change in bowel habit (constipation or diarrhoea). The most helpful physical sign is the profound drop in blood pressure when the patient quickly changes position from lying to standing (postural hypotension). Collapse and prostration may occur. As a result of a mineralocorticoid deficiency, serum potassium levels are actually elevated.

> **Dx** Differential diagnosis
> **Hyperadrenalism**
>
> - Iatrogenic, exogenous steroids
> - Bilateral adrenal hyperplasia
> - Benign autonomous adrenal adenoma
> - Malignant adrenal adenocarcinoma
> - Nonmetastatic tumour effect (e.g. lung cancer producing ACTH-like peptide)
> - Alcoholism causing pseudo-Cushing's syndrome

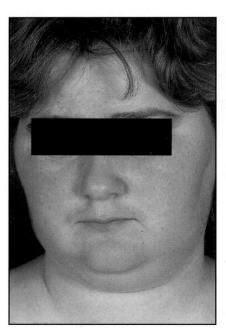

Fig. 2.42 Cushing's syndrome: plethoric 'moon-shaped' facies.

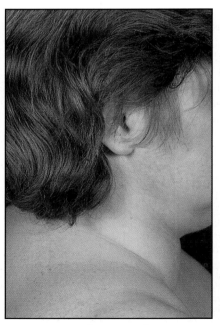

Fig. 2.43 Cushing's syndrome: typical buffalo hump. Recognised as fullness below the hairline, rather than an actual hump.

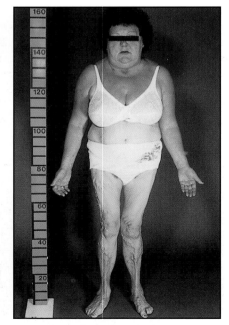

Fig. 2.44 Cushing's syndrome: proximal muscle wasting and central distribution of fat.

Symptoms and signs
Cushing's syndrome

- Round, moon-shaped, plethoric facies
- Hirsutes
- Acne
- Hypertension
- Buffalo hump on neck (fatty deposit)
- Central distribution of fat
- Proximal muscle weakness and wasting
- Purple skin striae

Differential diagnosis
Hypoadrenalism

Acute
- Rapid withdrawal after exogenous steroid treatment
- Failure to increase steroid dose when steroid-dependent patient is subjected to physiological stress
- Septicaemia (especially meningococcus)

Chronic
- Adrenal destruction
- Autoimmune (Addison's disease)
- Tuberculosis

In chronic, progressive adrenal failure there are usually clinical clues to the diagnosis. Increased pigmentation develops in the skin (especially sun-exposed areas, pressure points, areolae and skin creases) (Fig. 2.45) and mucous membranes (seen best in the buccal mucous membrane). In Addison's disease, patients may also develop characteristic symmetrical patches of depigmented skin (vitiligo). Vague abdominal pain, altered bowel habit, weight loss and weakness also occur. Like the acute disease, postural hypotension is a helpful clinical sign which, later in the course of the disease, may dominate the patient's symptoms.

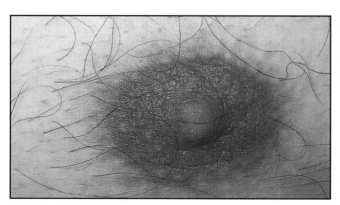

Fig. 2.45 Hyperpigmentation of the areola in Addison's disease.

Symptoms and signs
Presenting features of acute adrenal (Addisonian) crisis

- Profound dehydration, postural hypotension, shock
- Severe nausea and vomiting associated with unexplained weight loss
- Acute abdominal pain
- Unexplained hypoglycaemia
- Unexplained fever
- Hyponatraemia, hyperkalaemia, uraemia hypercalcaemia, eosinophilia
- Hyperpigmentation or vitiligo

STRUCTURE AND FUNCTION OF THE PITUITARY GLAND

The pituitary gland is suspended from the hypothalamus by the infundibulum and lies in the pituitary fossa at the base of the skull (Fig. 2.46). The hypothalamus communicates with the anterior pituitary (or adeno-

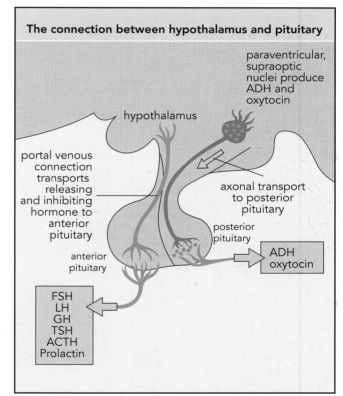

Fig. 2.46 The hypothalamus connects to the anterior pituitary by a portal venous network which carries releasing and inhibiting hormones to stimulate the release of hormones into the circulation. By contrast, the posterior pituitary hormones are synthesised in the supraoptic and paraventricular nuclei of the hypothalamus and transported to the posterior pituitary along axons which discharge directly into the systemic circulation.

hypophysis) via a unique portal blood system which transports chemical stimuli to the anterior pituitary. A different form of communication occurs with the posterior pituitary (or neurohypophysis). The supraoptic and paraventricular nuclei of the hypothalamus synthesise antidiuretic hormone (ADH) and oxytocin and these hormones flow along the axons to nerve endings in the posterior pituitary, where they are released into the circulation so that they can assert their distant effects.

Hormones synthesised and secreted by the anterior pituitary include follicle stimulating hormone (FSH), luteinising hormone (LH), growth hormone, prolactin, TSH and ACTH. These hormones are regulated by the secretion of specific releasing factors produced in the hypothalamus and transported to the pituitary by the hypothalamic–pituitary portal circulation (Fig. 2.47). The regulation of the anterior pituitary hormones is controlled by the balance between the stimulating effects of the release factors and the inhibitory feedback from the target circulating hormone. There are also inhibitory hypothalamic hormones (somatostatin and dopamine). Prolactin release is inhibited by hypothalamic dopamine; this neurotransmitter is secreted into the portal circulation, causing tonic inhibition of prolactin release (Fig. 2.48).

Hypothalamic osmoreceptors and volume receptors sense blood osmolality and effective circulating volume and regulate the secretion of ADH from the posterior pituitary. ADH reduces free water clearance by the distal tubules of the nephron, resulting in concentration of the urine and water conservation. Oxytocin from the posterior pituitary causes uterine contraction during childbirth. In addition, the

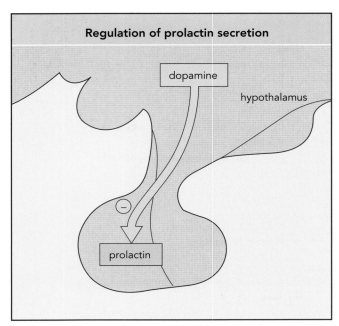

Fig. 2.48 Prolactin secretion from the anterior pituitary in inhibited by the tonic secretion of dopamine from the hypothalamus.

hormone promotes milk ejection during lactation by stimulating contraction of the smooth muscles surrounding the mammary gland ducts.

Pituitary tumours may cause overstimulation syndromes or destruction of the gland and deficiency syndromes. Both over- and understimulation cause recognisable clinical syndromes that can be identified on general examination. Remember that pituitary tumours may be associated with other endocrine adenomas, especially parathyroid adenomas, which cause hypercalcaemia. Diagnosis of pituitary disease depends on the responsiveness of stimulatory influences (e.g. effect of administration of hypothalamic releasing hormones or insulin-induced hypoglycaemic stress).

SYNDROMES ASSOCIATED WITH OVERPRODUCTION OF PITUITARY HORMONES

Acromegaly

Acidophil (or more rarely chromophobe) tumours of the anterior pituitary may cause inappropriate release of growth hormone, resulting in gigantism if the epiphyses have not fused and acromegaly in adults when fusion has occurred. Acromegalic patients may present complaining that their shoes, gloves or rings no longer fit or that they are aware of a change in facial appearance. There may also be symptoms suggestive of visual field defects. Ask for a previous photograph to compare physical features. On physical examination, a typical syndrome reflects the overgrowth of bone and other tissues resulting from growth hormone hypersecretion (Figs 2.49–2.51).

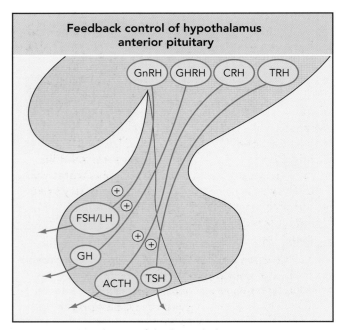

Fig. 2.47 Regulation of the hypothalamic–anterior pituitary endocrine axis.

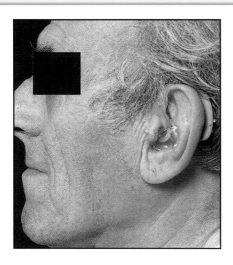

Fig. 2.49 Acromegaly: typical facial appearance.

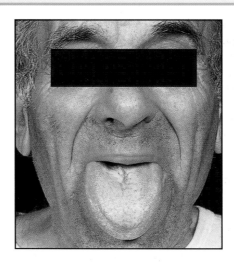

Fig. 2.50 Acromegaly: large tongue.

 Symptoms and signs
Acromegaly

- Coarse, prominent facial features
- Prognathoid jaw
- Prominent nose and forehead
- Thickened lips and large tongue
- 'Spade-shaped' hands
- Excessive sweating and greasy skin
- Kyphosis
- Hypertension
- Bitemporal hemianopia develops
- Carpal tunnel syndrome
- Impaired glucose tolerance

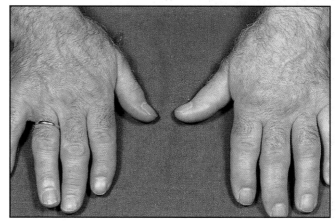

Fig. 2.51 Acromegaly: spade-shaped hands.

Hyperprolactinaemia

Disruption of the tonic inhibition of prolactin release by dopamine results in the syndrome of hyperprolactinaemia. The syndromes associated with the overproduction of prolactin may be dominated by either the effect of the prolactin or the destructive effect of the pituitary tumour. Breast secretion (galactorrhoea) may develop in both women and men. The usual presenting symptom in women is alteration in the menstrual pattern (usually oligomenorrhoea or amenorrhoea). Men may present with impotence or with symptoms of pituitary expansion and malfunction (headaches, visual defects, hypothyroidism, hypoadrenalism).

SYNDROMES ASSOCIATED WITH PITUITARY HYPOFUNCTION

Hypopituitarism

The syndrome of hypopituitarism may become recognisable if the pituitary is destroyed by a tumour, gran-

 Symptoms and signs
Hyperprolactinaemia

Women	Men
• present earlier	• present later
• galactorrhoea (<30%)	• galactorrhoea
• infertility	• importence
• menstrual disorders	• signs of pituitary tumour
	• visual field defects
	• anterior pituitary failure

 Symptoms and signs
Hypopituitarism

Women	Men
• amenorrhoea, infertility	• loss of libido or importence, infertility
• vaginal atrophy, dyspareunia	• soft atrophic testes and loss of secondary sexual characteristics
• atrophic breasts	
• loss of axillary and pubic hair	

- TSH deficiency, mild to moderate hypothyroidism
- ACTH defiency – weakness
  – postural hypotension
  – pallor
  – hypoglycaemia

ulomatous disease (e.g. sarcoidosis, tuberculosis, histiocytosis X), trauma or after a postpartum haemorrhage (Sheehan's syndrome). Secondary pituitary failure may also occur with disease of the hypothalamus. The clinical features progress in a characteristic sequence. Growth and luteinising hormone failure occurs first, followed by FSH and TSH and finally ACTH (Fig. 2.52).

Impaired ADH secretion causes a typical syndrome known as cranial diabetes insipidus. Patients have inappropriate polyuria and produce a dilute urine, even when deprived of water for prolonged periods. Often there is no obvious cause for the isolated defect. Head injury or cranial surgery may be complicated by posterior pituitary damage and diabetes insipidus. Other rare causes include pituitary tumours (e.g. destructive adenomas, craniopharyngiomas, metastases), granulomatous diseases (e.g. sarcoidosis, eosinophilic granulomas), infections (e.g. bacterial meningitis, tuberculosis) and familial disease. The symptoms of cranial diabetes insipidus can be confused with compulsive water drinking (i.e. when water deprivation causes appropriate urine concentration) and nephrogenic diabetes insipidus (i.e. when water deprivation is associated with dilute urine and high serum levels of ADH).

NUTRITION

Nutritional status may be an important marker of disease and the progression or regression of a disorder. Poor nutrition is readily treatable and nutritional support can hasten recovery and protect against compli-cations. Malnutrition may seriously impair immunological and healing responses and attention to nutritional status may positively influence the course of disease. In contrast, obesity is also associated with morbidity, so weight loss in these individuals can be advantageous.

ASSESSMENT OF NUTRITION

The clinical assessment of nutritional status includes overall appearance, weight, height, muscle and fat bulk and vitamin, mineral and haematinic status.

Either at the beginning or conclusion of the first examination, you should weigh the patient and measure the height. This provides useful baseline information, as standard growth charts are available to help you judge whether the patient falls within the normal range of weight for height (Fig. 2.53). Always adopt a standard procedure for weighing the patient. In the outpatient department, it is customary to weigh the patient in socks and basic clothing. Patients in hospital can be weighed either naked or with a light linen gown. Ensure that all subsequent weighings are performed in a standard manner. Standard weight charts indicating expected percentiles and norms for height assume that the patient has been weighed naked. Body mass index (BMI) is the preferred method for assessing weight as it considers both weight and height. This is calculated from the formula.

$$\frac{\text{weight (kg)}}{\text{height (m)}^2}$$

The normal BMI range is 20–25.

Standardise the method for measuring height. The height measurement is usually made on the vertical

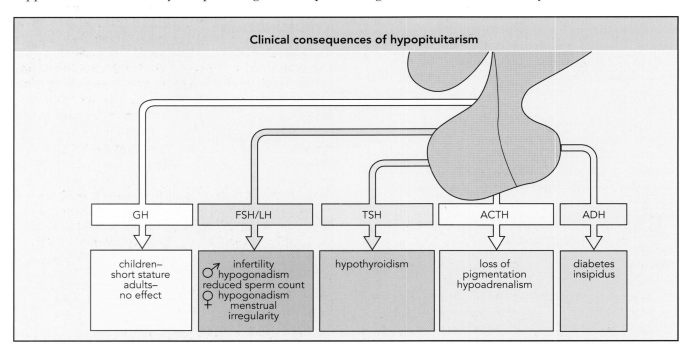

Fig. 2.52   Clinical consequences of pituitary failure. Diabetes insipidus is a rare manifestation of the hypopituitary syndrome. (GH, growth hormone; FSH, follicle stimulating hormone; LH, luteinising hormone; TSH, thyroid stimulating hormone; ACTH, adrenocorticotrophin; ADH, antidiuretic hormone).

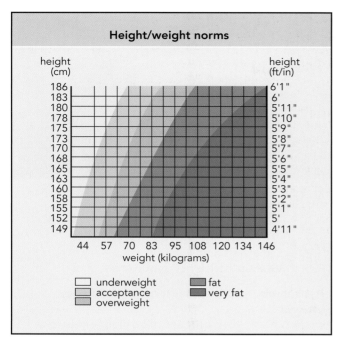

Height/weight norms

height (cm)		height (ft/in)

underweight   fat
acceptance   very fat
overweight

Fig. 2.53 Chart indicating height and weight norms in adults.

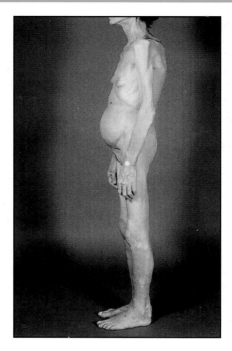

Fig. 2.54 Malnutrition in liver disease. Muscle wasting is readily recognised by the prominence of the skeleton due to loss of muscle bulk and fatty tissue.

height ruler attached to the scale. Ensure that the patient stands bolt upright with heels firmly on the surface and back flush against the rule. Measure the height by sliding the height marker to touch the crown. The sitting height is also useful; from the teens to adulthood, this height should be near 50% of the total height. In osteoporosis, the collapse of vertebrae causes shortening, which is reflected in a reduction of the sitting height. Arm span may occasionally be helpful. Ask the patient to extend the arms and hands fully and measure the distance between the tips of the middle fingers. This distance should equal the linear height. In Marfan's syndrome, the arm span exceeds the height.

When the patient is exposed during the course of the physical examination, take the opportunity to evaluate whether the patient is of usual body build, unusually thin or overweight. Weight loss and 'wasting' are suggested by indrawing of the cheeks and unusual prominence of the cheek-bones, head of humerus and major joints, the rib cage and bony landmarks of the pelvis (Fig. 2.54). Muscle wasting may exaggerate the skeletal prominence. Atrophy of the deltoid muscles may be particularly striking. Hypoalbuminaemia may cause white nails (leukonychia) and loss of capillary osmotic pressure results in pedal oedema. Iron deficiency may cause spooning of the nails (koilonychia). Other features of nutritional deficiency include inflammation and cracks at the angle of the mouth (angular stomatitis), a smooth tongue lacking in papillae (atrophic glossitis) (Fig. 2.55) and skin rashes (e.g. pellagra) (Fig. 2.56). Although a visual assessment provides a relatively accurate assessment of general nutritional status, more objective measures, both clinical and biochemical, are necessary, especially when it is important to establish a baseline for nutritional support and when progress needs monitoring.

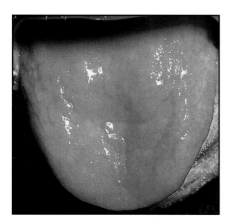

Fig. 2.55 Smooth shiny tongue of atrophic glossitis (especially iron deficiency).

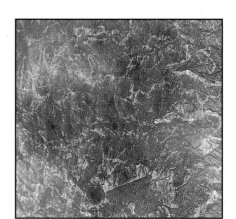

Fig. 2.56 Pellagra: photosensitive 'crazy- paving' skin rash.

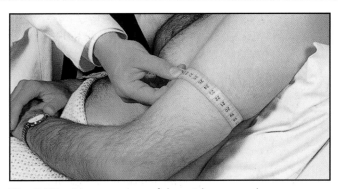

Fig. 2.57   Measurement of the midarm muscle circumference.

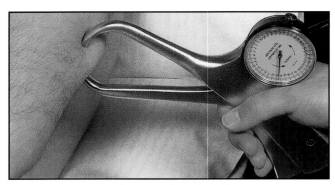

Fig. 2.58   Measurement of the triceps skinfold thickness.

Symptoms and signs
Biochemical and immunological markers of malnutrition

- Haemoglobin (iron, B$_{12}$, folate deficiency)
- Low serum albumin
- Low serum transferrin
- Reduced creatinine (reflects reduced muscle bulk)
- Creatinine:height ratio
- Reduced white cell count
- Impaired delayed cell-mediated immunity (skin tests)

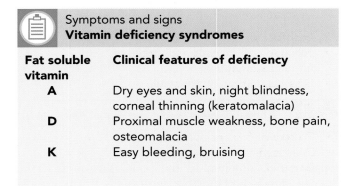

Symptoms and signs
Vitamin deficiency syndromes

Fat soluble vitamin	Clinical features of deficiency
A	Dry eyes and skin, night blindness, corneal thinning (keratomalacia)
D	Proximal muscle weakness, bone pain, osteomalacia
K	Easy bleeding, bruising

MIDARM MUSCLE CIRCUMFERENCE

This measurement provides an estimate of muscle and fat status. The standard position for measurement is the midpoint between the tip of the olecranon and acromial process. The patient's arm should be relaxed and flexed to a right angle. Take the measurement by wrapping the tape-measure around the upper arm midpoint (Fig. 2.57), taking care not to pull too tight or to leave excessive slackness. Take three measurements at the same point and calculate the average. The measurement is itself a useful baseline measure for follow-up purposes. In addition, the single measurement can be compared with percentiles in standard age and sex charts.

TRICEPS SKINFOLD THICKNESS

In adults, the skin overlying the triceps muscle can be lifted and subcutaneous tissue can be distinguished from the underlying muscle bulk. This fold of skin and subcutaneous tissue (the fatfold) provides an indirect assessment of fat stores. Measure the fatfold thickness from the patient's rear and make the measurement at the same midarm landmark used for measuring the midarm muscle circumference. It is useful to mark this point so that you can lift the skinfold between your thumb and index finger and position the jaws of the calipers on either side of the midarm mark on the raised skinfold (Fig. 2.58). As with the tape measurement of midarm muscle circumference, ensure that the

caliper jaws are neither too tight nor too loose. Repeat the measurement three times and take the average to compare with standard tables.

CLINICAL ASSESSMENT OF VITAMIN STATUS

Vitamins are essential cofactors obtained from the diet. Reduced dietary intake may result in recognisable deficiency syndromes. Specific deficiencies of the fat-soluble vitamins (A, D and K) occur in patients with chronic steatorrhoea due to chronic cholestasis and malabsorption syndromes complicated by steatorrhoea.

Deficiencies of water-soluble vitamins occur in all forms of malnutrition. The syndromes are especially prevalent in malnutrition due to famine, malnourished alcoholic patients, patients on chronic renal dialysis and in underdeveloped countries where processing of staple foods reduces vitamin content.

CLINICAL ASSESSMENT OF HYDRATION

Fluid and electrolyte balance is carefully regulated. The intake of fluid and electrolytes is closely matched

Symptoms and signs
Water-soluble vitamin deficiency

B₁ (thiamine)
- Wet beriberi
  - peripheral vasodilatation
  - high output cardiac failure
  - oedema
- Dry beriberi
  - sensory and motor peripheral neuropathy
- Wernicke's encephalopathy
  - ataxia, nystagmus, lateral rectus palsy
  - altered mental state
- Korsakoff's psychosis
  - retrograde amnesia, impaired learning
  - confabulation

B₂ (riboflavin)
- Inflamed oral mucous membranes
- Angular stomatitis
- Glossitis, normocytic anaemia

B₃ (niacin)
- Pellagra
- Dermatitis (photosensitive)
- Diarrhoea
- Dementia

B₆ (pyridoxine)
- Peripheral neuropathy
- Sideroblastic anaemia

B₁₂
- Megaloblastic, macrocytic anaemia
- Glossitis
- Subacute combined degeneration of the cord

Folic acid
- Megaloblastic, macrocytic anaemia
- Glossitis

C
- Scurvy
  - perifollicular haemorrhage
  - bleeding gums, skin purpura
  - bleeding into muscles and joints
- Anaemia
- Osteoporosis

Symptoms and signs
Measurement of postural change in blood pressure

- Lie the patient supine for 2 min
- Record pulse rate and blood pressure in supine position
- Ask the patient to stand upright
- Wait 1 min
- Measure standing heart rate and blood pressure at 1 and 3 min
- Heart rate normally increases by 8–12 beats/min
- Systolic blood pressure drops by 3–4 mmHg
- Diastolic blood pressure increases by 3–7 mmHg
- Postural hypotension when systolic drops by 20 mmHg and/or diastolic by 10 mmHg

Symptoms and signs
Measuring the capillary refill time

- Patient's hand placed level with the heart
- Distal phalanx of the middle finger compressed for 5 s
- Release pressure
- Measure time to regain normal colour (refill time)
- Normal filling time is 2–3 s (2–4 s in the elderly)

by loss in urine, stool and sweat. Dehydration can occur if there is a mismatch between fluid intake and loss. Ill patients may be anorexic and fail to take in the minimal fluid intake necessary to maintain fluid balance; the kidney may lose its ability to regulate the quality and quantity of urine; and there may be excessive gastrointestinal fluid loss (diarrhoea and vomiting) or abnormal sweating (pyrexia).

The history may be helpful when assessing hydration. Dehydration rapidly provokes thirst, the first clinical symptom of dehydration. Ask patients whether they feel abnormally thirsty and whether they have noticed a dry, parched mouth. Physical signs of dehydration are usually only apparent with moderate to severe dehydration. Inspect the tongue and note whether the mucosa is wet and glistening. Touching the tongue may help you assess its moistness. Look at the eyes, which should have a glistening, shiny appearance; this sparkle is lost as dehydration develops. With moderate dehydration, the eyes may appear sunken into the orbits; the pulse rate may increase to compensate for intravascular volume loss. Blood pressure falls in hypovolaemic patients and the demonstration of postural hypotension is a cardinal sign of significant intravascular fluid loss. In addition, the capillary refill time can be used to assess the circulatory effects of volume depletion.

With marked dehydration skin turgor is lost. This can be demonstrated by gently pinching a fold of skin on the neck or anterior chest wall, holding the fold for a few moments (Fig. 2.59) and letting it go. Well-hydrated skin immediately springs back to its original position, whereas in dehydration the skinfold only slowly returns back to normal. This sign is unreliable in elderly patients whose skin may have lost its normal elasticity. Urine output falls and the urine is concentrated. In severe dehydration, the patient may be profoundly hypotensive and anuric, and renal failure caused by tubular necrosis may occur.

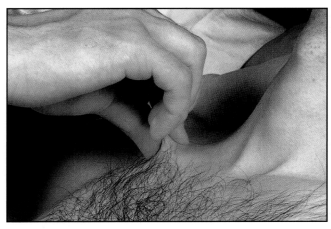

Fig. 2.59 To test for moderate to severe dehydration, assess skin turgor by lifting the skin, pinching it and observing the rate at which it springs back to its normal position.

 Differential diagnosis
Shock

- Hypovolaemic shock
  - GI bleeding
  - trauma
  - ruptured aneurysm
  - burns
  - haemorrhagic pancreatitis
  - fractures (e.g. neck of femur)
  - diarrhoea and vomiting
- Cardiogenic shock
  - acute myocardial infarction
  - acute arrhythmias
  - acute rupture of a valve cusp
  - pericardial tamponade
- Distributive shock
  - gram-negative sepsis
  - toxic shock syndrome
  - anaphylaxis
  - Addisonian crisis
  - spinal cord/major brain injury

 Emergency
Assessment of shock

- Early rise in pulse rate
- Reduced pulse volume/pulse pressure
- Orthostatic hypotension
- Recumbent hypotension
- Cool pale peripheries
- Delayed capillary filling time
- Dry mucous membranes
- Oliguria
- Altered mental state
- Signs of metabolic acidosis

CLINICAL ASSESSMENT OF SHOCK

The clinical presentation of shock varies both with the type and the cause, but there are several common features. Any patient suspected of developing shock should have continuous assessment of the peripheral and central circulation. In the earliest phase (pre-shock), the pulse rate rises and the blood pressure may be maintained by peripheral vasoconstriction, resulting in cool peripheries, skin pallor and reduced capillary refill time. Blood pressure measurement is very helpful in assessing shock, and postural (orthostatic) hypotension antedates the development of recumbent hypotension (systolic BP <90 mmHg or a drop of 40 mmHg in previous hypertensive patients). Once the blood pressure has fallen, oliguria develops. Cerebral hypoperfusion results in altered mental state, characterised initially be agitation and progressing to confusion, delirium, obtundation and coma. Initially patients might hyperventilate, causing a short, transient respiratory acidosis, but this is soon replaced by metabolic acidosis reflecting renal hypoperfusion and impaired clearance of lactate by the liver, kidney and muscle.

COLOUR

Once you have assessed nutrition and hydration, look at the patient's 'colour'. Look for pallor or plethora, central and peripheral cyanosis, jaundice and skin pigmentation.

PALLOR
The cardinal sign of anaemia is pallor. Severe anaemia may be readily recognised by a pale facial appearance and shortness of breath on exertion. The red colour of arterial blood is easiest to assess where the horny layer of the epidermis is thinnest; this includes the palpebral conjunctiva, nail bed, lips and tongue. Inspect the

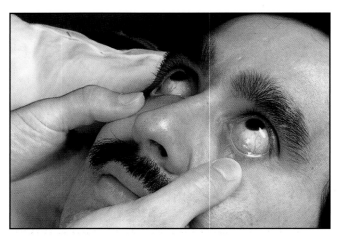

Fig. 2.60 Evert the lower lid to inspect the palpebral conjunctiva for pallor.

palpebral conjunctiva by gently everting the lower eyelid (Fig. 2.60). The palpebral conjunctiva is normally a healthy red colour but, in anaemia, it appears a pale pink.

Experience will teach you to distinguish normal from abnormal. Conjunctival pallor should be accompanied by pallor of the nail bed and palmar skin creases (only assess this if the hands are warm). Pallor is an unreliable sign in cold or shocked patients because peripheral vasoconstriction causes skin and conjunctival pallor even when not associated with blood loss.

PLETHORA

This refers to a ruddy 'weather beaten' facial appearance where the skin has an unusually red or bluish (cyanosed) appearance. Facial plethora is usually caused by an abnormally high haemoglobin concentration (polycythaemia). This is usually caused by chronic cyanotic lung disease in which hypoxia stimulates erythropoietin release from the macula densa of the proximal renal tubule cells. This hormone stimulates the marrow to increase red cell production with consequent increase in haemoglobin concentration. The plethora causes a bloated facial appearance and, together with the cyanosis, these patients have a typical 'blue bloater' appearance.

Polycythaemia rubra vera is a myeloproliferative disorder that causes very high haemoglobin levels and plethora occurs in the absence of hypoxic cyanosis. The conjunctiva has a characteristic 'plum' colour and on fundoscopy the increased blood viscosity causes the venules to assume a thickened 'sausage-shaped' appearance.

CYANOSIS

Cyanosis refers to a bluish or purplish discoloration of the skin or mucous membranes caused by excessive amounts of reduced haemoglobin in blood. At least 5 g/dl of reduced haemoglobin is necessary for cyanosis to appear. In peripheral cyanosis, the extremities are cyanosed (Fig. 2.61) but the tongue retains a healthy pink colour. This is caused by any condition resulting in slowing of the peripheral circulation. In cold weather, there is reflex peripheral vasoconstriction with slowing of the circulation, allowing more time for the extraction of oxygen from haemoglobin. A similar mechanism accounts for peripheral cyanosis in heart failure, peripheral vascular disease, Raynaud's phenomenon and shock. A reduction in arterial oxygen saturation results in central cyanosis. The extremities are cyanosed and the tongue and mucous membranes also have a bluish or purple discoloration. Central cyanosis may develop in any lung disease in which there is a mismatch between ventilation and perfusion. In right-to-left shunts caused by congenital heart disease, the admixture of venous blood to the systemic circulation causes cyanosis.

JAUNDICE

Skin pigmentation influences the ease with which jaundice can be detected. The yellow discoloration is most easily recognised in fair-skinned individuals and is more difficult to detect in darkly pigmented patients. Bilirubin has a high affinity for elastic tissue. This, together with the sclera's white colour, makes the sclera the most sensitive area for looking for the yellow discoloration of jaundice.

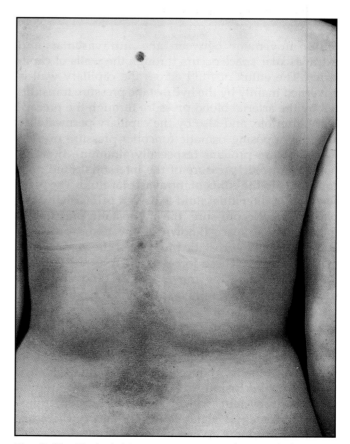

Fig. 2.62 Typical skin pigmentation in chronic cholestasis (primary biliary cirrhosis).

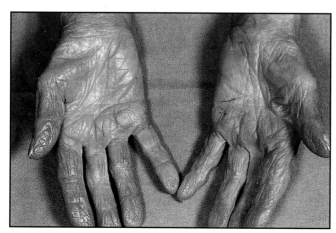

Fig. 2.61 Peripheral cyanosis; note the blue discoloration of the fingers.

Differential diagnosis
Hypothermia

- Environmental exposure
- Hypothyroidism
- Increased cutaneous heat loss – burns, toxic epidermal necrolysis
- Drugs (alcohol, opiates, barbiturates, phenothiazines, lithium)
- Altered thermoregulation (sepsis, hypothalamic disease, spinal cord injury)

myxoedema, pituitary dysfunction, Addison's disease and abuse of drugs or alcohol. Patients are pale, the skin feels cold and waxy and the muscles are stiff. Consciousness is depressed and when the temperature drops to below 27°C, consciousness is lost. A special low-reading thermometer is required to establish the baseline temperature. The most convenient measuring device is a rectal probe (thermocouple) which provides real-time temperature measurement.

EXAMINATION OF THE LYMPHATIC SYSTEM

As the lymphoreticular system is widespread, it is convenient to consider its examination in the general examination. You may choose to examine for enlargement of the lymph nodes (lymphadenopathy) as part of the preliminary general examination, although most clinicians integrate the examination into the regional examination of the head and neck, chest and abdomen.

STRUCTURE AND FUNCTION OF THE LYMPHATIC SYSTEM

The lymphatic system drains the interstitial space, facilitates antigen presentation, produces antibodies and phagocytes and provides a pathway for chylomicron absorption from enterocytes. It comprises the lymphatic ducts, lymph nodes, spleen, tonsils, adenoids and the thymus gland (Figs 2.67, 2.68). Lymphoid tissue is also present in the Peyer's patches of the terminal ileum. The lungs contain significant islands of lymphoid tissue and the hepatic reticuloendothelial cells are an integral component of the lymphoreticular system.

A network of lymphatic ducts accompany the blood vessels; these lymphatics transport lymph from the interstitial tissues to the lymph nodes. Lymph is an opalescent fluid derived from the protein-rich fluid, enriched with lymphocytes, which bathes the interstitial space. The lymphatic vessels drain distinct regions of the body into groups of regional lymph nodes. Efferent lymph vessels leave the regional nodes,

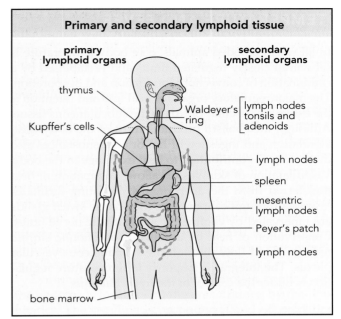

Fig. 2.67 The primary lymphoid organs include bone marrow (which produces B lymphocytes) and the thymus (which produces T lymphocytes). The secondary lymphoid organs provide a 'base camp' for interaction between lymphocytic subtypes and antigens (i.e. macrophages, antigen presenting cells, T and B lymphocytes). The immune response is generated in the secondary lymphoid tissues.

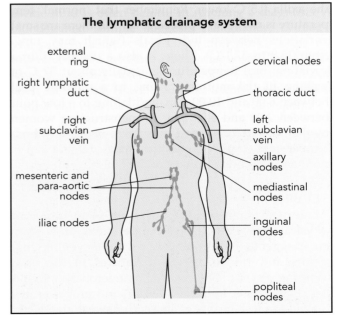

Fig. 2.68 Regional drainage of the lymphatic system. The right upper quadrant drains via the right thoracic duct into the right subclavian vein. The remainder of the lymphatic network drains into the left subclavian vein via the thoracic duct.

converging to form larger vessels. Ultimately, the larger lymphatic vessels converge into two main lymph vessels; the lymphatic trunk drains the right upper body into the right subclavian vein, with the remainder of the body ultimately draining to the thoracic duct, which drains into the left subclavian vein (Fig. 2.68). Fat from the small intestine is not absorbed into the portal circulation. Triglyceride in the enterocyte is coated with protein to form chylomicrons and these are absorbed into mesenteric lymphatics which drain through the thoracic duct into the systemic circulation.

The lymph nodes are comprised of lymphocyte-rich lymphoid follicles and sinuses that are lined with reticuloendothelial cells (histiocytes and macrophages). The follicles in the cortex of the node have a germinal centre populated by rapidly dividing B lymphocytes and macrophages. The germinal centre is surrounded by a cuff of T lymphocytes. Antigens from a distant region drain through the lymphatic vessels into the regional nodes, where they are presented to the lymphocytes, which respond by proliferating into antibody-producing B lymphocytes or antigen-specific T lymphocytes (Fig. 2.69).

Lymphadenopathy may be caused by proliferation of cells in response to antigen challenge. Abnormal cells may populate the nodes. Malignant transformation of the lymphoid cells in lymphomas may cause lymphadenopathy. The glands may become populated by leukaemic cells or metastatic carcinoma. In the lipid storage diseases, lipid-laden macrophages may infiltrate and enlarge the nodes.

Before setting out to examine the lymphatic system, it is important to know the regional arrangement of the major groups of superficial nodes (Fig. 2.68).

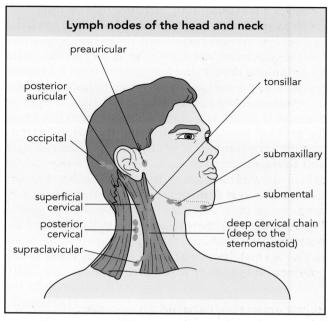

Fig. 2.70 Horizontal ring of facial nodes and the vertical chain of cervical neck nodes.

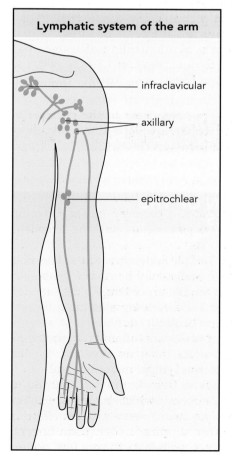

Fig. 2.71 Lymphatic drainage of the arm.

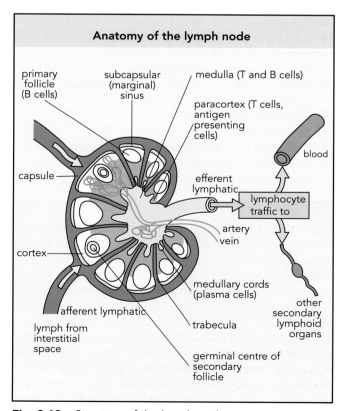

Fig. 2.69 Structure of the lymph node.

this muscle. Conclude the examination by probing for the supraclavicular nodes which lie in the area bound by the clavicle inferiorly and the lateral border of sternocleidomastoid medially (Fig. 2.75). A palpable left supraclavicular node (Virchow's node) should always alert you to the possibility of stomach cancer.

EPITROCHLEAR AND AXILLARY NODES

To palpate the epitrochlear node, passively flex the patient's relaxed elbow to a right angle. Support this position with one hand while feeling with your fingers for the epitrochlear nodes which lie in a groove above and posterior to the medial condyle of the humerus (Fig. 2.76). The axillary group includes anterior, posterior, central, lateral and brachial nodes. Examine the axillary nodes from the patient's front. The technique for examining this region is described in Chapter 8.

INGUINAL AND LEG NODES

Examine these nodes with the patient lying down (Fig. 2.77). The superficial inguinal nodes run in two chains. Palpate the horizontal chain which runs just below the line of the inguinal ligament and the vertical chain which runs along the saphenous vein. Relax the posterior popliteal fossa by passively flexing the knee. Explore the fossa for enlarged popliteal nodes by wrapping the hands around either side of the knee and exploring the fossa with the fingers of both hands (Fig. 2.78).

Remember that the spleen and liver are important components of the lymphoreticular system. Both may enlarge in lymphoreticular diseases. The examination of these organs is covered in Chapter 6.

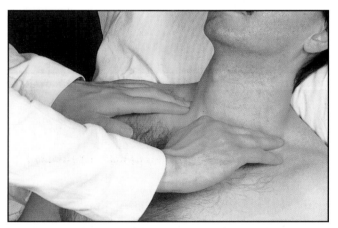

Fig. 2.75 Palpation of the supraclavicular nodes in the supraclavicular fossa.

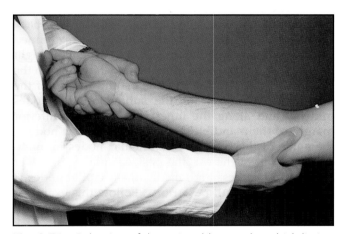

Fig. 2.76 Palpation of the epitrochlear nodes which lie in a groove above and posterior to the medial condyle of the humerus.

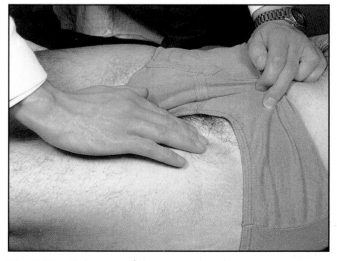

Fig. 2.77 Palpation of the inguinal nodes.

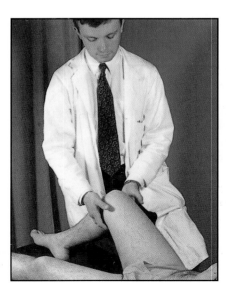

Fig. 2.78 Palpation of the popliteal nodes.

Review
Framework for choreographing the physical examination

General examination
- First impressions
- Clinical syndromes (including endocrinopathies)
- Nutritional status
- Hydration
- 'Colour'
- Oedema
- Temperature
- Lymphoreticular examination

Skin examination
- Skin inspection
- Palpation
- Description of lesions
- Hair
- Nails

Ears, nose and throat examination
- Inspection outer ear, drum, test hearing and balance
- Inspection of nose and palpation/percussion of sinuses
- Inspection of lips, teeth, tongue, oral cavity and pharynx, inspection and palpation of salivary glands
- Palpation of regional lymph nodes

Cardiovascular examination
- Hands (splinters, clubbing)
- Pulses
- Blood pressure
- Jugular venous pressure
- Heart (inspect, palpate, auscultate)
- Lungs (basal crackles, effusions)
- Abdomen (liver pulsation)
- Extremities (peripheral circulation, oedema)

Respiratiory examination
- Hands (clubbing, cyanosis, CO_2 retention)
- Blood pressure (pulsus paradoxus)
- Neck (JVP, trachea)

- Lungs (inspect, palpate, percuss, auscultate)
- Heart (evidence of cor pulmonale)

Abdominal examination
- Hands (flapping tremor, nails, palms)
- Jaundice and signs of liver failure
- Parotids
- Mouth and tongue
- Chest (gynaecomastia, spiders, upper border of liver)
- Abdomen (inspect, palpate, percuss, auscultate)
- Groins
- Rectal examination

Male genitalia
- Sexual development
- Penis
- Scrotum
- Testes and spermatic cord
- Inguinal region

Female breasts and genitalia
- Sexual development
- Breast (inspection, palpation)
- Vulva (inspection, palpation)
- Vagina (inspection, palpation)
- Uterus and adnexae (palpation)

Musculoskeletal examination
- Proximal and distal muscles (inspection, palpation)
- Large joints
- Small joints
- Spine

Neurological examination
- Psychological profile
- Mental status
- Cranial nerves
- Motor and sensory examination (central and peripheral), cerebellar examination
- Autonomic nervous system

Examination of elderly people
Nutrition in the elderly

- Elderly at special risk of nutritional compromise
- Contributory factors
  - socioeconomic
  - inability to shop
  - loneliness
  - loss of smell, taste and teeth
- Age-related norms for height, weight, midarm muscle circumference and triceps skinfold thickness unavailable for elderly people
- Nutrition best assessed by careful dietary assessment (using 3rd party to validate information), and the use of haematological and biochemical markers
- Assessment of hydration affected by loss of elastic tissue in skin

3.
Skin, Nails and Hair

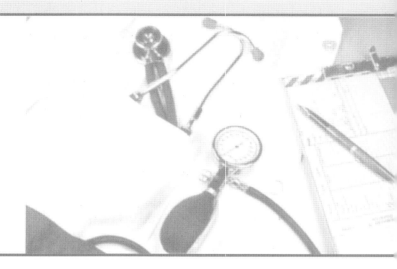

This section aims to familiarise you with the clinical features of skin disease and illustrates some of the more common skin disorders.

The relatively sparse distribution of hair in the human species contrasts starkly with most other mammals and reflects an evolutionary event that must, in some way, have been advantageous. Perhaps human nakedness provided a strong stimulus for developing alternative 'coats' and from this emerged the creative attributes that characterise the species.

The environment in which we live is harsh, variable and unpredictable. In contrast, the efficiency with which the body operates is set within narrow limits of temperature and hydration. Skin has evolved to encapsulate, insulate and thermoregulate. Recently, other functions have been recognised: the skin is an important link in the immune system, and the Langerhans cells of the dermis are closely related to monocytes and macrophages and are probably important in delayed hypersensitivity reactions and allograft rejection. Skin also has an important endocrine function, being responsible for the modification of sex hormones produced by the gonads and adrenals. In addition, skin is the site of vitamin D synthesis.

STRUCTURE AND FUNCTION

SKIN

The skin comprises two layers: the epidermis, derived from embryonic ectoderm; and the dermis and hypodermis, derived from mesoderm.

Epidermis

This layer consists of a modified stratified squamous epithelium and arises from basal, germinal columnar keratinocytes that evolve as they migrate towards the surface through a prickle cell layer (where the cells acquire a polyhedral shape) and a granular cell layer (where the nucleated cells acquire keratohyalin granules) and eventually form the superficial keratinised layer (horny layer of the stratum corneum) where the

cells lose their nuclei and form a tough superficial barrier (Fig. 3.1). The migratory cycle from the basal to horny layer takes approximately 30 days, with the cornified cells shedding from the surface some 14 days later. Abnormalities of this transit time may lead to certain skin diseases such as psoriasis, in which the

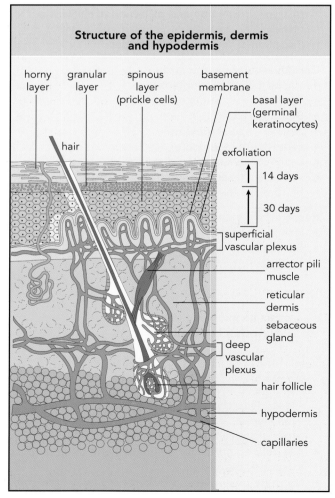

Fig. 3.1 Section through full thickness of skin showing the structure of the epidermis, dermis and hypodermis.

migration rate is greatly accelerated. Epidermal cells are linked by structures known as desmosomes. The epidermis rests on a thin basement membrane and is anchored to the dermis by hemidesmosomes and other anchor proteins such as laminin, basement membrane proteoglycan and type IV collagen. These and other proteins are of importance in the pathogenesis of diseases occurring at the epidermal–dermal junction (e.g. bullous pemphigoid and epidermolysis bullosa).

Melanocytes develop among the basal cells. These cells are derived from neural crest cells and synthesise melanin pigment which is transferred to keratinocytes through dendritic processes. Melanin is responsible for skin and hair pigmentation. The pigment protects the skin from the potentially harmful effects of ultraviolet irradiation. Skin colour is determined by the total number, size and distribution of melanin granules, not the number of melanocytes. Hereditary failure to synthesise melanin results in albinism.

Dermis

This layer provides the supporting framework on which the epidermis rests and consists of a fibrous matrix of collagen and elastin set in a ground substance of glycosaminoglycans, hylauronic acid and chondroitin sulphate (Fig. 3.1). The skin appendages are set in the dermis. Nerves, blood vessels, fibroblasts and various inflammatory cells also populate this layer. The dermis is divided into two layers: the papillary dermis apposes the undulating dermal–epidermal junction, whereas the reticular dermis lies beneath, forming the bulk of collagen, elastic fibres and ground substance. Dermal fibroblasts synthesise and secrete the dermal collagen subtypes (I and III) and elastin. If there is disruption of dermal elastin, disorders such as wrinkles and a loose skin syndrome (cutis laxa) occur.

Hypodermis

The dermis rests on the hypodermis, which is the subcutaneous layer of fat and loose connective tissue. This layer serves both as a fat store and an insulating layer.

SKIN APPENDAGES

Sebaceous glands

Skin sebaceous glands can function throughout life, although activity is latent between birth and puberty. These glands are partly responsible for the production of vernix caseosa which covers and waterproofs the fetus during the latter stages of gestation. The glands become particularly active during puberty. The secretion is holocrine (i.e. caused by complete degeneration of the acinar cells) and is stimulated by androgens and opposed by oestrogens. Sebaceous glands are absent from the palms and soles and are concentrated on the face, scalp, midline of the back and the perineum. Sebum contains triglyceride, scalene and wax esters and functions to waterproof and lubricate the skin, as well as inhibiting the growth of skin flora and fungi. Skin disorders such as acne vulgaris and rosacea occur in areas where sebaceous glands concentrate.

Apocrine and eccrine glands

The apocrine glands are concentrated in the axillae, areolae, nipples, anogenital regions, eyelids and external ears. These glands become functionally active at puberty and are responsible for an odourless secretion which is acted on by skin flora, causing characteristic body odour to develop. The eccrine sweat glands are widely distributed and are extremely important in heat regulation and fluid balance. Whereas the eccrine cells secrete an isotonic fluid, the duct cells modify the fluid to render it hypotonic. Secretion and its modification is under cholinergic and hormonal control. Sweating in response to temperature change is under hypothalamic control.

HAIR

In most mammals, hair is important in the control of temperature. In humans, however, hair is mainly important as a tactile organ which also has a sensual function, important in both sexual attraction and stimulation. Hair covers all of the body except the palms, soles, prepuce and glans and inner surface of the labia minora. During gestation the fetus is covered by a fine coat of lanugo hair which is lost shortly before birth, except for the scalp, eyebrows and lashes. Hair may be vellus, which is short, fine and unpigmented, or terminal hair, which is thicker and pigmented. Puberty is characterised by the development of coarse, pigmented hair in a pubic, axillary and facial distribution.

Hair is formed by specialised epidermal cells that invaginate deep into the dermal layer. Hair develops from the base of the hair follicle where the papilla, a network of capillaries, supports the nutrition and growth of the hair. Hair growth is cyclical: the active growth phase is termed anagen; involution of the hair, catagen; and the resting phase, telogen.

The hair shaft consists of a cuticle, cortex and medulla. The arrectores pilorum muscles anchor in the papillary dermis and insert into the perifollicular tissue (Fig. 3.1). Contraction of these muscles causes goose pimples (cutis anserina) to occur. Hair colour is determined by the density of melanosomes within the cortex of the hair shaft; none is present in white hair, whereas grey hair has a reduced number. Red hair has different melanosomes to black hair, both chemically and structurally.

THE NAIL

Nail is a specialised skin appendage derived from an epidermal tuck that invaginates into the dermis. The highly keratinised epithelium is strong but flexible and provides a sharpened surface for fine manipulation, clawing, scraping or scratching.

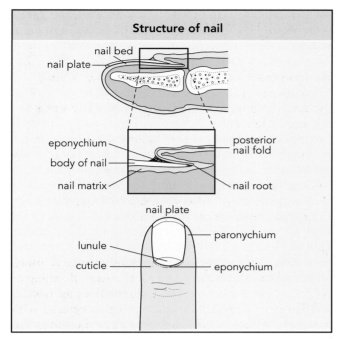

Structure of nail

nail bed
nail plate

eponychium
body of nail
nail matrix
posterior nail fold
nail root

nail plate
lunule
cuticle
paronychium
eponychium

Fig. 3.2 Structure of nail.

Questions to ask
Skin history

- Was the onset sudden or gradual?
- Is the skin itchy or painful?
- Is there any associated discharge (blood or pus)?
- Where is the problem located?
- Have you recently taken any antibiotics or other drugs?
- Have you used any topical medications?
- Were there any preceding systemic symptoms (fever, sore throat, anorexia, vaginal discharge)?
- Have you travelled abroad recently?
- Were you bitten by insects?
- Any possible exposure to industrial or domestic toxins?
- Any possible contact with sexually transmitted disease or HIV?
- Was there close physical contact with others with skin disorders?

Dx Differential diagnosis
Systemic diseases causing pruritus

- Intrahepatic and extrahepatic biliary obstruction (cholestasis)
- Diabetes mellitus
- Polycythaemia rubra vera
- Chronic renal failure
- Lymphoma (especially Hodgkin's disease)

The nail has three major components: the root, the nail plate and the free edge (Fig. 3.2). The proximal and lateral nail folds overlap the edges of the nail and a thin cuticular fold, the eponychium, overlies the proximal nail plate. The lunula is the crescent-shaped portion of the proximal nail formed by the distal end of the nail matrix. The free margin of the distal nail is continuous along its undersurface with the hyponychium, a specialised area of thickened epidermis. The nail plate lies on the highly vascularised nail bed, which gives the nail its pink appearance. The paroncyhium is the soft, loose tissue surrounding the nail border; it is particularly susceptible to bacterial or fungal infection infiltrating from a breach in the eponychium (a paronychia). Fingernails grow approximately 0.1 mm per day, with more rapid growth in summer compared with winter.

SYMPTOMS OF SKIN DISEAS

The history should evaluate possible precipitating factors and determine whether the skin problem is localised or a manifestation of systemic illness.

The skin is readily examined and for this reason the history often assumes less importance than with other systems. However, a thorough history may unearth crucial information to aid diagnosis. Attempt to gain some insight into the patient's social conditions, as overcrowding and close physical contact are important when considering infectious disorders such as scabies and impetigo. Enquire in some depth about possible precipitating factors, especially contact with occupational or domestic toxins or chemicals. Ask whether waterproof gloves are worn when washing dishes or dusting and cleaning the home. Question the patient about recent exposure to medicines, especially antibiotics which often cause skin rashes. Cosmetics are an important cause of skin sensitisation so enquire about the use of new soaps, deodorants and toiletries. Ask about hobbies (e.g. gardening, model building and photographic developing), foreign travel and insect bites. Ascertain whether or not the skin complaint is seasonal.

Systemic disorders may also present with skin symptoms. Infectious diseases often present with skin rashes or lesions. Ask about a recent sore throat, as streptococcal infection may be accompanied by typical rash (scarlet fever), painful red nodules on the extensor surface (erythema nodosum) or guttate psoriasis. In a cutaneous candidal infection, the patient often complains of an itchy rash and sore tongue or, in women, a vaginal discharge. *Candida albicans* infection often follows a course of broad-spectrum antibiotics. Skin rashes developing in sun-exposed areas (in the absence of strong sunburn, these are known as photosensitive rashes) should raise the possibility of systemic lupus erythematosis, porphyria or drugs. If the patient complains of skin lesions around the genitalia, enquire about possible contact with sexually transmitted disease. AIDS may present with the nodular lesions characteristic of Kaposi's sarcoma or thrush affecting the mucosa or skin. Therefore, it is important to take a history of risk factors (e.g. male homosexuality, high-risk heterosexual contact, blood transfusion and intravenous drug abuse). Skin itching (pruritus) in the absence of an obvious rash should alert you to an underlying systemic disorder.

Topical steroids and other topical substances are commonly prescribed to treat a variety of skin lesions. Always ask about topical treatment as this may alter the appearance of a skin lesion, making the diagnosis more difficult.

SYMPTOMS OF HAIR DISEASE

HAIR THINNING
Balding (alopecia) worries patients and you will often be asked to assess scalp hair loss. Male pattern baldness is common; the patient will note the slow onset of hair loss with the hairline receding from the frontal and temporal scalp and crown. Ask about a family history of baldness as male alopecia is an expression of autosomal dominance and may begin early in life. After the menopause, many women note thinning of the hair (Fig. 3.3); this is often associated with growth of facial hair.

Hair loss may also be a feature of disease and the characteristics of the alopecia may be helpful. Patients complaining of localised alopecia (alopecia areata) (Fig. 3.4) may have an autoimmune disease (e.g. Hashimoto's thyroiditis with myxoedema). Patients

Questions to ask
Hair history

- Was the hair loss sudden or gradual?
- Does the loss occur only on the scalp or is the body hair involved as well?
- Is the baldness localised or general, symmetrical or asymmetrical?
- Is there a family history of baldness (especially in men)?
- What drugs have you taken recently?
- Any recent illnesses, stress or trauma?
- Are there other systemic symptoms (e.g. symptoms of hypothyroidism)?

with stress or anxiety neurosis may nervously pluck hair from the scalp, causing a local area of thinning or baldness. Severe illness and malnutrition, as well as sudden psychological shock, may be associated with hair loss, which usually recovers once the stress has been resolved.

ABNORMAL HAIR GROWTH
Remember to warn patients undergoing cytotoxic treatment for cancer that they can expect generalised hair loss. Failure to develop axillary and pubic hair at the expected time of puberty should alert you to the possibility of pituitary or gonadal dysfunction.

Abnormal facial hair growth (hirsutism) is a distressing symptom in women. It is important to recognise that a certain degree of facial hair growth occurs naturally in postpubertal women. There are racial differences: physiological hirsutism is least apparent in Japanese and Chinese women and most apparent in women of Mediterranean, Middle Eastern, Indian and Negroid extraction. The unexpected occurrence of hirsutism, especially if accompanied by other symptoms and signs of virilism, should alert you to the possibility of a hormonal imbalance.

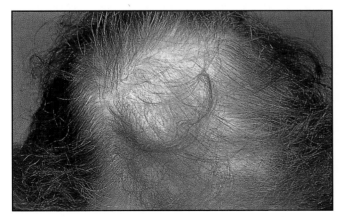
Fig. 3.3 Alopecia.

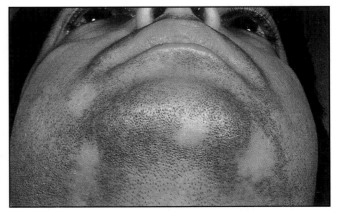
Fig. 3.4 Alopecia areata characterised by localised patches of hair loss.

Differential diagnosis
Hirsutism

- Racial variation in hair distribution
- Hormonal imbalance
  - polycystic ovaries
  - ovarian failure or menopause
  - virilising adrenal tumours
- Drugs
  - phenytoin
  - progestogens
  - anabolic steroids
  - ciclosporin

Questions to ask
Hirsutism

- Is there a family history of hirsutism?
- Are your menstrual periods normal or absent (or scanty)?
- Is there a history of primary or secondary infertility?
- Do you experience visual disturbances or headaches (pituitary disease)?
- What medications do you take (e.g. phenytoin, anabolic steroids, progestogens)?

SYMPTOMS OF NAIL DISEASE

Whereas examination of the nails may be very revealing, nail-related symptoms are usually nonspecific. Patients may relate symptoms suggestive of bacterial infection along the nail edge; these include intense pain, swelling and often a purulent discharge. Complaints of brittleness, splitting or cracking provide little diagnostic information. Ask specifically about skin disease that may affect the nail, such as psoriasis, severe eczema, lichen planus or a susceptibility to fungal skin infection.

EXAMINATION OF THE SKIN, NAILS AND HAIR

EXAMINING THE SKIN

When examining the skin, there is a tendency to focus on the local area noticed by the patient. Nonetheless, you should consider the skin as an organ in its own right and, like any other examination, the whole organ should be examined to gain maximum information. The patient should be stripped to the underwear, covered with a gown or blanket and the examination area should be well lit (preferably natural daylight or fluorescent light).

Inspection and palpation

Scan the skin, looking for skin lesions and noting both position and symmetry. Remember to expose hidden areas like the axillae, inner thighs and buttock with its natal cleft. Many skin lesions can be diagnosed by their appearance and localisation. Unlike any other organ system, the examination relies almost entirely on careful inspection and meticulous use of descriptive terminology.

Measurement of the length and breadth of skin lesions is useful, especially when monitoring progression or regression. A broad beam torch or electric light helps to define the outline of the border of a skin lesion; a thin beam is helpful if you wish to check whether or not a lesion transilluminates. A fluid-filled but not solid lesion emits a red glow when the torch light shines through it. A Wood's lamp helps to distinguish a fluorescing lesion; by shining the lamp at a suspect lesion, it may be possible to show the characteristic blue–green fluorescence of fungal infections.

Skin colour

Skin colour varies between individuals and races and is usually even and symmetrical in distribution. Normal variations occur in freckling and sun-exposed areas. During pregnancy, there may be darkening of the skin overlying the cheek bones (melasma) and the areolae surrounding the nipple (chloasma).

Abnormal skin colour

Generalised changes in skin colour occur in jaundice, iron overload, endocrine disorders and albinism. The yellow tinge of jaundice is best observed in good daylight, appearing initially as yellowing of the sclerae and then as a yellow discoloration on the trunk, arms and legs. Jaundice is less apparent in unconjugated as opposed to conjugated hyperbilirubinaemia. In long-standing, deep obstructive jaundice, the skin may turn a deep yellow–green. Remember that people eating large quantities of carrots or other forms of vitamin A may develop yellow skin pigmentation (carotenaemia) and that the absence of scleral discoloration distinguishes this syndrome from jaundice.

Iron overload (haemosiderosis and haemochromatosis) causes the skin to turn a slate-grey colour. The astute observer may recognise this metabolic disease by the characteristic skin pigmentation. Addison's disease (autoimmune adrenal destruction) is characterised by darkening of the skin, occurring first in the skin creases of the palms and soles, scars and other skin creases. The mucosa of the mouth and gums also becomes pigmented. Striking pigmentation also arises after bilateral adrenalectomy for adrenal hyperplasia: this syndrome (Nelson's syndrome) is caused by unopposed pituitary over-stimulation. In hypopituitarism, the skin is soft, pale and wrinkled.

Albinism is an autosomal recessive disorder caused by failure of melanocytes to produce melanin. The skin and hair are white and the eyes are pink because of a lack of pigmentation of the iris (there may also be nystagmus).

Common localised abnormalities of skin pigmentation include vitiligo (Fig. 3.5), café au lait spots (Figs 3.6, 3.7), pityriasis versicolor and idiopathic guttate hypomelanosis. Erythema of the skin is caused by capillary dilatation; when pressure is applied the red lesion blanches and reforms. When examining a patient, you may notice an erythematous flush in the necklace area which is caused by anxiety. Purpura is the term used for red-purplish lesions of the skin caused by seepage of blood from skin blood vessels. Unlike erythema, these lesions do not blanch with pressure. If the lesions are small (< 5 mm) they are called petechiae (Fig. 3.8), whereas larger lesions are purpura. Traumatic bruises are called ecchymoses. Telangiectasia refers to fine blanching vascular lesions caused by superficial capillary dilatation (Fig. 3.9).

Localised skin lesions

Careful descriptions of size, shape, colour, texture and position of lesions are helpful in skin diagnosis. Try to ascertain a primary and secondary description of the skin lesion. To establish the primary nature of the skin lesion decide whether the lesion is flat, nodular or fluid-filled. Flat circumscribed changes in colour are termed macules if less than 1 cm or patches if more than 1 cm. If the lesion is raised and can be palpated, assess whether the mass is a papule, plaque, nodule, tumour or wheal. If a circumscribed elevated lesion is fluctuant and fluid-filled, describe whether it is a vesicle, bulla or pustule (Fig. 3.10). If possible, describe the arrangement of the lesions; that is, whether linear, annular (ring-shaped) or clustered. In shingles (herpes zoster), the rash occurs in the distribution of one or more skin dermatomes.

Add to the primary description any secondary characteristics such as superficial erosions, ulceration, crusting, scaling, fissuring, lichenification, atrophy, excoriation, scarring, necrosis or keloid formation.

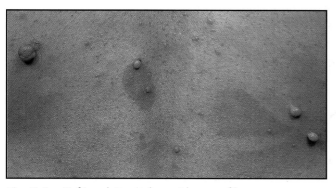

Fig. 3.5 Depigmented skin (vitiligo): white discoloration of brown hand.

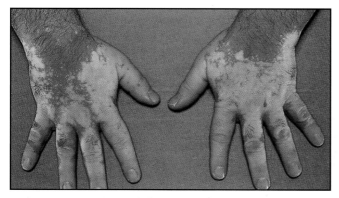

Fig. 3.6 Café au lait patches with neurofibromas.

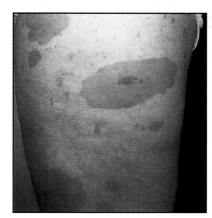

Fig. 3.7 Café au lait patches in neurofibromatosis.

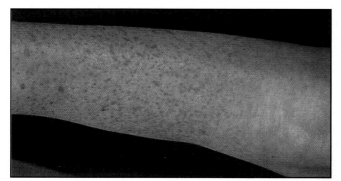

Fig. 3.8 Typical appearance of petechial haemorrhage in a patient with thrombocytopenia.

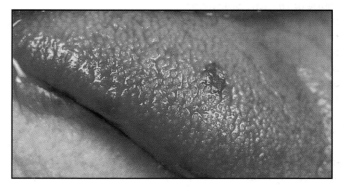

Fig. 3.9 Telangiectasia on the tongue.

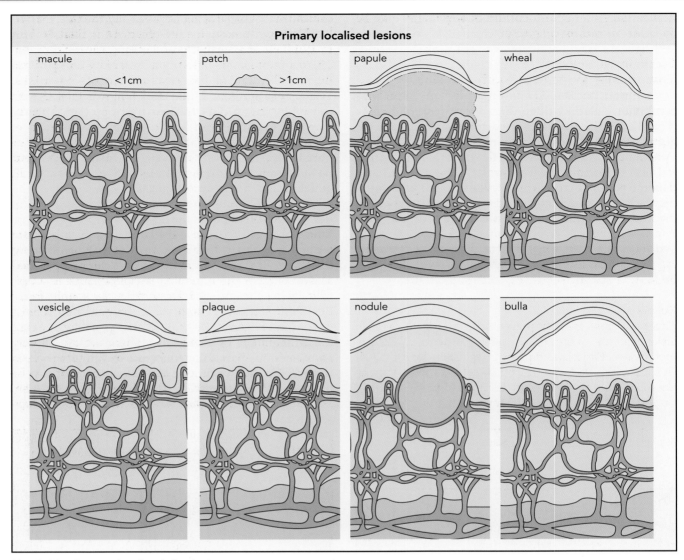

Fig. 3.10 *Primary localised skin lesions.*

Palpation is used to decide whether a lesion is flat, raised or tender. Compression may be helpful (e.g. demonstration of the characteristic arteriolar dilatation of spider naevi occurring in decompensated liver disease) (Fig. 3.11). Use the back of your hand to assess temperature. Inflamed lesions (e.g. cellulitis) are hotter than surrounding tissue, whereas skin overlying a lipoma (subcutaneous fat tumours) is cooler than adjacent tissue. Skin turgor may be used as a measure of moderate to severe hydration. Pinch a small area of skin between index finger and thumb. Hold firmly for 2–3 s and then release. Healthy, well-hydrated skin immediately springs back into its resting position. In significant dehydration or when skin elastic tissue is lost (e.g. ageing), the skin behaves like putty and only slowly reshapes to its resting position. Skin oedema can be demonstrated by pressing your thumb or fingers into the skin, maintaining the pressure for a short while and then releasing. Your thumb or finger impression will remain indented in the skin if there is excessive fluid ('pitting' oedema).

Although most disorders can be diagnosed from their appearance, special techniques such as microscopy of skin biopsies or skin scrapings, immuno-

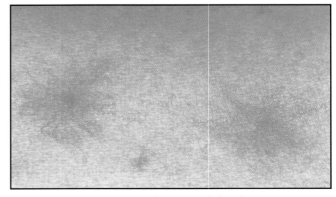

Fig. 3.11 Spider naevi in hepatocellular disease.

fluorescent staining and culture of specimens may be required to confirm diagnosis.

Common skin lesions

Skin lesions are often readily recognisable and you should be able to distinguish some common conditions.

Acne vulgaris

This common disorder of the pilosebaceous unit occurs at puberty. Plugging of the duct, increased sebum production, bacterial growth and hormonal changes all predispose to the condition. Acne presents with greasy skin, blackheads (comedones), papules, pustules and scars (Fig. 3.12). The lesions are common and vary in severity and most teenagers recognise the problem before visiting the doctor. The disorder affects the face, chest and back. Acne usually subsides in the third decade.

Rosacea

This facial rash usually presents in the fourth decade, although, in women, it may present after the menopause. Papules and pustules erupt on the forehead, cheeks, bridge of the nose and the chin. The erythematous background highlights the rash (Figs 3.13, 3.14). Comedones do not occur, distinguishing the condition clinically from facial acne. Occasionally, the rash may be localised to the nose. Eye involvement is characterised by grittiness, conjunctivitis and even corneal ulceration. There appears to be vasomotor instability and patients flush readily in response to stimuli such as hot drinks, alcohol and spicy foods. If this disorder is treated with potent topical corticoids there may be a temporary response, but a marked relapse occurs on cessation of treatment. It is important to check carefully whether or not steroids have been applied and to dissuade your patient from using this treatment (like acne vulgaris, antibiotics are the treatment of choice).

Drug reactions

Drugs are probably the most common cause of acute skin disease and your history must include a complete history of all drugs the patient may have been exposed to over the preceding month. Antibiotics such as ampicillin, penicillin and sulphonamides commonly cause drug rashes. It may be difficult to distinguish between a drug reaction and the manifestations of the disease under treatment. In addition, drug reaction may closely mimic skin diseases. Diagnosis may be further confused in patients taking more than one drug, because it may be difficult to decide which is the offending agent. Also, remember that drugs may cause secondary skin erup-

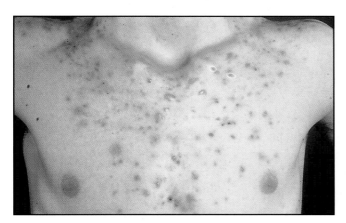

Fig. 3.12 Papules, pustules and scarring in acne vulgaris.

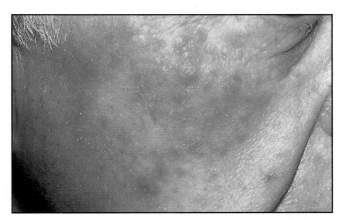

Fig. 3.13 Rosacea: papules and pustules occur on the face.

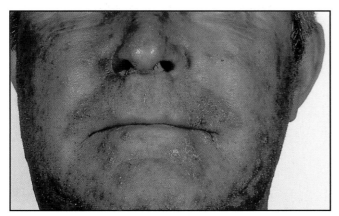

Fig. 3.14 Rosacea: lesions occur on the nose, cheeks and chin.

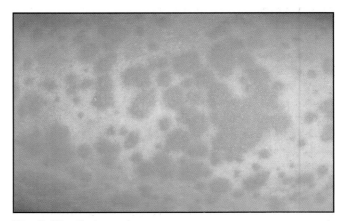

Fig. 3.15 Toxic erythema.

tions: broad-spectrum antibiotics may encourage the growth of candida, which, in turn, can present as a 'drug-related' skin rash. Drug reactions may occur within minutes or hours of taking the medication but there may also be delays of up to 2 weeks for the reaction to manifest. This may even follow the discontinuation of the drug (well known with ampicillin). It is important to recognise different expressions of drug sensitivity.

Toxic erythema

Profuse eruptions affect most of the body. Red macules appear and overlap and coalesce to give the appearance of diffuse erythema (Fig. 3.15). The erythematous skin desquamates as it heals. This condition is most often caused by ampicillin but also by sulphonamides (including co-trimoxazole), phenobarbital and infections.

Exfoliative dermatitis

Also known as erythroderma, this form of dermatitis is characterised by diffuse erythema and desquamation of the epithelium. If severe, the patient may lose both

heat and fluids. Many drugs are implicated, although barbiturates, sulphonamides, streptomycin and gold are especially predominant.

Urticaria

This presents with intense itching and localised swellings of the skin that may occur anywhere on the body. Typically, wheals occur that are red at the margins with paler centres (Fig. 3.16). The characteristic feature of the rash is its tendency to disappear within a few hours. Angio-oedema usually occurs in association with urticaria and is characterised by swelling of the face and hands.

Erythema nodosum

Symmetrical in distribution, the acute crops of painful, tender, raised red nodules usually affect the extensor surfaces, especially the shins but also the thighs and upper arms (Figs 3.17, 3.18). Over 7–10 days, the lesions change colour from bright red through shades of purple to a yellowish area of discoloration. Ery-

 Differential diagnosis
Skin lesions associated with drug sensitivity

- Toxic erythema
- Exfoliative dermatitis
- Urticaria
- Angioneurotic oedema
- Erythema nodosum
- Erythema multiforme
- Fixed drug reaction
- Photosensitive drug reactions
- Pemphigus

 Questions to ask
Exfoliative dermatitis

- Is there any loss of hair or nails?
- Have you ever had psoriasis or eczema?
- What drugs have you taken recently (barbituates, sulphonamides, phenylbutazone, streptomycin)?
- Do you have a fever?

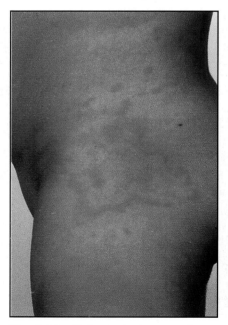

Fig. 3.16 Urticaria: lesions vary in size and shape.

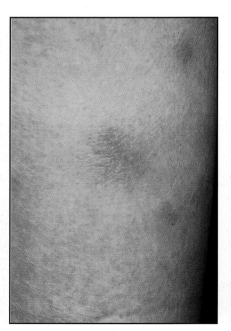

Fig. 3.17 Erythema nodosum: painful, smooth red nodules on the lower leg.

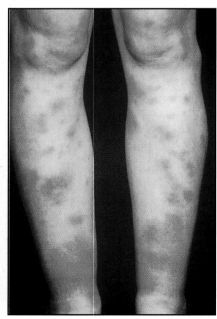

Fig. 3.18 Erythema nodosum: the nodules are raised and tender.

thema nodosum is caused by vasculitis, may be recurrent and is most commonly associated with sulphonamides, oral contraceptives and barbiturates.

Erythema multiforme

This is characterised by symmetrical, round (annular) lesions occurring especially on the hands and feet but which may extend more proximally (Figs 3.19, 3.20). Central blistering may occur, giving the appearance of 'target' lesions. In severe forms, bullae may appear. This skin disease occurs with drugs, vaccination and, frequently, with a herpes simplex infection.

Stevens–Johnson syndrome

This is a severe blistering form of erythema multiforme with blistering and ulceration affecting the mucous membranes of the mouth and often affecting the eyes and nasal and genital mucosa (Fig. 3.21).

Fixed drug eruption

This presents with one or more red blotches that may become swollen and even bullous. The rash always

 Differential diagnosis
Erythema nodosum

Infections
- Streptococcal infections
- Tuberculosis
- Leprosy
- Syphilis
- Deep fungal diseases

Drugs
- Sulphonamides
- Barbiturates
- Oral contraceptives

Systemic diseases
- Sarcoidosis
- Inflammatory bowel disease

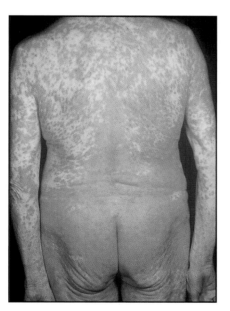

Fig. 3.19 Erythema multiforme: the lesions are widespread on this patient.

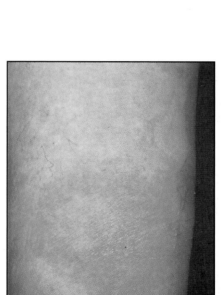

Fig. 3.20 Erythema multiforme.

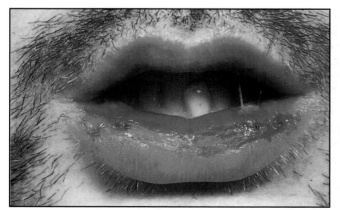

Fig. 3.21 Stevens–Johnson syndrome: ulceration is present on the lips and in the mouth.

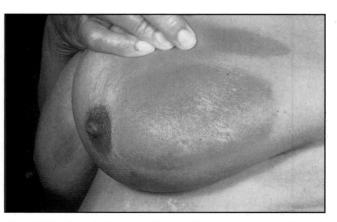

Fig. 3.22 Fixed drug eruption, with hyperpigmentation of the breasts.

recurs in the same anatomical site: usually the mouth, a limb or genital area. The rash fades, leaving an area of skin discoloration (Fig. 3.22). Associated with many drugs but especially phenolphthalein (common in laxatives), sulphonamides, tetracycline and barbiturates.

Photosensitive drug rashes

This rash occurs in sun-exposed areas (face, necklace region and extensor surfaces of limbs). It may appear as erythema, oedema, blistering or an eczematous rash.

Eczema

This common skin abnormality is caused by a number of different mechanisms and the disease may be acute, subacute or chronic, all of which may coexist. Itching is a major symptom. Acute eczema is characterised by oedema, vesicle formation (Fig. 3.23), exudation (weeping) (Fig. 3.24) and crusting. In chronic eczema there are dry, scaly, hyperkeratotic patches and thickening and fissuring of the skin (Fig. 3.25). The appearance of eczema is often modified because the patient scratches, causing secondary changes such as excoriation and secondary infection. The boundaries of an area of chronic eczema are less well defined than psoriasis and this may be a helpful sign in the differential diagnosis (Fig. 3.26).

Discoid (nummular) eczema Unlike other forms of eczema, this subtype has a well-defined, coin-shaped (L. nummularius = of money) outline and may be confused with psoriasis. However, nummular eczema tends to occur on the back of the fingers and hands. It also weeps and does not have the characteristic scales typical of psoriasis.

Atopic eczema This usually presents in infancy, although it does occasionally present for the first time

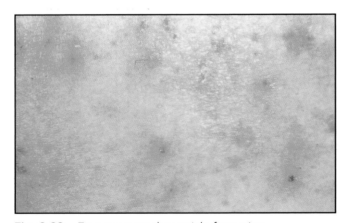

Fig. 3.23 Eczema: note the vesicle formation.

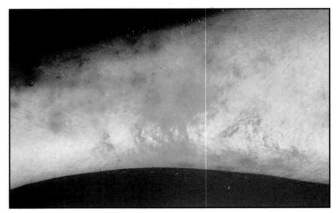

Fig. 3.24 Acute eczema: red exudative eruption which is painful.

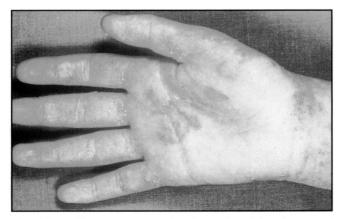

Fig. 3.25 Chronic eczema: the skin is dry and scaly.

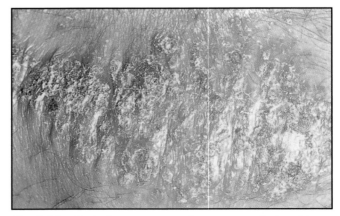

Fig. 3.26 Typical appearance of eczematous lesion. Note that the boundary is less distinct than plaques of psoriasis.

in adulthood. There is normally a family history of eczema or some other atopic disorder (e.g. asthma, hay fever, urticaria). The rash is symmetrical, usually starting on the face and migrating to the trunk and limbs (where it tends to affect the flexures of the elbows, knees, wrists and ankles).

Contact dermatitis This variant of eczema is caused by an exogenous irritant (Fig. 3.27). The lesion may be a primary irritant phenomenon, occurring almost predictably when skin contact is made with a concentrated toxic agent, or an allergic contact dermatitis which only occurs in patients who generate a delayed

(type IV) immune response to a substance in contact with the skin. The distribution of the eczema may provide an important clue to the nature of the topical irritant. Individuals who regularly immerse their hands in water containing detergents or other sensitising substances will present with the rash restricted to the hands. Jewellery may cause an allergic contact dermatitis; nickel is an important sensitising agent. Rubber, dyes, cosmetics and industrial chemicals are common allergens implicated in this immune-mediated form of eczema. Plants such as primulas and chrysanthemums have also been implicated.

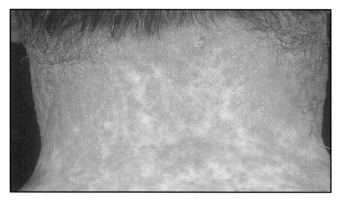

Fig. 3.27 Contact dermatitis caused by shampoo.

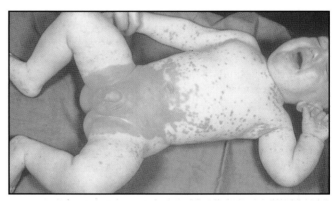

Fig. 3.28 Seborrhoeic dermatitis in an infant.

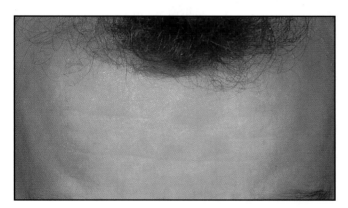

Fig. 3.29 Seborrhoeic dermatitis occurs most commonly on the face.

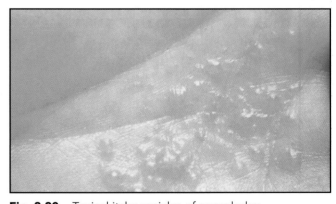

Fig. 3.30 Typical itchy vesicles of pompholyx.

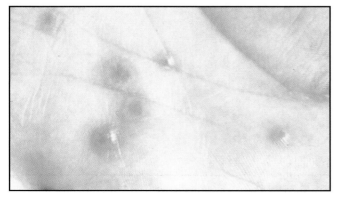

Fig. 3.31 Pompholyx: pruritic vesicles on the hand.

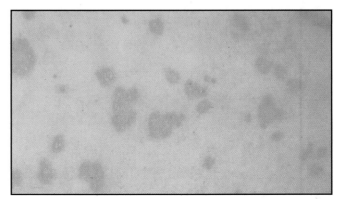

Fig. 3.32 Guttate (teardrop) psoriasis.

Seborrhoeic dermatitis This is an eczematous condition occurring in infants (Fig. 3.28), adolescents and young adults. There is erythema and scaling with a symmetrical rash (Fig. 3.29). Secondary infection may occur, altering the appearance of the primary lesion. The scalp is most commonly involved and the condition is distinguished from dandruff by the associated erythema of the skin due to inflammation. Other regions involved include the central areas of the face, eyelid margins, nasolabial folds, cheeks, eyebrows and forehead. Involvement of the outer ear occurs (otitis externa). The vulva may also be affected.

Pompholyx Pompholyx is another variant of eczema affecting the hands and feet (Figs 3.30, 3.31). This variant is characterised by the eruption of itchy vesicles, especially on the lateral margins of the fingers and toes, as well as the palms and soles.

Varicose eczema This subtype occurs in patients with longstanding varicose veins. The eczematous patches affect the lower leg and may or may not be associated with other skin disorders caused by varicose veins; for example, venous ulcers that occur in the region of the medial maleolus, pigmentation and oedema.

Psoriasis

The lesions are well-defined, slightly raised and erythematous. In the chronic phase, silvery scales cover the surface. The lesions vary in size from small (guttate) (Figs 3.32, 3.33) to large plaques (Figs 3.34, 3.35). These guttate (1–3 cm) lesions are widely distributed over the body and may either resolve or persist as chronic psoriasis. Guttate psoriasis may follow streptococcal pharyngitis.

Chronic psoriasis The plaques of chronic psoriasis have a predilection for the scalp, elbows, knees, perineum, umbilicus and submammary skin. The lesions are usually symmetrical. A characteristic feature of psoriasis is the development of new psoriatic lesions where the skin is traumatised (the Koebner phenomenon). If you gently scratch the surface of a psoriatic plaque, tiny bleeding points appear.

Pustular psoriasis Pustular psoriasis is a variant, usually confined to the palms (Fig. 3.36) and soles, although some are occasionally more diffuse. The pustules, 2–5 mm in diameter, are yellow (Fig. 3.37). On the palms and soles they become pigmented and hyperkeratotic. Rarely, psoriasis may be so extensive that most of the skin is involved and exfoliation occurs.

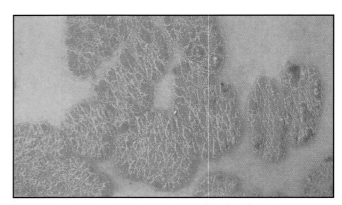

Fig. 3.35 Psoriatic plaque. Note the scaly, shiny surface and the sharp border.

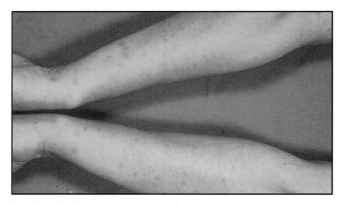

Fig. 3.33 Acute guttate psoriasis.

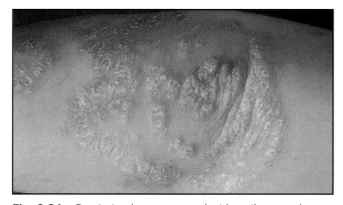

Fig. 3.34 Psoriatic plaque covered with a silvery scale.

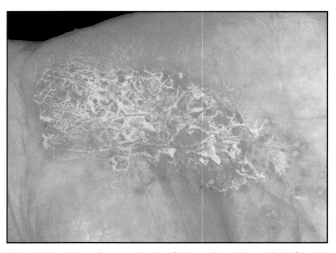

Fig. 3.36 Pustular psoriasis of the palm with well-defined scaling and erythema.

Psoriatic arthropathy In psoriatic arthropathy, the distal interphalangeal joints are affected. Large joints may also be affected, either singly or symmetrically. Rarely, patients may have sacroiliitis or even spinal ankylosis. The nails may be involved even in the absence of skin disease. The typical features include pinpoint pitting of the nail (Fig. 3.38) and onycholysis (lifting of the distal nail from the nail bed). Unlike fungal nail lesions, nail psoriasis is symmetrical. Severe nail dystrophy may occur.

Pityriasis rosea

This is a common skin disorder in the younger patient. A single patch rash occurs days or even weeks before the more general eruption. This 'herald patch' may be confused with ringworm. The full blown rash affects the upper arms, trunk and upper thighs ('shirt and shorts' distribution). Pink papules evolve into 1–3 cm itchy oval macules (Fig. 3.39) that scale near the edge, giving a characteristic appearance (Figs 3.40, 3.41). The rash resolves spontaneously within approximately 6 weeks.

Lichen planus

This is another itchy rash that can usually be diagnosed at the bedside by its typical appearance (Fig. 3.42). Occasionally, a lichenoid rash may be associated with systemic disorders (e.g. primary biliary cirrhosis, chronic graft versus host disease) or drugs (e.g penicillamine and gold) but most commonly there is no associated disease.

The rash affects both the skin and mucous membranes. It has a predeliction for the volar (front) aspect of the forearm and wrists, the dorsal (back) surface of the hands, the shins, ankles and lower back region. The rash is symmetrical and characterised by small, shiny, purple or violaceous papules which have a polygonal rather than rounded outline. A network of white lines on the surface of the papules are termed Wickham's striae (best seen after coating the lesion with mineral oil). As the

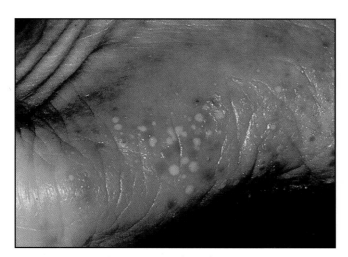

Fig. 3.37 Pustular psoriasis of the foot. The yellow pustules turn brown.

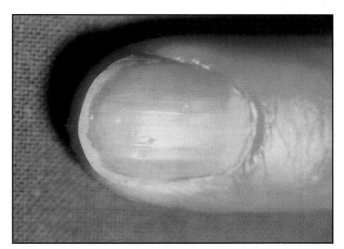

Fig. 3.38 Pitting of the nails in psoriasis.

Fig. 3.39 Pityriasis rosea: the pink papules become oval macules.

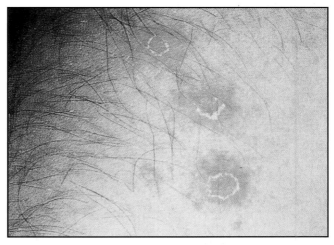

Fig. 3.40 In pityriasis rosea, the typical lesions are ovoid macules with scaling.

papules resolve, the affected skin becomes pigmented. Eruptions occur after trauma (Koebner phenomenon) (Fig. 3.43) and linear lesions are tell-tale signs occurring in scratched areas. The buccal mucous membrane is commonly involved (Fig. 3.44). Use a spatula and light to inspect the mouth, looking for the lace-like network of white lines or spots. The scalp is usually, although not always, spared. The disease may affect the nails and penis.

SKIN INFECTIONS

BACTERIAL

Impetigo

This is a highly contageous skin lesion caused by β-haemolytic streptococci. The face is most commonly infected (Fig. 3.45). The lesions start as a papular eruption around the mouth and nose that then evolves into a vesicular eruption and spreads locally. The lesion breaks down to leave a typical honey-coloured crust. Secondary infection with *Staphylococcus aureus* is common.

Furuncle (boil)

A furuncle is an infection of a hair follicle, caused by *S. aureus*, that spreads locally into the surrounding tissue. A head of pus may be obvious at its apex. Furuncles usually affect adolescents. A local collection of furuncles is called a carbuncle. A stye (or hordeolum) is a small furuncle affecting an eyelash.

Erysipelas and cellulitis

Infection of the superficial skin layers by *Streptococcus pyogenes* is termed erysipelas, whereas an infection of the deeper skin layers is called cellulitis. The lower limbs are most commonly affected. Erysipelas is characterised by the abrupt onset of a well-demarcated slightly raised and tender erythematous rash (Fig. 3.46). Left untreated, the margins of the lesion advance rapidly. The patient is usually pyrexial and toxic. The infection responds quickly to antibiotics. The margin of an area of cellulitis is less well defined than erysipelas; in addition, superficial bullae may develop in the centre of an affected area of skin (Fig. 3.47).

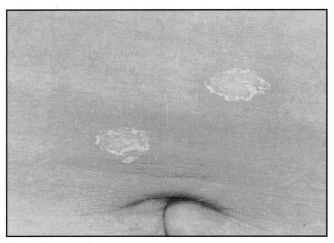

Fig. 3.41 Pityriasis rosea with obvious scaling.

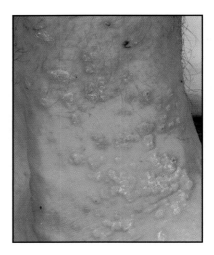

Fig. 3.42
Polygonal papules in lichen planus.

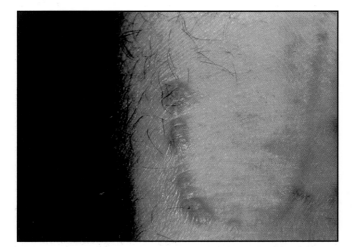

Fig. 3.43 Lichen planus: linear lesion of the Koebner syndrome.

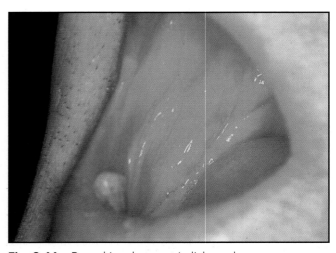

Fig. 3.44 Buccal involvement in lichen planus.

Syphilis

There are numerous skin manifestations of syphilis and you should always suspect this disease when confronted with an unexplained, nonitchy rash, especially when the patient is generally unwell or when there is a high risk of sexually transmitted disease. In primary syphilis, a painless ulcer with an indurated edge (primary chancre) (Figs 3.48, 3.49) appears at the site of infection (usually on the genitalia but occasionally on the lips or even fingers). Approximately 2 months after the appearance of the chancre, the secondary rash appears: a pink macular rash on the trunk (Fig. 3.50) that becomes papular, affecting the genital skin, palms and soles. In the anal and groin regions, the moistness may cause erosions (condylomata accuminata) (Fig. 3.51). Raised oval patches occur in the mucous membrane of the mouth (snail-track ulcers). In the tertiary stage, granulomas form (gummas); these can be felt as skin nodules which are prone to degenerate and ulcerate.

VIRAL

Warts

Common warts caused by papilloma viruses are self-limiting and generally occur in the young patient.

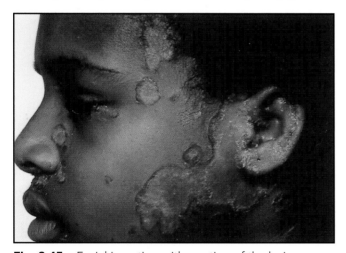

Fig. 3.45 Facial impetigo with crusting of the lesion.

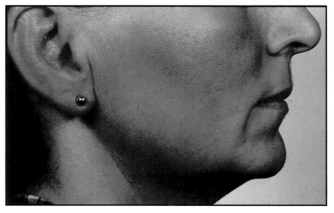

Fig. 3.46 Erysipelas. Note the erythema and oedema.

Warts usually occur on the fingers and hands as discrete papules with a typical irregular surface (Fig. 3.52). Plantar warts occur on the pressure-bearing areas of the feet and are consequently flattened rather than raised.

Molluscum contagiosum

This is a common infection caused by a member of the pox virus group. The lesions appear as flesh-coloured, dome-shaped papules varying in size from pinpoint to 1 cm in diameter. The most characteristic feature of the lesion is umbilication (a central depression of the surface). In children, the lesions are especially common on the face and trunk, whereas in adults, the genitalia may be affected. As the lesions resolve, an area of induration often develops in the surrounding skin.

Herpes simplex

There are two types of herpes simplex virus (HSV). Type 1 virus normally affects the mouth and lips (Fig. 3.53), whereas type 2 usually affects the genitals. Crossover infections do sometimes occur. The primary HSV infection presents with crops of painful superficial vesicles surrounded by an area of erythema. The vesicles erode superficially then crust and finally heal without scarring. After the primary infection, the virus lies dormant in the dorsal root nerve ganglion, with recurrences occurring predictably in the same area as the initial infection. Reactivation is heralded by a tingling sensation in the skin which is followed within 1–2 days by the eruption of a crop of vesicles. Exacerbations may be precipitated by infection, stress, fever (hence the term fever blisters), abnormal exposure to sunlight, menstruation and trauma. Often, no obvious precipitating cause is discovered.

Herpes zoster (shingles)

After an attack of chicken pox, the varicella-zoster virus lies dormant in a dorsal root or cranial nerve ganglion. Reactivation of the virus causes a localised eruption called shingles. The cause of reactivation is often not apparent, although immunosuppression, lymphomas and ageing may be implicated.

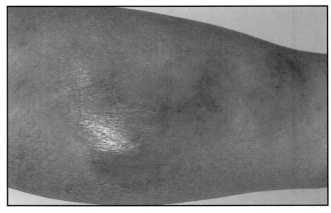

Fig. 3.47 Erythema and oedema associated with cellulitis.

The patient complains of pain or discomfort in a localised area of skin and, within a few days, a crop of vesicles appear in a characteristic dermatomal distribution (Fig. 3.54). Over 2–3 weeks, the vesicles evolve into pustules, scab, then heal. Often there is some residual scarring. In order of frequency, the thoracic, cervical, lumbar and sacral dermatomes are affected. If the ophthalmic branch of the trigeminal nerve is involved, there may be serious damage to the cornea. This is associated with a typical distribution of the vesicles on the tip and side of the nose. Involvement of the geniculate ganglion of the facial nerve causes a facial palsy with involvement of the outer ear (Ramsay Hunt syndrome). The most debilitating long-term effect of shingles, even when healing has occurred, is chronic pain and hyperaesthesia in the affected dermatome.

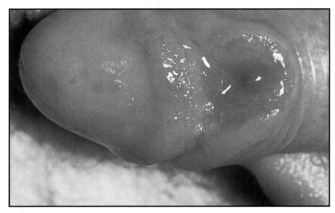

Fig. 3.48 Primary chancre in syphilis.

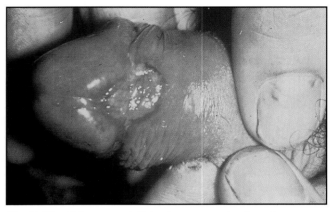

Fig. 3.49 Primary syphilitic chancre on the frenulum.

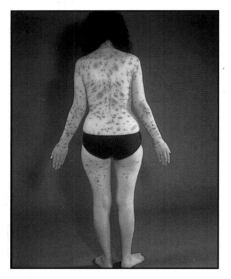

Fig. 3.50 The maculopapular rash of secondary syphilis.

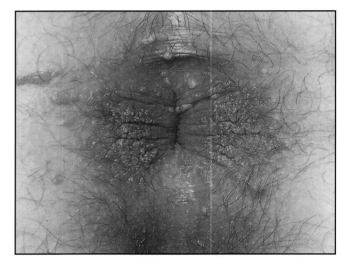

Fig. 3.51 Condylomata accuminata.

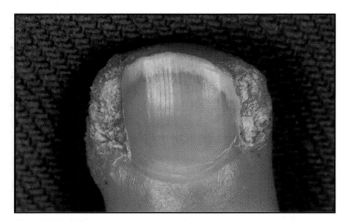

Fig. 3.52 Finger warts.

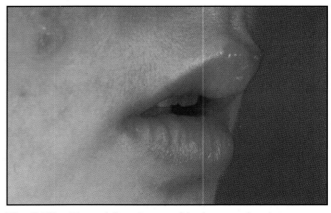

Fig. 3.53 'Fever blister' caused by herpes simplex.

FUNGAL

Candida albicans

This is a common infection of the skin and mucous membranes. Oral candidosis tends to occur in immunosuppressed patients and diabetics and after treatment with antibiotics. Candidosis is a major manifestation of AIDS. Look for candidosis in the mouth; the oral infection is characterised by white or off-white plaques that can be scraped off, leaving a raw red base. Other manifestations include angular stomatitis, vulval and vaginal infections and involvement of contact surfaces (e.g. the natal cleft, inner thighs, scrotum and inframammary fold (intertrigo)).

Pityriasis versicolor (tinea versicolor)

This common condition of young adults is caused by *Malassezia furfur* and presents as small pigmented or hypopigmented macules on the upper trunk and arms. The macules tend to coalesce, resulting in lesions that vary in size and shape. Scales can be demonstrated by scraping or teasing the lesions with a scalpel blade. In sunburnt areas, the lesions appear to be hypopigmented in comparison to the surrounding skin.

Dermatophytes (tinea)

The dermatophytes inhabit the stratum corneum and the dead keratin of the nails and hair. Hair infection (tinea capitis) presents with localised patches of hair loss and skin inflammation. Skin infection (tinea corporis) affects the unhairy parts of the body. This presentation is often referred to as 'ringworm', because the lesion has an inflamed annular edge with a paler central area of healing (Fig. 3.55). Athlete's foot (tinea pedis) appears as a scaling erythematous rash between the toes. A nail infection (tinea unguium) is often asymmetrical and affects the toenails more often than the fingernails. The nail becomes yellow and thick; there is onycholysis and, at a later stage, the nail crumbles and breaks. If suspected, take nail clippings for mycology.

INFESTATIONS

Pediculosis

Infestation with lice causes skin irritation. Headlice infestation (pediculosis capitis) is common in children. The diagnosis is made by careful inspection of the hair for eggs (nits) which, unlike dandruff, cannot be shaken off the hair. Scratching may give rise to secondary inflammation and itching. Body lice infestation (pediculosis corporis) is rare and almost always occurs in malnutrition and when hygiene is poor. Infection of the pubic hair (pediculosis pubis) is caused by the crab louse and is usually sexually transmitted. Like other lice infections, the infestation causes intense pruritus and the nits (and lice) are seen with the naked eye.

Scabies

Consider scabies in any patient presenting with widespread pruritus. The mite (*Sarcoptes scabei*) burrows into the skin, where the female lays her eggs. The burrows can be seen on inspection; look for these along the sides of the fingers, the webs (Fig. 3.56) and the wrist. The burrows are linear and just palpable and the white dot of the mite can often be seen. The lesions may develop into inflamed papules and may affect the elbows, axillae and genitalia. Scratching causes secondary excoriation and infection.

BLISTERING LESIONS

Bullous pemphigoid

This disorder occurs most commonly in elderly people. The lesions are itchy and appear as tense, mainly sym-

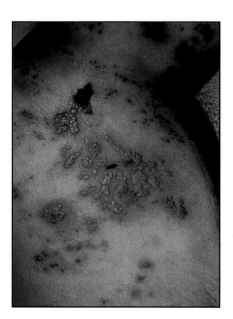

Fig. 3.54 Herpes zoster: note the haemorrhagic lesions (distribution of L2).

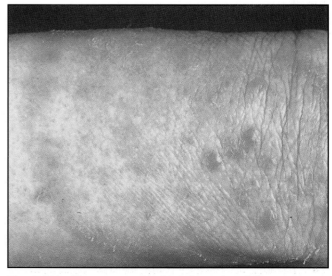

Fig. 3.55 Ringworm rash with inflamed periphery.

metrical blisters overlying and surrounded by an area of erythema (Fig. 3.57). The blisters are initially small but enlarge to a considerable size over a few days (Fig. 3.58). Although truncal involvement also occurs, the blisters appear mainly on the limbs, especially along the inner aspects of the thighs and arms. The blisters become haemorrhagic and then degenerate, causing erosions that are susceptible to secondary infection (Fig. 3.59). Healing occurs without scarring.

Pemphigus

This autoimmune disorder occurs most commonly in middle-aged Ashkenazi Jews. The onset is usually insidious and the earliest lesions often start in the mouth or genital mucous membrane; however, patients usually present to the doctor once the skin is involved. Pemphigus is characterised by painful, flaccid blisters that rupture to reveal a raw base that heals slowly (Figs 3.60, 3.61). The skin adjacent to the bullous lesion slides over the underlying dermis (Nikolsky's sign). The umbilicus, trunk, intertrigenous areas and scalp are most commonly affected. The clinical diagnosis is confirmed by typical immunofluorescent staining, which shows immunoglobulin G (IgG) and complement deposition in the epidermis.

Dermatitis herpetiformis

This disorder usually occurs in the third and fourth decades and is characterised by strikingly symmetrical groups of intensely itchy vesicles which most commonly erupt on the elbows, below the knees, buttocks, back and scalp (Fig. 3.62). Scratching causes local excoriation. Healing leaves tell-tale areas of hyperpigmentation. The disorder is almost always associated with gluten-sensitive enteropathy (coeliac disease). Although almost all patients have villous atrophy, it is unusual for them to present with features of malabsorption.

Naevi

There are numerous skin blemishes collectively called naevi. Pigmented naevi cause the greatest concern because of the seriousness of malignant change. The

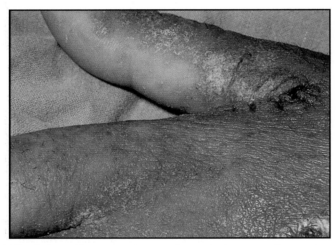

Fig. 3.56 Chronic scabies in the webs between fingers.

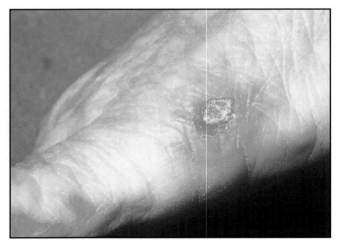

Fig. 3.57 Bullous pemphigoid with surrounding erythema.

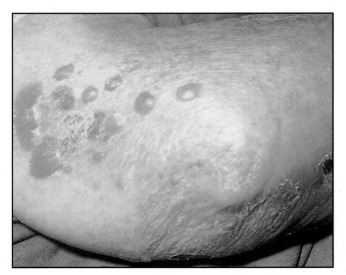

Fig. 3.58 Tense blisters of bullous pemphigoid.

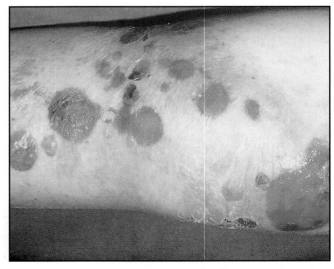

Fig. 3.59 Haemorrhagic blisters of bullous pemphigoid.

junctional naevus is distinguished as a flat or slightly raised smooth lesion which has a uniform colour and varies in size up to about 1 cm (Fig. 3.63). A compound naevus is a raised, rounded, pigmented papular lesion from which hairs may project (Fig. 3.64). Dermal naevi are raised, flesh-coloured, dome-shaped lesions with a wrinkled surface, occurring most commonly on the face (Fig. 3.65).

Café au lait patches

These are flat, coffee-coloured patches, usually centimetres in size, which may occur as a benign blemish or a marker of neurofibromatosis (Von Recklinghausen's disease). The presence of five or more of these patches is a sure sign of the disorder. Neurofibromas appear as soft, sessile, pedunculated lesions or discrete subcutaneous nodules.

TUMOURS

Squamous cell carcinoma

There is usually a risk factor predisposing to this cancer. Consider excessive sun exposure, carcinomatous change in a chronic leg ulcer and areas of leuko-

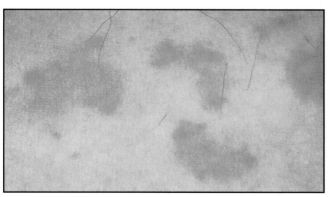

Fig. 3.60 Skin pemphigus.

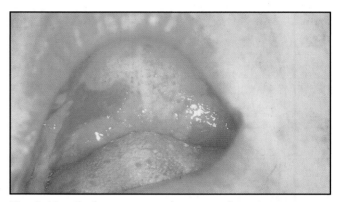

Fig. 3.61 Oral mucous membrane involvement in pemphigus.

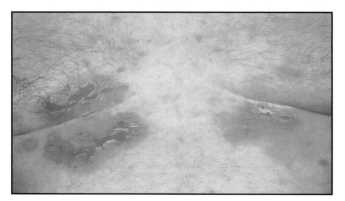

Fig. 3.62 The skin lesions of dermatitis herpetiformis.

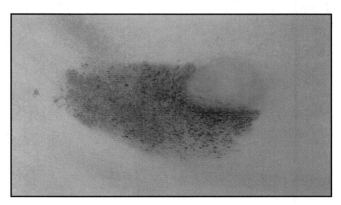

Fig. 3.63 Junctional naevus.

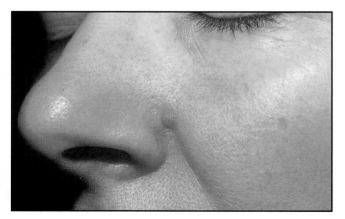

Fig. 3.64 Cellular naevus.

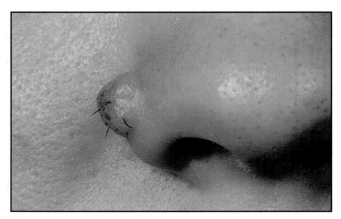

Fig. 3.65 Dermal naevus.

plakia. The tumour presents as an ulcer or nodule with a firm indurated margin; the ulcer margin is often everted (Fig. 3.66). The cancer usually occurs in sun-exposed areas (face, back of the hands and forearm) or, in women, in an area of vulval leukoplakia (Fig. 3.67).

Basal cell carcinoma

This tumour most commonly affects the face and, like squamous carcinoma, sun-exposure is an important predisposing factor. The 'rodent' ulcer starts as a small painless papule (Fig. 3.68) which ulcerates. The ulcer margin is well-defined and rolled at the edges. The tumour bleeds and scabs. Your index of suspicion must be aroused if any skin ulcer fails to heal.

Malignant melanoma

This is less common than squamous or basal cell carcinoma but is the most serious, because it spreads by the lymphatics and blood. Most lesions are not associated with a pre-existing pigmented lesion but approximately one-third are associated with a junctional pigmented naevus. The tumour is usually pigmented and presents either as a nodule or a spreading area of pigmentation (Fig. 3.69). Consider the diagnosis if a pigmented lesion is nodular, grows, darkens in colour, changes shape or bleeds. The back is a common site in men, whereas in women the legs are the most common site.

Kaposi's sarcoma

This tumour was once restricted to equatorial black Africans (Fig. 3.70) and elderly Ashkenazi Jews (Fig. 3.71). Immunosuppression is an important predisposing factor and the sarcoma occurs in transplant recipients on immunosuppressive drugs and is particularly associated with AIDS (Fig. 3.72). The Kaposi's lesion is characterised by red–blue nodules, especially affecting the lower legs but also involving the hands.

 Risk factors
Malignant melanoma

- New mole, change in pre-existing mole
- Prior melanoma or family history of melanoma
- Caucasian
- Oral psoralens and PUVA for psoriasis
- Immunosuppression
- Excessive sun exposure
- Red hair, blond hair, green or blue eyes

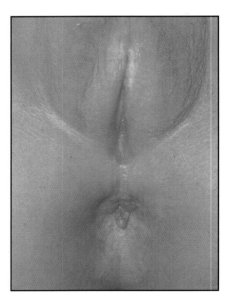

Fig. 3.67 Leukoplakia of the vulva. (The pubic area has been shaved.)

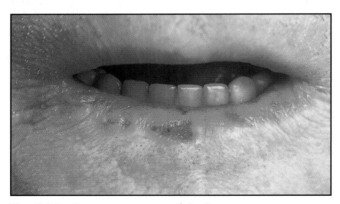

Fig. 3.66 Squamous cancer of the lip.

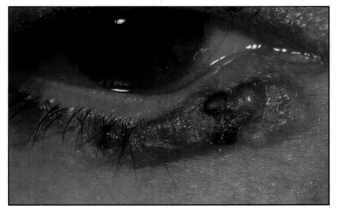

Fig. 3.68 Papular form of basal cell carcinoma.

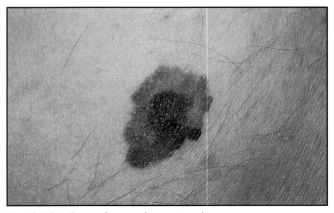

Fig. 3.69 Spreading malignant melanoma.

NAIL DISORDERS

Examination of the nails can provide useful and often diagnostic physical signs. Patients often complain of cracking, ridging and brittleness of the nail. This may be caused by nail-biting, picking and poor nail care rather than disease. In addition, nails may have white spots which have no significance. First examine the nail face-on. Asymmetrical splinter-like lesions (splinter haemorrhages) may indicate microemboli from infected heart valves (subacute bacterial endocarditis) or vasculitis. Remember that manual labourers may have traumatic nail lesions that resemble splinter haemorrhages. Pitting of the nail occurs in psoriasis (Fig. 3.73) and may even occur in the absence of the typical skin rash. Premature lifting of the distal nail is called onycholysis (Fig. 3.74). This occurs in many chronic nail disorders and is also associated with hyperthyroidism (Plummer's nails). White nails with loss of the lunule (leukonychia) is typical of hypo-albuminaemia and severe chronic ill-health (Fig. 3.75).

Acute severe illness may be associated with the later appearance of transverse depressions in the nail (Beau's lines) (Fig. 3.76) which grow out with normal nail growth on recovery. Infection of the skin adjacent to the nail is called paronychia and is characterised by pain, swelling, redness and tenderness of the skin at its interface with the nail (Fig. 3.77). Fungal infection of the nail causes opacification and distortion of the nail.

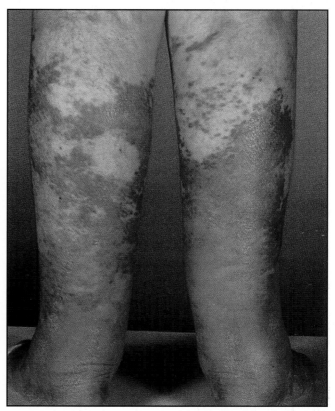

Fig. 3.71 Kaposi's sarcoma in an Ashkenazi Jew. The purple plaques particularly occur on the lower legs and feet.

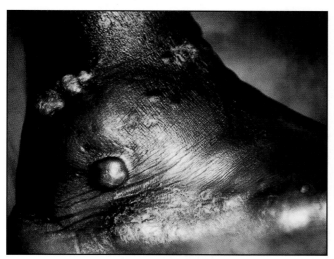

Fig. 3.70 Kaposi's sarcoma in a black African. The nodules are mutiple and dark blue in colour.

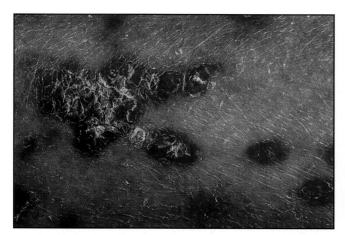

Fig. 3.72 Kaposi's sarcoma in an immunosuppressed AIDS patient.

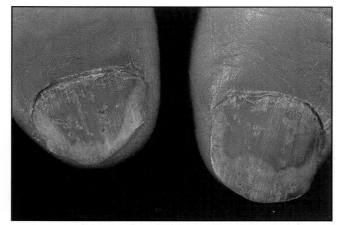

Fig. 3.73 Pitting and onycholysis of the nail caused by psoriasis.

Spooning of the nail (koilonychia) occurs in iron deficiency (Figs 3.78, 3.79).

Always examine the lateral outline of the nails and fingertip to check for clubbing. The normal angle between the fingernail and nail base is 160° (Fig. 3.80)

and the base is firm to palpation. Clubbing occurs when abnormal connective tissue and capillaries fill this angle. In early clubbing, the angle increases and if you press the nail base the nail appears to 'float'. In severe clubbing, such as occurs with lung cancer,

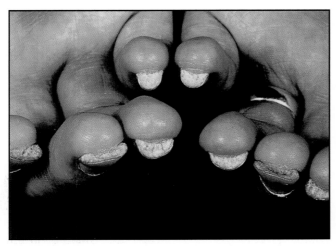

Fig. 3.74   Onycholysis caused by hyperkeratotic psoriasis beneath the nail.

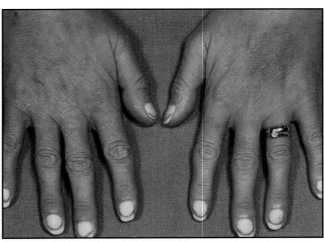

Fig. 3.75   Leukonychia in a patient with liver disease and hypoalbuminaemia.

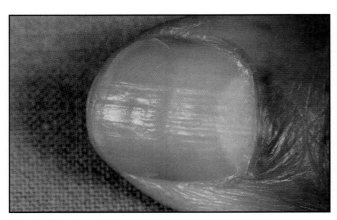

Fig. 3.76   Beau's lines.

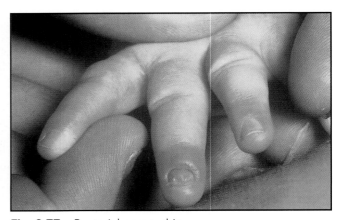

Fig. 3.77   Bacterial paronychia.

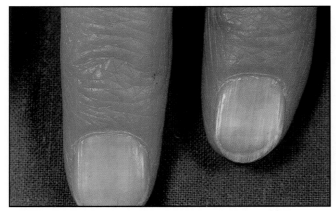

Fig. 3.78   Koilonychia with spooning of the nail in a patient with chronic iron deficiency anaemia.

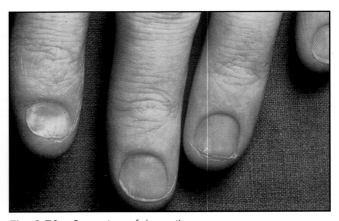

Fig. 3.79   Spooning of the nails.

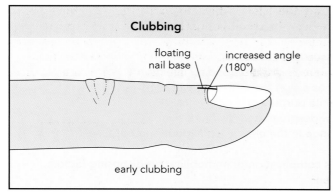

Clubbing

floating nail base

increased angle (180°)

early clubbing

Fig. 3.80 Clubbing. The angle is increased and filled in and the nail base has a spongy consistency.

 Differential diagnosis
Finger clubbing

Lung disease
- Pyogenic (abscess, bronchiectasis, empyema)
- Bronchogenic carcinoma
- Fibrosing alveolitis

Heart disease
- Cyanotic congenital heart disease
- Subacute bacterial endocarditis

Gastrointestinal
- Cirrhosis
- Ulcerative colitis
- Crohn's disease

Idiopathic/congenital

SKIN MANIFESTATIONS OF SYSTEMIC DISEASE

the fingers may have a drumstick appearance and may be associated with wrist pain and tenderness due to periostitis (hypertrophic pulmonary osteo-arthropathy).

Many systemic disorders involve the skin and careful examination of the skin often helps in diagnosis.

 Symptoms and signs
Skin manifestations of systemic disease

Disease	Skin findings
Sarcoidosis	Erythema nodosum, lupus pernio, nodules in scars
Systemic lupus erythematosus	Facial 'butterfly' rash (malar erythema over cheeks and bridging nose); occurs in 50% of patients on exposure to UV rays. Also alopoecia areata and discoid lupus
Scleroderma	Thickened tight skin (especially fingers), skin telangiectasia, calcified skin nodules
Hyperlipidaemia	Xanthelasmata of eyelids, xanthomas of elbows, knuckles, buttock, soles and palms, and Achilles tendon
Diabetes mellitus	Necrobiosis lipoidica – symmetrical plaques on shins with atrophic, yellow appearance and waxy feel; cutaneous candida, ulcers on feet
Hyperthyroidism	Pretibial myxoedema – thickened skin on front of skin, clubbing
Cushing's syndrome	Purple striae, thin skin, easy bruising
Ulcerative colitis/ Crohn's disease	Pyoderma gangrenosum – large ulcer
Dermatomyositis	Oedema and mauve discoloration of eyelid, erythema of the knuckles and other bony parts such as elbow and shoulder tip; photosensitive 'butterfly rash' on face
Cancer	Acanthosis nigricans – brown, velvet-like thickening of skin in axilla and groin; tylosis – thickening of palms/soles; ichthyosis – fish-skin appearance

HOARSE VOICE

The majority of patients with a hoarse voice have an inflammatory disorder of the larynx (laryngitis). However, any patient with hoarseness that has not resolved after 3 weeks should have the larynx visualised. If hoarseness is associated with upper airway obstruction (stridor), emergency referral to an ENT surgeon is required.

The history will often give the examiner a good idea of the diagnosis. Any alteration in the smooth lining of the true vocal cords (vocal folds) will give rise to hoarseness. If one of the vocal folds is paralysed or if there is inadequate apposition of the vocal folds, a more 'breathy' quality of the voice is noted and is more accurately called dysphonia; it requires considerable experience to make the distinction between hoarseness and dysphonia on merely listening to the patient speak. A preceding upper respiratory tract infection will usually point to a diagnosis of laryngitis, as may excessive voice abuse (traumatic laryngitis). A history of excessive smoking, alcohol (especially spirits) and poor periodontal and dental hygiene should alert you to the possibility of a malignancy. The causes of hoarseness also vary in different age groups.

OBSTRUCTED AIRWAY

Patients with any difficulty in breathing may not be able to indicate the exact anatomical level of the obstruction. With upper airway obstruction they may point to the throat or neck or describe a feeling of 'tightness' in the throat. The causes of an obstructed upper airway differ according to the age of the patient.

Snoring is also caused by an obstructed airway. The obstruction may be nasal, postnasal (e.g. enlarged adenoid), oropharyngeal (e.g. tonsils, lax palate and faucial pillars) or laryngeal (e.g. congenital abnormalities in children). If snoring is severe it may be associated with apnoeic episodes during sleep. This in turn may lead to daytime irritability and somnolence. The hypoxic episodes during sleep may lead to cardiorespiratory abnormalities.

DIFFICULTY IN SWALLOWING

For a discussion of difficulty in swallowing (dysphagia) see Chapter 7.

Differential diagnosis
Hoarseness or dysphonia

Neonate (abnormal cry)	Congenital abnormality Neurological disorder
Infant	Congenital abnormality Neurological disorder Inflammation (croup or upper respiratory tract infection (URTI))
Toddler	Inflammation (croup or URTI)
Child	Inflammatory (laryngitis) Vocal nodules (voice abuse)
Adult	Inflammatory and traumatic laryngitis Vocal nodules (voice abuse) Dysphonia (voice abuse or misuse) Carcinoma

Emergency
Upper airway obstruction

Symptoms and signs
- Patient distressed/anxious
- Tachypnoea (rapid rate of breathing)
- Excess salivation/drooling
- Stridor (noise of upper airway obstruction)
- Pulsus paradoxus

Differential diagnosis
Obstructed upper airway

Neonate	Congenital abnormality
Infant	Congenital abnormality Inflammation (croup)
Toddler	Inflammation (croup or supraglottis) Foreign body Congenital abnormality
Child	Inflammation (croup or supraglottis) Foreign body
Adult	Inflammatory (supraglottis) Carcinoma (usually over 50 years old)

Risk factors
Carcinoma of the larynx, mouth and tongue

- Cigarette smoking
- Excessive alcohol consumption
- Poor oral and dental hygiene
- Older patient

Questions to ask
Hoarse voice

- How long has the hoarseness been present?
- Has there been any previous upper respiratory tract infection?
- Have you abused your voice, for example, shouting at sports events or singing at a party or concert?
- Do you smoke; if so, how many a day?
- How much alcohol do you drink?
- What type of work do you do?

PAIN ON SWALLOWING

Painful swallowing is called odynophagia. Swallowing is usually painful in the presence of inflammation in the hypopharynx or oesophagus (e.g. candidiasis) but rarely is the presenting complaint in oesophageal carcinoma. These patients usually present initially with dysphagia before the act of swallowing becomes painful. However, carcinoma of the piriform fossa or posterior one-third of the tongue may present with odynophagia.

LUMP IN THE NECK

Patients with a lump in the neck have either felt the lump themselves or it has been noticed by someone else. Most neck lumps are due to enlarged lymph nodes, in which case questioning is directed to a potential source of origin (Fig. 4.11). Enlarged lymph nodes in the neck may arise from sources in the head and neck or they may arise from disease in the chest and abdomen (carcinoma). Enlarged neck nodes may also be part of generalised disease of the lymphatic system, such as lymphoma. Thyroid swellings would require a history of symptoms of hyperthyroidism or hypothyroidism. Most neck lumps are painless unless there is associated inflammation or abscess formation.

Questions to ask
Lump in the neck

- How long has it been present?
- Has the lump changed in size?
- Is the lump painful?
- Do you sweat at night?
- Have you lost weight recently?
- Do you have thyroid problems?
- Do you have a cough?
- Is there anything abnormal about your mouth or throat?
- Are you generally well?

Lymphatic drainage in the head and neck

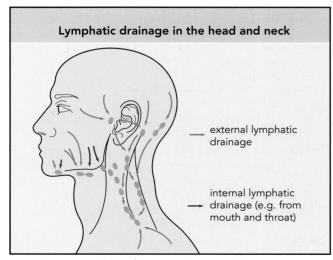

external lymphatic drainage

internal lymphatic drainage (e.g. from mouth and throat)

Fig. 4.11 Lymphatic drainage of the head and neck.

HALITOSIS

Bad breath may arise from a variety of sources. The most common cause of halitosis is probably poor dental and oral hygiene. Paranasal sinus infection with a purulent postnasal discharge may lead to halitosis, as may tonsillar crypts. Infection of the oral cavity, the gums in particular (gingivitis), may give rise to foul-smelling breath.

SYMPTOMS OF NASAL DISORDERS

Nasal disorders may present with local symptoms or symptoms some distance from the nose.

BLOCKED NOSE

The examiner must establish whether the patient is describing true nasal obstruction or the physiological nasal cycle with alternating vasoconstriction and vasodilatation of the nasal vasculature. Mechanical abnormalities (e.g. a deviated septum or enlarged turbinates or nasal polyps) will usually cause constant obstruction, whereas the nasal cycle and seasonal allergic rhinitis are usually intermittent, the former alternating between left and right sides.

RUNNY NOSE (RHINORRHOEA)

It is important to ascertain whether there is associated nasal obstruction and whether the discharge is constant (as in parasympathetic-dominant vasomotor rhinitis seen in elderly people) or intermittent (as in seasonal rhinitis associated with sneezing and nasal obstruction). The discharge may be watery or mucoid, purulent in the presence of infection or a foreign body (children or mentally handicapped adults) and blood-

Risk factors
Rhinitis

- Family history
- Atopic patient (associated asthma, eczema)

Questions to ask
Blocked nose

- Is the nose blocked constantly or only some of the time (day or night)?
- Does it vary with the seasons?
- Is there any associated nasal discharge?
- Are both nostrils affected or only one?
- What aggravates and what relieves the condition?
- Do you use nose drops?
- Do you sniff glue or illicit substances (e.g. cocaine)?
- Have you had previous nose surgery?
- Do you suffer from asthma?

stained in the presence of a tumour or foreign body. In addition, if rhinorrhoea is associated with an itchy nose, sneezing and itchy eyes, a diagnosis of allergic rhinitis can easily be made.

INJURED NOSE

The importance of the history in the acute injury of the nose relates to the timing of any fracture reduction, if necessary, and to medicolegal implications if a report is required.

BLEEDING NOSE (EPISTAXIS)

Patients either give a history of intermittent nose bleeds, possibly with a precipitating cause, or they actually present with a bleeding nose. If the patient is actively bleeding, necessary treatment may precede the history-taking or this can be done while staunching the flow! A history of a bleeding disorder is relevant, as is a history of previous nasal surgery: septal perforations often crust and bleed. Nose bleeds may be caused by excessive nasal picking or an injury to the nose. Hypertension per se is not a cause of epistaxis but an elevated venous or arterial pressure will prolong any established epistaxis.

NASAL DEFORMITY

Patients complaining about the shape of their nose may or may not have associated nasal obstruction. Nasal 'deformity' may be traumatic or congenital in origin.

'NONSMELLING' NOSE

Patients may complain of a diminished sense of smell (hyposmia) or no sense of smell (anosmia). There may be a history of head injury, although this needs to have been severe to tear the olfactory fibres emerging through the cribriform plate. Some patients may report a loss of the sense of smell after an upper respiratory tract infection (so-called 'postinfluenza neuritis'). Patients with mechanical obstruction of the upper part of the nose (e.g. caused by nasal polyps or mucosal oedema in allergic rhinitis) will also complain of anosmia. In many patients the cause is unknown.

Nasal and paranasal disorders may also be present with 'regional' symptoms such as headache, facial pain, epiphora (excessive tear production) if the naso-lacrimal duct is obstructed, diplopia (double vision), proptosis (bulging eyes) and orbital pain (if a tumour invades the orbit).

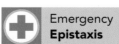

Emergency
Epistaxis

Symptoms and signs
- Blood from nostrils
- Swallowing and spitting blood
- Anxious patient
- Tachycardia

SYMPTOMS OF EAR DISORDERS

PAINFUL EAR (OTALGIA)

Pain in the ear arises from the ear itself or is referred from several other anatomical sites. The sensory nerve supply of the ear is, therefore, very important as the same sensory derivations apply to other areas of the head and neck (Fig. 4.8). Thus, disorders of the nose and sinuses, nasopharynx, teeth, jaws, temporo-mandibular joints, salivary glands and ducts, oropharynx, laryngopharynx and hypopharynx, tongue and cervical spine may all give rise to earache. The history must establish the nature of the pain, its radiation and aggravating factors.

DISCHARGING EAR (OTORRHOEA)

Discharge from the ear may contain mucus or pus, and it may be bloodstained. The questions to ask the patient are similar to those asked in cases of earache; the two symptoms, earache and discharge, often coexist.

HEARING LOSS OR DEAFNESS

It is more appropriate to talk of hearing loss than deafness, as the latter often implies a total lack of hearing and also has a certain stigma attached to it. Hearing loss can be qualified as being mild, moderate, severe or profound, according to the degree measured in decibels.

The age of onset of the hearing loss is important, as is the suddenness of its onset. The more likely causes of hearing loss in the different age groups are indicated in the differential diagnosis box. In patients whose hearing loss is severe and occurred before their acquisition of language, speech will be unusual (prelingual speech). The family history is relevant, for syndromal disorders may have some hereditary basis. In ostosclerosis, in which the stapes footplate is fixed, there may also be a family history of the same disorder. If the hearing loss follows trauma, this may be caused by blood in the external auditory meatus, a perforation of the tympanic membrane or disruption of the ossicular

Questions to ask
Otalgia

- Where does it hurt?
- Does the pain spread?
- What exacerbates the pain?
- Is there a discharge?
- Have you ever had an ear operation or your ears syringed?
- Do you use cotton buds?
- Have you hurt your ear recently?
- Have you been swimming or on an aeroplane recently?
- Is your hearing ability affected?

chain. In addition, the inner ear may have been damaged, especially in fractures of the temporal bone.

Discharge from the ear may cause a hearing loss from the accumulation of debris in the external ear. In chronic inflammation, the hearing loss may be associated with a tympanic membrane perforation or disruption of the ossicular chain. Certain drugs (e.g. the aminoglycoside antibiotics, some diuretics, cytotoxics) may damage the inner ear and a history of the use of such drugs or the illnesses requiring them is impor-tant; for example, tuberculosis (streptomycin), severe septicaemic illness (aminoglycosides) and cancer (cytotoxics). Previous ear surgery may have resulted in a reduction in hearing.

Eighth nerve involvement by syphilis was seen more commonly in the past but this is now rare. Patients should be asked about prolonged exposure to loud noise, either in their employment or in the armed services, in case they have suffered some noise-induced hearing loss. Finally, children with a hearing loss caused by secretory otitis media (glue ear) may present with problems related to a hearing loss but when hearing loss itself is not the presenting com-plaint. They may present with delay in language development, inattention at school or poor scholastic performance.

Questions to ask
Hearing loss

- How long have you noticed a hearing loss?
- Is it partial or complete?
- Are both the ears affected or just one?
- Is there a family history of hearing problems?
- Have you had an injury or surgery to your ears?
- Have you had any serious illnesses such as tuberculosis or septicaemia (ototoxic drugs)?
- Have you been exposed to loud noise for any length of time?
- Is there associated vertigo?

Differential diagnosis
Hearing loss

Infants	Congenital Secretory otitis media ('glue ear')
Toddlers and young children	'Glue ear' Congenital Postinfective (measles, mumps, meningitis)
Teenagers and adolescents	Congenital Malingering Postinfective Noise induced (often temporary in this age group)
20–40 years old	Otosclerosis Postinfective Noise induced Acoustic neuroma Ménière's disease
40–60 years old	Otosclerosis Noise induced Early presbycusis Acoustic neuroma Ménière's disease
Above 60 years old	Presbycusis Noise induced Acoustic neuroma

'NOISY' EAR (TINNITUS)

Tinnitus is the perception of abnormal noise in the ear or head. Tinnitus may be subjective, that is, only the patient can hear it (this is the commonest form of tin-nitus), or objective, that is, the patient and the exam-iner can hear it. The latter is much less common and usually arises from arteriovenous malformations or clicking muscles in the middle ear or palate.

Tinnitus usually presents as buzzing, whistling, hissing, ringing or pulsating and must be distin-guished from complex noises (e.g. voices, music), as these constitute auditory hallucinations, an indication of a psychiatric disorder. Tinnitus is usually asso-ciated with a degree of hearing loss, yet it may occur without any hearing loss. The cause and site of origin of the noise in subjective tinnitus is usually unknown.

Ask questions similar to those asked for patients with a hearing loss. In addition, aspirin overdosage can cause reversible tinnitus. It is important to ask how much the tinnitus bothers the patient, that is, if it keeps the patient awake at night or interferes with daily living. Any history of ear disease is relevant because these are the few patients in whom, if the disease is treated, tinnitus may disappear.

DEFORMED EAR

Patients may complain of deformity of the ear arising from congenital causes and trauma. Congenital ear deformities include complete or partial absence of the pinna (anotia or microtia). This may be associated with middle and inner ear abnormalities. There may be accessory auricles, often seen just anterior to the tragus (Fig. 4.12), or there may be a preauricular sinus (Fig. 4.27). The latter may become infected and require excision if it is troublesome.

Patients may also complain about the size or shape of their ears, particularly if the ears protrude: 'bat ears'. This may result in children being teased at school and may cause social embarrassment. This condition can be corrected surgically.

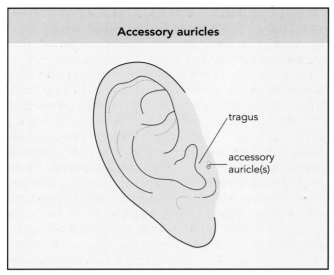

Accessory auricles

tragus

accessory
auricle(s)

Fig. 4.12 Site of accessory auricles.

INJURY TO THE EAR

Injury to the ear may be blunt or sharp. Patients who have had an ear injury may have sustained trauma to the pinna resulting in a haematoma auris. Trauma may have occurred in the external meatus, ususally self-inflicted (e.g. with cotton buds, hairgrips or pencils). These objects may also injure the tympanic membrane and ossicles but rarely the inner ear. Blunt trauma in the form of a blow to the side of the head or in diffuse head injury may rupture the tympanic membrane, dislocate the ossicles and cause damage to the inner ear. Any of these injuries may result in hearing loss, dizziness and damage to the facial nerve as it passes through the temporal bone. The damage can be either temporary or permanent.

VERTIGO

Dizziness is a common complaint and means different things to different people. The key to making a diagnosis in the dizzy patient involves taking a good history. It is imortant to establish exactly what the patient means by feeling dizzy. The aim is to find out whether the dizziness is in fact true vertigo (see also Ch. 11). Vertigo is an hallucination of movement. Feelings of 'light headedness', 'about to black out or faint', do not constitute true vertigo. Although the hallucination of movement is not always rotatory, this is often the complaint mentioned by the patient. Once the symptom of vertigo is verified, establish whether it is of central origin or arising from peripheral receptors (e.g. the vestibule of the inner ear).

Encourage the patient to describe in detail a typical atack of dizziness in his or her own words. This is better than suggesting sensations like 'feeling faint' or asking if the room spins around.

In general terms, central causes of vertigo are more constant and are progressive, whereas vestibular causes tend to be intermittent and paroxysmal (sudden or intensified) and are not usually progressive. However, the symptoms of peripheral causes of vertigo (e.g. the vomiting and the vertigo itself) may be as severe as in central causes.

FACIAL PAIN

Facial pain is a common complaint and arises from many different sources. The source may be relatively obvious (e.g. the patient may say 'I have toothache') or the pain may be referred from a distant site (e.g. the patient with tonsillitis who complains of earache). It is important to remember that not all facial pain is caused by sinusitis and not all earache is caused by ear disease.

FACIAL NERVE PALSY

Patients may present with an isolated facial nerve palsy or the palsy may be part of a more generalised neurological disorder (e.g. a cerebrovascular accident). The suddenness of onset and any association with other neurological complaints should be elicited. A history of ear disease is particularly relevant because the facial nerve makes a considerable journey through the temporal bone, crossing the medial wall of the middle ear, the mastoid, before making its exit at the stylomastoid foramen. Questions relating to the function of branches of the facial nerve, such as dry eyes (if the greater superficial petrosal nerve is involved) or altered taste (if the chorda tympani is involved) can give you an idea of the level of nerve disruption.

Questions to ask
Vertigo

- Can you describe the dizziness? N.B. Don't ask leading questions.
- How long does it last?
- Does anything precipitate the attack?
- Is there associated nausea or vomiting?
- Does rapid head movement cause dizziness?
- Is there associated hearing loss or tinnitus?
- Are you on any medication (e.g. hypertensive)?
- Have you ever had ear problems or ear surgery?

Questions to ask
Facial pain

- Where does it hurt?
- How long has your face been painful?
- What is the pain like (e.g. throbbing, piercing)?
- What aggravates and what relieves the pain?
- Do you have any dental problems?
- Do you ever have trouble with your jaw or with eating?
- Any ENT disease in the past?
- Do you suffer from migraine headache?

EXAMINATION OF THE MOUTH AND THROAT

To perform an adequate examination of this system requires certain basic instruments (Fig. 4.13), a good light source and a systematic approach, as in any other organ system. The patient and the doctor should be sitting opposite each other. The ideal situation involves using a head light or head mirror because this leaves the examiner with both hands free.

Observe the patient's face and facial expression for any immediately obvious abnormalities: these may include lumps and bumps, scars, deformities and facial asymmetry.

Conveniently, the mouth and throat are examined first. Examine the lips for telangiectasia, ulcers, pigmentation and cracks. Also look for evidence of previous surgery (e.g. the repair of a 'harelip'). Ask the patient to open the mouth; inspect the buccal mucosa, gums and teeth. If the patient wears dentures, these should be removed. Note the state of periodontal hygiene and any evidence of gingivitis (inflammation of the gums). Look for ulceration, nodules and pigmentation. Inspect the hard palate for evidence of a cleft palate or a repaired cleft and for telangiectasia.

Next, examine the tongue and floor of the mouth. Ask the patient to protrude the tongue. This not only allows more of the tongue to be seen but also gives an indication of XIIth nerve function. Ask the patient to touch the palate with the tongue to allow you to see the floor of the mouth with the submandibular ducts opening on either side of the frenulum. Look for ulcers, nodules, furring and leukoplakia (white patches) on the tongue. Then, ask the patient to say 'aaah'. This will allow you to see the tonsils, the posterior pharyngeal wall and the movement of the soft palate (the Xth cranial nerve is the motor supply). You

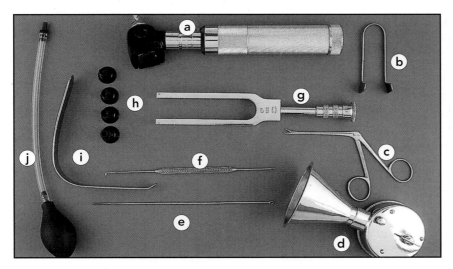

Fig. 4.13 Basic instruments necessary for the ear, nose and throat examination: (a) auroscope, (b) Thudicum speculum, (c) crocodile forceps, (d) Barany noise-box, (e) Jobson–Horne or ring probe, (f) wax hook, (g) 512 Hz tuning fork, (h) aural specula, (i) tongue depressor and (j) auroscope puffer.

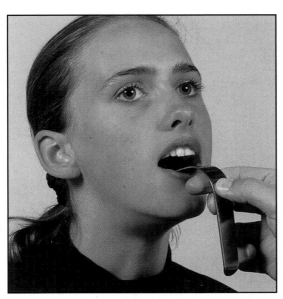

Fig. 4.14 Examining the mouth using a tongue depressor.

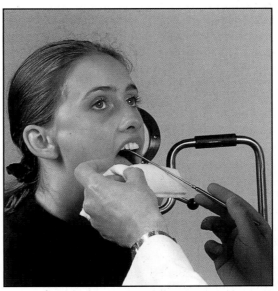

Fig. 4.15 Technique of indirect laryngoscopy.

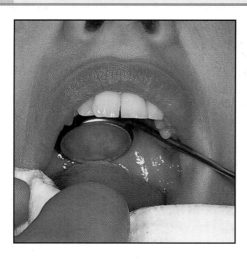

Fig. 4.16
Technique of
indirect
laryngoscopy.

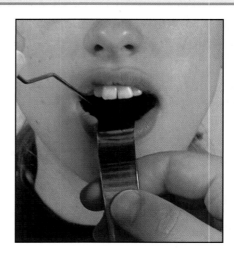

Fig. 4.17
Technique of
mirror
examination of
postnasal space
(posterior
rhinoscopy).

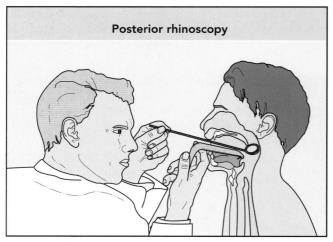

Posterior rhinoscopy

Fig. 4.18   Posterior rhinoscopy.

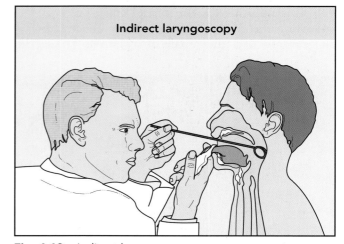

Indirect laryngoscopy

Fig. 4.19   Indirect laryngoscopy.

may require a tongue depressor to obtain an adequate view of the posterior aspects of the oral cavity and oropharynx (Fig. 4.14).

Finally, put on a glove and feel any suspicious areas within the mouth. This often gives a better idea of a lesion than inspection alone. At this stage of the examination, the ENT surgeon would perform an indirect laryngoscopy (Figs 4.15, 4.16) and examination of the postnasal space (posterior rhinoscopy) using appropriate mirrors (Figs 4.17–4.19). These techniques are only expected to be part of the clinical expertise of ENT surgeons.

EXAMINATION OF THE NOSE

First, observe the external appearance of the nose because this may give an indication of a more generalised skin disorder or deformity of the nasal skeleton and may point to previous injury as the cause of nasal obstruction. Second, examine the nasal vestibule. In children, the cartilages of the nasal tip are soft and a good view of the nasal vestibule, anterior end of the septum and anterior ends of the inferior turbinates can

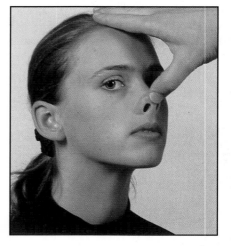

Fig. 4.20
Anterior
rhinoscopy by
elevating the tip
of the nose.

be obtained by simply elevating the tip of the nose (Fig. 4.20). In adults, the cartilages are firmer and the use of a Thudicum speculum is usually necessary to obtain a similar view (Fig. 4.21).

A more detailed view of the nasal cavities can be obtained using rigid Hopkins rod telescopes or a flexible nasendoscope (Fig. 4.22), which can then be advanced through the nasal cavity to view the postnasal space (Fig. 4.23) and larynx (Fig. 4.24). There are significant advantages in viewing the larynx by this method. If the patient gags on indirect laryngoscopy, this is minimised by flexible nasendoscopy. When performing indirect laryngoscopy using a laryngeal mirror, the examiner must hold the tongue (Fig. 4.15); consequently, this permits only limited phonation by the patient. This method is suitable for seeing laryngeal tumours and other obvious laryngeal pathology. Nevertheless, the more subtle changes of dysphonia can be better diagnosed by using the flexible nasendoscope.

On anterior rhinoscopy, the nonspecialist should be able to comment on deflection of the nasal septum and

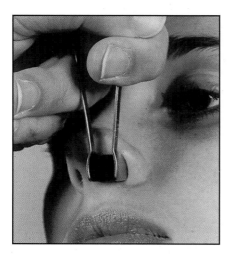

Fig. 4.21 Anterior rhinoscopy using a Thudicum speculum.

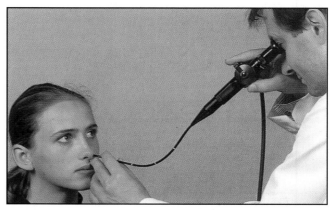

Fig. 4.22 Examination of the nose, postnasal space and larynx using a flexible nasendoscope.

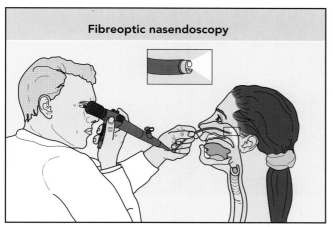

Fig. 4.23 Fibreoptic examination of the postnasal space (transnasal).

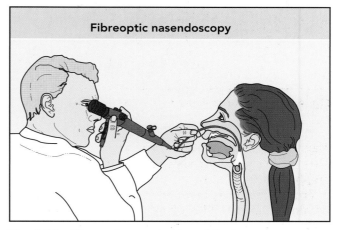

Fig. 4.24 Fibreoptic examination of the larynx (transnasal).

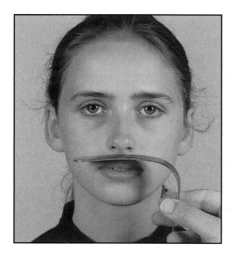

Fig. 4.25 Assessment of nasal airflow on breathing out.

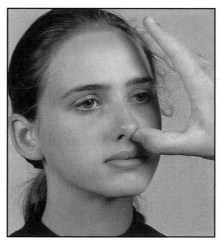

Fig. 4.26 Assessing nasal inspiratory airflow by occluding one nostril at a time.

the state of the inferior turbinates (both size and colour) and identify abnormal lesions (e.g. papillomata and polyps). Assessment of the nasal airflow follows next. Ask the patient to breath out nasally and observe the resultant moisture on a silver tongue depressor or mirror positioned at the anterior nares (Fig. 4.25). The inspiratory flow can be assessed crudely by occluding the undersurface of one nasal cavity at a time and asking the patient to sniff inwards (Fig. 4.26). To assess the sense of smell ask the patient to identify the smells from simple smell bottles, although this is not particularly reliable. Objective and quantitative tests of smell are not yet available for clinical practice.

EXAMINATION OF THE EAR

Examine the pinna, note its shape, size and any deformity. Look for pits (preauricular sinuses) just inferior and anterior to the origin of the helix (Fig. 4.27). Look behind the ear for any scars from previous surgery and note whether or not the patient wears a hearing aid. This will obviously need removal before examination. Tug gently on the pinna; tenderness here will be the result of external ear disease or of temporomandibular joint pain. Feel for preauricular, postauricular and infra-auricular lymph nodes, again the result of external ear disease, not middle or inner ear disease.

Observe the meatus. If this is particularly wide it may be the result of previous mastoid surgery in which a meatoplasty was fashioned. An auroscope with a puffer attached is then used to examine the deep meatus and tympanic membrane. Ensure the light works properly and the batteries are not too old! Apply gentle traction on the ear to straighten the external ear canal (exert the traction in whichever direction serves to straighten the canal) and gently insert the auroscope. Use a black speculum (grey specula lose

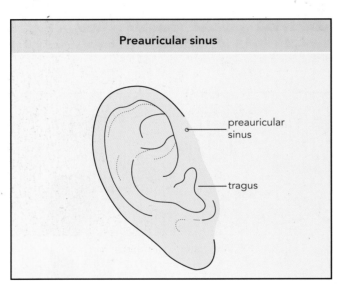

Fig. 4.27 Site of preauricular sinus.

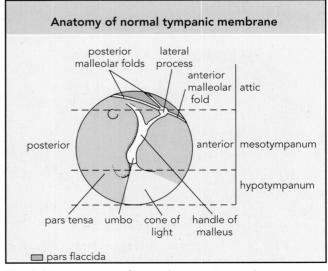

Fig. 4.28 Examination of the ear using an auroscope. Note the position of the right hand against the patient's face.

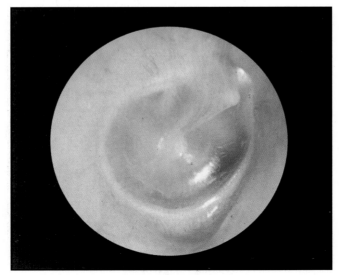

Fig. 4.29 Normal tympanic membrane.

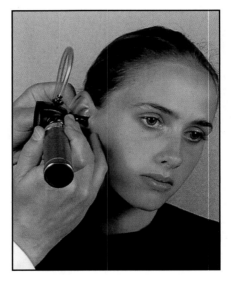

Fig. 4.30 Anatomy of normal tympanic membrane.

too much light) and use the biggest speculum that will fit the ear canal because this will permit you to see in your visual field as much of the topographical anatomy as possible. Always use the longer variety of aural speculum to allow adequate vision of the deep canal and tympanic membrane. A larger diameter speculum facilitates an air-tight seal when using the puffer. It is important to hold the auroscope correctly (Fig. 4.28). This guards against injury, particularly in children, if the patient suddenly moves.

Introduce the auroscope and look at the canal wall skin for otitis externa and exostoses (bony outgrowths from the deep canal wall). Severe otitis externa or a boil (furuncle) of the external meatus may totally occlude the meatus, making visualisation impossible. At this stage the canal and tympanic membrane may be obscured by wax. Wax is a normal phenomenon and

is not 'dirt', as believed by many patients. Gently remove the wax by using a ring probe, a wax hook (Fig. 4.13) or a suction apparatus under the operating microscope or by syringing of the ear.

If removing wax causes pain or bleeding, STOP! If the wax is very hard, it may be possible to use a wax softener (e.g. olive oil or sodium bicarbonate ear drops) for a few days before attempting its removal. If wax cannot be removed without the risk of damage to the ear, a specialist referral is necessary. Do not syringe an ear if there is a history of a perforated tympanic membrane as this may introduce infection into the middle ear.

The tympanic membrane is inspected next (Fig. 4.29). All anatomical features of the drum should be actively sought and noted (Fig. 4.30). there are great variations of normality and accurate assessment comes

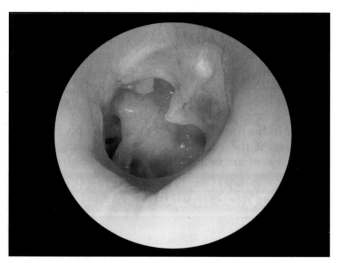

Fig. 4.31 Large tympanic membrane perforation. Incudostapedial joint just visible posterosuperiorly; round window visible posteriorly.

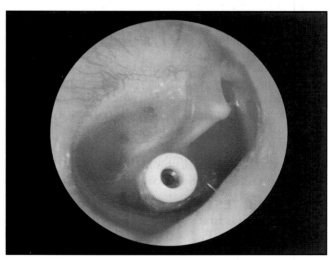

Fig. 4.32 Ventilation tube (grommet) in situ.

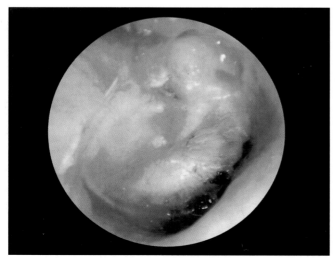

Fig. 4.33 Cholesteatoma in attic region. Note perforation of tympanic membrane in this area as well as erosion of bony outer attic wall.

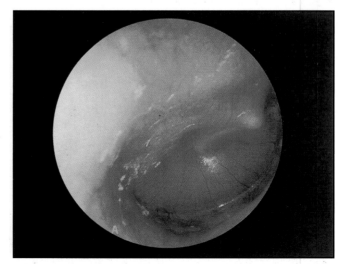

Fig. 4.34 Middle ear effusion ('glue ear').

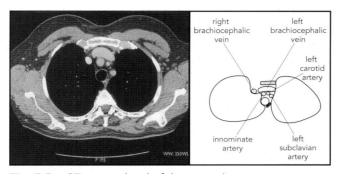

Fig. 5.5   CT scan at level of thoracic inlet.

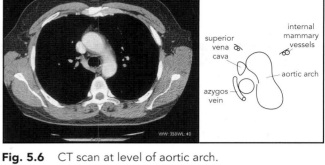

Fig. 5.6   CT scan at level of aortic arch.

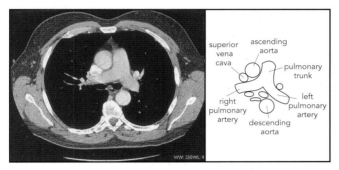

Fig. 5.7   CT scan at level of carina.

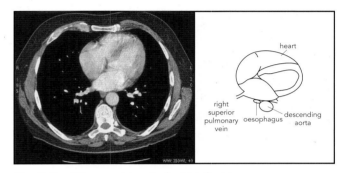

Fig. 5.8   CT scan at level of mid left atrium.

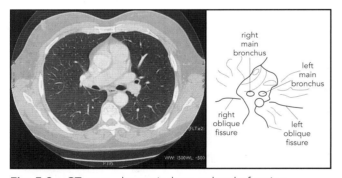

Fig. 5.9   CT scan – lung windows at level of carina.

LUNG DEFENCE AND HISTOLOGY

The lung is exposed to 6 litres of potentially infected and irritant-laden air every minute. There are, therefore, numerous defence mechanisms to ensure survival. The nose humidifies, warms and filters the air and contains lymphocytes of the B series which secrete immunoglobulin A. The epiglottis protects the larynx from inhalation of material from the gastrointestinal tract.

The cough reflex is both a protective and a clearing mechanism. Cough receptors are found in the pharynx, larynx and larger airways. A cough starts with a deep inspiration followed by expiration against a closed glottis. Glottal opening then allows a forceful jet of air to be expelled.

The main clearance mechanism is the remarkable mucociliary escalator. Bronchial secretions from

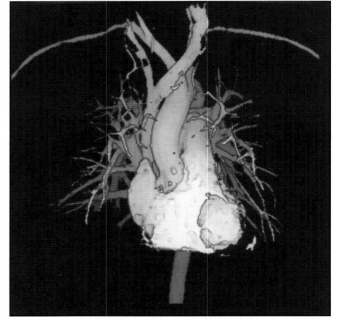

Fig. 5.10   Shaded surface display of reconstruction of dynamic magnetic resonance angiography of pulmonary and great vessels.

bronchial glands and goblet cells, together with secretions from deeper in the lungs, form a sheet of fluid which is propelled upwards continuously by the beat of the cilia lining the bronchial epithelium (Figs 5.13, 5.14). This cilial action can fail either from the rare

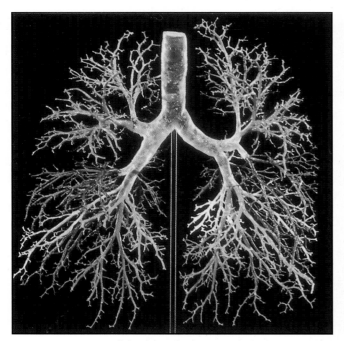

Fig. 5.11 A cast of the bronchial tree with the segments outlined in different colours.

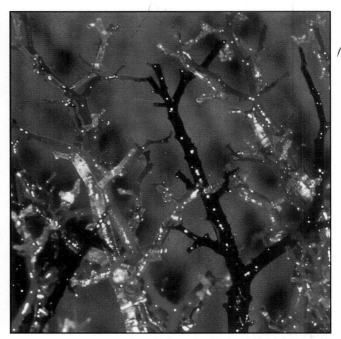

Fig. 5.12 Injection model showing bronchi (white), arteries (red but carrying deoxygenated blood) and veins (blue but carrying oxygenated blood).

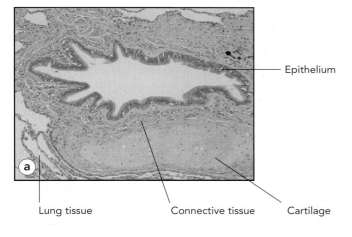

Epithelium

Lung tissue   Connective tissue   Cartilage

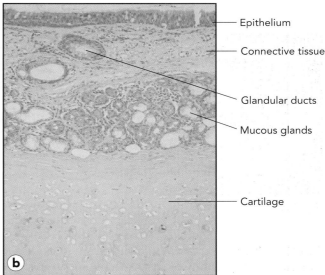

Epithelium

Connective tissue

Glandular ducts

Mucous glands

Cartilage

Fig. 5.13 (a) Low-power photomicrograph of a bronchus. (b) High-power photomicrograph of normal bronchial wall.

immotile cilia syndromes or commonly from cigarette smoke.

The chief defence of the alveoli is the alveolar macrophage (Fig. 5.15), which, in conjunction with complement and immunoglobulin, ingests foreign material that is then transported either up the airways or into the pulmonary lymphatics. T and B lymphocytes are present throughout the lung substance and most of the immunoglobulin in the lung is made locally. The blood supplies neutrophils that pass into the lung structure in inflammation.

LUNG FUNCTION

The function of the lung is to oxygenate the blood and to remove carbon dioxide. To achieve this, ventilation of the lungs is performed by the respiratory muscles under the control of the respiratory centre in the brain. The rhythm of breathing depends on various inhibitory and excitatory mechanisms within the brainstem. These can be influenced voluntarily from higher centres and from the effect of chemoreceptors. The medullary or central chemoreceptors in the brainstem respond to changes in partial pressure of carbon

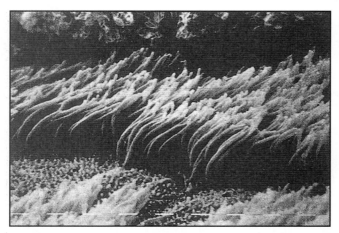

Fig. 5.14 Electronmicrograph of bronchial cilia and the mucus sheet.

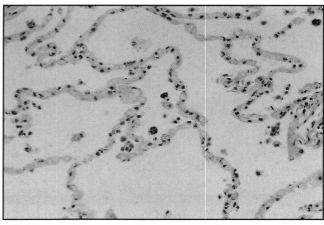

Fig. 5.15 Normal lung. Occasional pigment-containing macrophages are present within the alveolar spaces. Haematoxylin and eosin stain ($\times$ 25).

dioxide in the blood ($P\text{CO}_2$). Chemoreceptors in the aortic and carotid body respond to low partial pressure of oxygen ($P\text{O}_2$) but only when this falls below 8 kPa. Thus, alteration in $P\text{CO}_2$ is the most important factor in respiratory control in health.

The sensitivity of the medullary chemoreceptor to $P\text{CO}_2$ can be reset either upwards in prolonged ventilatory failure or downwards, as when a patient is placed on a mechanical ventilator. The first situation is most commonly seen in chronic airflow limitation (chronic obstructive lung disease) when patients may become dependent on hypoxic drive to maintain respiration. The injudicious administration of oxygen can then lead to ventilatory failure and death. In the second situation, 'weaning' a patient away from a ventilator is difficult because the medullary centre demands a low $P\text{CO}_2$ that cannot be maintained by the patient unaided.

Ventilation is largely performed by nerve impulses in the phrenic nerve acting to contract the diaphragm and expand the volume of the chest. Scalene and intercostal muscles act mainly by stabilising the chest wall. The result is to decrease the pressure in the pleura (already less than atmospheric). As the air inside the airways is at atmospheric pressure, the lungs must follow the chest wall through pleural apposition and expand, sucking in air. Expiration is largely a passive process: when the muscles relax the lung recoils under the influence of its own elasticity. Ventilation is, therefore, much more than just forcing air through tubes. Higher brain centres, the brainstem, spinal cord, peripheral nerves, intercostal muscles, spine, ribs and diaphragm are all involved. Moreover, the lung tissue itself must overcome its own inertia and stiffness. Malfunction of any of these can lead to respiratory failure.

Diaphragm function is in two parts: contraction leads to descent of the diaphragm and the costal parts elevate the lower ribs. A common consequence of chronic airflow limitation and hyperinflation is a low flat diaphragm which may pull the ribs inwards rather than out.

ASSESSING RESPIRATORY FUNCTION

As the function of the lungs is to add oxygen to the blood and to remove carbon dioxide, it might be thought that measurement of the $P\text{O}_2$ and $P\text{CO}_2$ in the blood would be an adequate assessment of its efficiency. However, the lung has such an enormous reserve capacity that it can sustain considerable damage before blood gases are affected. There are, nonetheless, a number of other tests of lung function that are briefly described here. These are tests of static lung volumes, ventilation or dynamic lung volumes and gas exchange across the alveolar–capillary membrane.

Static lung volumes

When attempting to take as deep an inspiration as possible we are eventually stopped, partly by the resist-

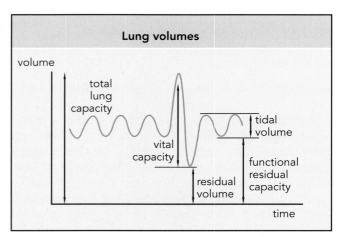

Fig. 5.16 Subdivisions of lung volume.

ance of the chest wall to further deformation and partly by the inability to stretch the lung tissues any further (Fig. 5.16). Total lung capacity (TLC) at one end is, therefore, largely influenced by this 'stretchability' or elasticity of the lung. The stiffer the lung, as in fibrosis or scarring, the less distensible it will be. Conversely, damage to the elastic tissue of the lung (e.g. emphysema) with destruction of the alveolar walls will make it more distensible, leading to an increase in TLC. TLC is also high is some patients with asthma and chronic obstructive bronchitis, probably because the lungs are overexpanded in an attempt to widen the airways.

As already indicated, breathing out from TLC is largely passive by progressive retraction of the lung; this process will end at functional residual capacity (FRC) when the tendency of the lung to contract is balanced by the thorax resisting further deformation. This point is also the end of normal expiration. Further expiration is an active process involving expiratory muscles. By using these muscles, more air can be forced out until, at least in older individuals, the limiting factor is closure of the small airways which have been getting smaller along with the alveoli. Beyond this the lungs can only become smaller by direct compression of gas (Boyle's law) by the expiratory muscles. At this point, the amount of air left in the lung is designated residual volume (RV).

In chronic bronchitis, the small airways are narrowed and inflamed; in emphysema, the elastic tissue supporting the small airways is lost and they collapse in expiration. Both mechanisms lead to an increase in RV. Conversely, if the lungs are stiffer (fibrosis), the increased tension in the lung tissue holds the airways open with closure occurring later in expiration, thus reducing the RV.

In summary, stiff lungs from fibrosis cause a low TLC and low RV, emphysema causes a high TLC and a high RV and chronic bronchitis causes a high RV. Vital

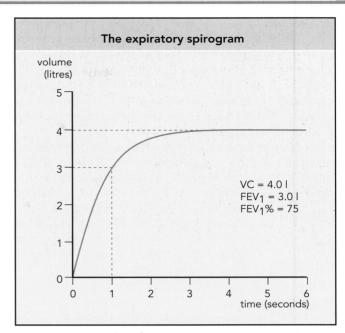

Fig. 5.17 Normal expiratory spirogram.

capacity (VC) depends on the relative changes in RV and TLC but usually the overall effect in lung disease is a reduction.

Dynamic lung volumes

Assessment of airflow involves measuring the volume exhaled in unit time by use of a spirometric trace (Fig. 5.17). This is produced by a forced exhalation from TLC to RV. The conventional parameters derived from this trace are the forced vital capacity (FVC) and the forced expiratory volume in 1 s (FEV_1). FVC is the amount exhaled forcefully from a single deep inspiration, FEV_1 is the fraction of that volume exhaled in the

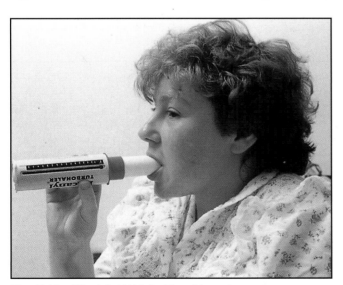

Fig. 5.18 The Mini-Wright Flow Meter in use.

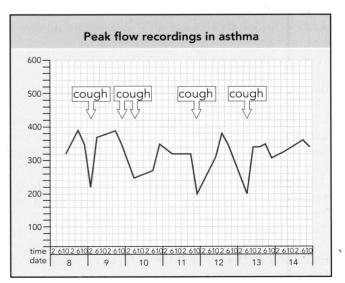

Fig. 5.19 Peak flow chart in a child with asthma whose main symptom was cough. The dips coincide with the symptoms.

first second. These are then expressed as a ratio of the FEV_1 over the FVC ($FEV_1\%$). This is normally approximately 75%, which indicates that a normal person can exhale forcibly three-quarters of their VC in 1 s. VC and FVC, one in slow expiration and the other in fast expiration, give similar results in normal individuals, although FVC is reduced because of premature airway closure in many disease states.

In diseases causing airways obstruction, the proportion of the VC that can be exhaled in 1 s is reduced and the $FEV_1\%$ falls. Conversely, in restrictive lung disease the airways are held open by the stiff lungs and the $FEV_1\%$ is normal, even increased. Nevertheless, the FVC will be reduced because the TLC is reduced. In restrictive lung disease, FEV_1 is reduced in proportion to FVC; in airways obstruction, it is reduced disproportionately.

Peak flow

The peak expiratory flow rate (PEFR) is the flow generated in the first 0.1 s of a forced expiration; the resulting figure is extrapolated over 1 min. It can be measured easily by a variety of portable devices (Fig. 5.18) and serial recordings can be very useful in the diagnosis and monitoring of asthma (Fig. 5.19).

Gas exchange

The transfer factor (TF) is a measurement of gas transference across the alveolar–capillary membrane. For technical reasons carbon monoxide is used as the test gas but oxygen is affected in a similar way. TF is reduced when there is destruction of the alveolar–capillary bed, as in emphysema, and also when there is a barrier to diffusion. This may occur when the alveolar–capillary membrane is thickened or where there is lack of homogeneity in the distribution of blood and air at alveolar level. Both mechanisms are important in lung fibrosis.

The TF will naturally be reduced if the lungs are small or if one has been removed (pneumonectomy). The transfer coefficient (KCO or D_LCO divided by alveolar volume, calculated separately) is a more useful measurement because it reflects the true situation in the ventilated lung.

LUNG VOLUMES IN DISEASE

In summary, it is possible to distinguish two main patterns of abnormal lung function. An 'obstructive pattern' is seen in asthma, chronic obstructive bronchitis and emphysema. FVC, FEV_1 and $FEV_1\%$ are all reduced and RV increased; TLC is often reduced but high in emphysema. TF is low in emphysema but otherwise normal. A 'restrictive pattern' is seen in lung fibrosis, such as occurs in cryptogenic fibrosing alveolitis. TLC, VC, FEV_1, RV and TF are all reduced but $FEV_1\%$ is normal or high.

When other results do not give a clear pattern, RV can be very helpful, being high in airways obstruction and low in fibrosis.

DISTRIBUTION OF VENTILATION AND PERFUSION

Distribution of air within the lung is best assessed for clinical purposes by radioactive isotopes. The usual tracer gas is radioactive xenon. The measurement of radioactivity over the lung gives a measure of the distribution and also the rate at which gas enters and leaves various parts of the lung. Thus, it can be used to detect 'air trapping' or absence of ventilation. Perfusion of blood can be measured in a similar way, usually by microaggregates of albumin labelled with technetium-99m, and injected into a peripheral vein. These microaggregates form small emboli within the lung and the radioactivity they give off is a measure of blood distribution. These tests are most useful in the diagnosis of pulmonary embolism when perfusion to an area of lung is reduced but ventilation is maintained (Fig. 5.20). If both ventilation and perfusion are reduced, then the defect probably lies within the airways and is a failure of ventilation with secondary changes in the blood supply.

BLOOD GASES

Blood gases can be measured directly by electrodes in blood obtained by arterial puncture. The results are expressed as partial pressure of gas in the plasma (PO_2 and PCO_2). It is important to realise that this is not the same as the amount of gas carried by the blood. If all the red cells were removed, the PO_2 would be unchanged, yet the patient would be in a perilous state. The haemoglobin in the red cell packages and

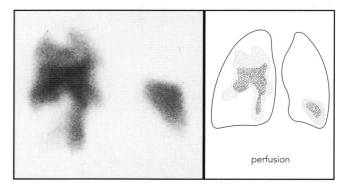

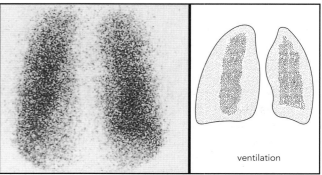

Fig. 5.20 Perfusion (upper) and ventilation (lower) scans in pulmonary emboli. Note the multiple perfusion defects but the normal ventilation pattern.

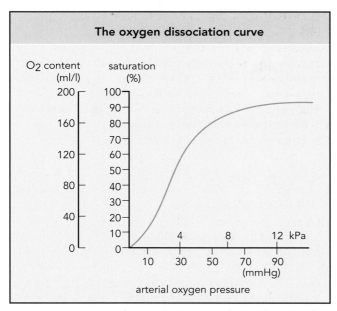

Fig. 5.21 Oxygen dissociation curve relating the partial pressure of oxygen in the blood to saturation of haemoglobin and amount of oxygen carried (assuming haemoglobin is normal).

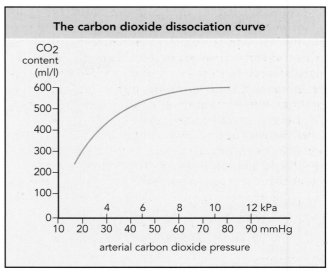

Fig. 5.22 Carbon dioxide dissociation curve relating partial pressure of gas in the blood to amount carried.

transports oxygen and carbon dioxide just as a subway train packages and transports passengers.

The relationship between P_{O_2} and saturation of the haemoglobin by oxygen (and hence the volume of oxygen carried) is given by the oxygen dissociation curve (Fig. 5.21). It will be seen that the P_{O_2} can drop significantly before there is a drop in the saturation, clearly a good thing in the early stages of lung disease. Nevertheless, it means that overventilation of the lung's good parts cannot fully compensate for underventilation of bad parts because the good parts on the flat part of the curve cannot increase the carriage of oxygen in the blood supplied to them beyond a certain maximum. Thus, when there is a shunt of blood from the right to the left heart, either directly through the heart or through unventilated lung, then the total amount of oxygen carried is bound to be reduced and cannot be restored to normal either by increasing ventilation or administering oxygen.

The steep part of the curve indicates that a small increase in inspired oxygen gives a large increase in the amount of oxygen carried: clearly useful for oxygen therapy in sick patients. It also indicates how readily hypoxic tissues can remove large amounts of oxygen from the blood.

The dissociation curve for carbon dioxide is very different to that of oxygen; lowering the P_{CO_2} continuously lowers the saturation and hence the volume of gas carried (Fig. 5.22). This means that overventilation in one part of the lung can compensate for underventilation elsewhere. Arterial P_{CO_2} is a good measure of overall alveolar ventilation, being increased in alveolar hypoventilation (e.g. severe chronic airflow limitation)

and decreased in alveolar hyperventilation (e.g. anxiety states, heart failure, pulmonary embolus, asthma), in which hypoxia and other factors stimulate an increase in ventilation.

The lungs help to regulate the acid–base balance by their ability to excrete or to retain carbon dioxide. In cases of metabolic acidosis (e.g. diabetic ketoacidosis, renal failure), the lungs can 'blow off' carbon dioxide to restore the pH towards normal. In cases of metabolic alkalosis (e.g. prolonged vomiting with loss of acid from the stomach), the retention of carbon dioxide again restores the pH towards normal. Retention or secretion of carbon dioxide as a result of lung disease (respiratory acidosis and alkalosis) alters pH, which is then secondarily restored by excretion or retention of bicarbonate by the kidney. Thus, changes in arterial P_{CO_2} (whether primary or secondary) can be regarded as functions of the lung, and changes in bicarbonate (again, either primary or secondary) can be regarded as functions of the kidney.

SYMPTOMS OF RESPIRATORY DISEASE

History-taking must follow the principles outlined earlier. Here, we are concerned with the analysis of the main symptoms of respiratory disease in turn. These are dyspnoea, cough, sputum, haemoptysis, pain and wheeze.

DYSPNOEA
Most lung diseases will cause dyspnoea or difficulty in breathing. Patients will express this in different ways as 'shortness of breath', 'shortwindedness', 'can't get my breath' or in terms of functional disability ('can't do the housework').

Differential diagnosis
Some causes of breathlessness

Control and movement of the chest wall and pleura
- Hyperventilation syndrome
- Hypothalamic lesions
- Neuromuscular disease
- Kyphoscoliosis
- Ankylosing spondylitis
- Pleural effusion and thickening
- Bilateral diaphragm paralysis

Diseases of the lungs
- Airways disease
  - chronic bronchitis and emphysema
  - asthma
  - bronchiectasis
  - cystic fibrosis
- Parenchymal disease
  - pneumonia
  - cryptogenic fibrosing alveolitis
  - extrinsic allergic alveolitis
  - primary and secondary tumour
  - sarcoidosis
  - pneumothorax
  - pulmonary oedema
- Reduced blood supply
  - pulmonary embolism
  - anaemia

Differential diagnosis
Duration of breathlessness

Immediate (minutes)
- Pulmonary embolism
- Pneumothorax
- Pulmonary oedema
- Asthma

Short (hours to days)
- Pulmonary oedema
- Pneumonia
- Asthma
- Pleural effusion
- Anaemia

Long (weeks to years)
- Chronic airflow limitation
- Cryptogenic fibrosing alveolitis
- Extrinsic allergic alveolitis
- Anaemia

Some patients will talk about 'tightness'. It may not be immediately clear whether they are describing breathlessness or pain. If the complaint is really a pain then this may well be angina, which is in itself associated with breathlessness. If asked directly, patients can

Questions to ask
Dyspnoea

- Is the breathlessness recent or has it been present for sometime?
- Is it constant or does it come and go?
- What can't you do because of the breathlessness?
- What makes the breathing worse?
- Does anything make it better?

usually tell you whether their tightness means pain or breathlessness. Some patients with pleuritic pain complain of breathlessness, but what they really mean is that they are unable to take a deep breath because of pain. It is of interest to consider why patients complain of breathlessness. Most normal people do not regard themselves as ill when they are short of breath, say when running for a bus. It seems probable that the sensations reported by patients are the same as the rest of us but they recognise that the work the lungs are being asked to do is disproportionate to the task the body is performing, that is, it feels inappropriate.

Causes of breathlessness
The causes of breathlessness may be listed as those to do with the control and movement of the chest wall, lung disease itself and problems with the blood and its supply to the lungs. The control of breathing can start with psychological factors in the brain, problems with the control centre in the medulla (rare) and the increased effort needed to overcome the effects of spinal cord disease (trauma or degeneration), neuropathies (e.g. Guillain–Barré syndrome), myopathies and chest wall problems (e.g. kyphoscoliosis, ankylosing spondylitis).

Lung diseases may require more work to overcome obstruction to airflow (e.g. chronic obstructive bronchitis, emphysema, asthma) or to stretch stiff lungs (e.g. pulmonary oedema, lung fibrosis).

Hypoxia needs to be severe to stimulate respiration but may be the mechanism in pneumonia, severe heart failure and other causes of pulmonary oedema. Pulmonary embolism leads to wasted ventilation in the affected area. Severe anaemia reduces the oxygen-carrying capacity of the blood.

J receptors are vagal nerve endings and are adjacent to pulmonary capillaries. Stimulation of these by pulmonary oedema, fibrosis and lung irritants is an additional mechanism causing breathlessness.

Duration of dyspnoea
The duration of dyspnoea may give a clue to the cause and can conveniently be divided into immediate (over minutes), short (hours to days) and long (weeks to years). There is some overlap but contrast, for example, the patient with a large pulmonary embolism who collapses in minutes in acute distress compared with the progressive relentless disability extending

over a decade in the patient with smoking-related airflow limitation. Some patients find it difficult to remember duration accurately. Many report symptoms as lasting for only 'a few weeks' when they mean 'worse for a few weeks'. A question like 'when could you last run for a bus' may indicate problems stretching back for years. A spouse is often more accurate in this respect than the patient.

Variability of dyspnoea

Questions about variability can be couched as 'does it come and go or is it much the same' or 'do you have good days and bad days or is it much the same from one day to another'. A reply suggesting variability is highly characteristic of variable airflow limitation, that is, asthma. If asthma is suspected, this can be followed-up by questions on aggravating factors. Follow this up with some more directed questions about particular factors. These are important not only as potentially preventable causes but because positive replies strengthen the diagnosis. The house dust mite is the most common allergen; patients will report worsening of symptoms on sweeping, dusting or making the beds. Exercise, at least in children, is a potent trigger of asthma but exercise will also make other forms of breathlessness worse. The difference is that in asthma the attack is caused by the exercise, may indeed follow it and may last for 30 min or more. In other causes of breathlessness, recovery starts as soon as exercise stops.

Asthma

Asthma due solely to emotional causes probably does not exist; nonetheless, most patients who have asthma are worse if emotionally upset. Patients may feel that admitting to stress is respectable when they would deny other emotions. Nocturnal asthma is very common. Few asthmatics smoke because they know it makes them worse. Ask what happens if they go into a bar. Many will say they are unable to do so because of smoke. The response to household aerosol sprays can be helpful. Many breathless patients with a variety of illnesses will think it logical, rightly or wrongly, that 'dust' or 'fumes' will make them worse but only true asthmatics seem to notice a deterioration with the ubiquitous domestic spray can.

Severity of dyspnoea

Severity can be assessed by rating scales, although it is much better to use some functional measure. Ask the patient in what way their breathlessness restricts their activities: can they go upstairs, go shopping, wash the car or do the garden? If they are troubled with stairs, how many flights can they manage? Do they stop half way up or at the top? Questions about gardening are useful, at least in the summer, as it is possible to grade activity from pulling out a few weeds to digging the potato patch. It is important to be certain that any

Questions to ask
Asthma

- Does anything make any difference to the asthma?
- What happens if you are worried or upset?
- Does your chest wake you at night?
- Does cigarette smoke make any difference?
- Do household sprays affect you?
- Have you lost time from work/school?
- What happens when sweeping or dusting the house?
- Does exposure to cats or dogs make any difference?

restriction is caused by breathlessness and not some other disability (e.g. an arthritic hip or angina).

Orthopnoea and paroxysmal nocturnal dyspnoea

Orthopnoea and paroxysmal nocturnal dyspnoea need special consideration. Both are usually regarded as manifestations of left ventricular failure, yet this is an oversimplification. Orthopnoea is defined as breathlessness lying flat but relieved by sitting up. It is common in patients with severe fixed airways obstruction, as in some chronic bronchitics who may admit to not having slept flat for years. Normal people, when they lie flat, breathe more with the diaphragm and less with the chest wall. In patients with airways obstruction, the diaphragm is often flat and inefficient and may even draw the ribs inwards rather than out. Thus, when they lie down the diaphragm cannot provide the ventilation required.

The term paroxysmal nocturnal dyspnoea is self-explanatory and is a feature of pulmonary oedema from left ventricular failure. However, many asthmatics develop bronchoconstriction in the night and wake with wheeze and breathlessness very similar to the symptoms of left ventricular failure. In contrast, patients with severe fixed flow limitation usually sleep well even if they do have to be propped up.

The hyperventilation syndrome

The hyperventilation syndrome is more common than is generally realised but produces a distinct pattern of symptoms. It is usually associated with anxiety and patients overbreathe inappropriately. The initial complaint is often, although not always, of breathlessness. The hyperventilation is the response to this sensation. It may be described by the patient as a 'difficulty in breathing in' or an inability to 'fill the bottom of the lungs'. The hyperventilation induces a reduction in the $P\text{CO}_2$, creating a variety of other symptoms: paraesthesiae in the fingers, tingling around the lips, 'dizziness', 'lightheadedness' and sometimes frank tetany. Chest pain is the probable consequence of increased chest wall movement. The onset is often triggered by some life event; especially work related (e.g. redundancy or dismissal). The diagnosis can be confirmed by the

Symptoms and signs
Features suggestive of the hyperventilation syndrome

- Breathlessness at rest
- Breathlessness as severe with mild exertion as with greater exertion
- Marked variability in breathlessness
- More difficulty breathing in than out
- Paraesthesiae of the fingers
- Numbness around the mouth
- 'Lightheadedness'
- Feelings of impending collapse or remoteness from surroundings
- Chest wall pain

Symptoms and signs
Allergic and nonallergic factors in asthma

Allergic
- House dust mite
- Animals (especially cats)
- Pollens (especially grass)

Nonallergic
- Exercise
- Emotion
- Sleep
- Smoke
- Aerosol sprays
- Cold air
- Upper respiratory tract infections

'20 deep breaths test', which will reproduce the symptoms.

Dyspnoea and hypoxia

Dyspnoea should be distinguished from tachypnoea (increased rate of breathing) and from hypoxia. It is a symptom, not a sign, nor is it necessarily an indication of lung disease. Psychological factors, such as the hyperventilation syndrome, and acidosis from diabetic ketosis or renal failure may produce tachypnoea which may be felt as dyspnoea. Many patients think that if they are short of breath, they must be short of oxygen. This is sometimes the case but, as mentioned earlier, hypoxia only stimulates respiration when relatively severe. To illustrate the distinction between hypoxia and dyspnoea, consider that many patients with airflow limitation from chronic bronchitis have hypoxia severe enough to cause right-sided heart failure, yet they have relatively little dyspnoea (blue bloaters). In contrast, some patients with emphysema seem to need to keep their blood gases normal by a heroic effort of breathing (pink puffers); they are very dyspnoeic.

COUGH

Cough arises from the cough receptors in the pharynx, larynx and bronchi; cough, therefore, results from irritation of these receptors from infection, inflammation, tumour or foreign body. Cough may be the only symptom in asthma, particularly childhood asthma. Cough in children occurring regularly after exercise or at night is virtually diagnostic of asthma. Many smokers regard cough as normal: 'only a smokers cough' or may deny it completely despite having just coughed in front of the examiner. In these patients, a change in the character of the cough can be highly significant.

Patients can often localise cough to above the larynx ('a tickle in the throat') or below. Postnasal drip from rhinitis can cause the former and may be accompanied by sneezing and nasal blockage.

Laryngitis will cause both cough and a hoarse voice. Recurrent laryngeal nerve palsy causes a hoarse voice and an ineffective cough because the cord is immobile. The usual cause is involvement of the left recurrent laryngeal nerve by tumour in its course in the chest. Cough from tracheitis is usually dry and painful. Cough from further down the airways is often associated with sputum production (bronchitis, bronchiectasis or pneumonia). In the latter, associated pleurisy makes coughing very distressing and reduces its effectiveness. Other possibilities are carcinoma, lung fibrosis and increased bronchial responsiveness (this is an inflammatory condition of the airways, thought to be part of the mechanism underlying asthma and often made worse by the factors in the symptoms and signs box on allergic and nonallergic factors in asthma). An uncommon cause of cough and often overlooked is aspiration into the lungs from gastro-oesophageal reflux or a pharyngeal pouch. Cough will then follow meals or lying down. Prolonged coughing bouts can cause both unconsciousness from reduction of venous return from the brain (cough syncope) and also vomiting. Sometimes the history of cough is omitted, making diagnosis difficult!

SPUTUM

Patients may understand the term 'phlegm' better than sputum. It is the result of excessive bronchial secretion; itself a manifestation of inflammation and infection. Like cough, smokers may not acknowledge its existence. Children usually swallow their sputum. It is essential to be certain that the complaint relates to the chest, because some patients have difficulty in distinguishing sputum production from gastrointestinal reflux, postnasal drip or saliva. Sometimes asking the patient to 'show me what you have to do to get phlegm up' can be helpful. If the patient denies sputum, a cough producing a rattle (a 'loose cough') suggests that it is present.

Sputum caused by chronic irritation is usually white or grey, particularly in smokers; if infected, it

Differential diagnosis
Sputum

White or grey
- Smoking
- Simple chronic bronchitis
- Asthma

Yellow or green
- Acute bronchitis
- Acute on chronic bronchitis
- Asthma
- Bronchiectasis
- Cystic fibrosis

Frothy, blood-streaked
- Pulmonary oedema

Questions to ask
Sputum

- What colour is the phlegm?
- How often do you bring it up?
- How much do you bring up?
- Do you have trouble getting it up?

Differential diagnosis
Haemoptysis

Common
- Infection including bronchiectasis
- Bronchial carcinoma
- Tuberculosis
- Pulmonary embolism and infarction
- No cause found

Uncommon
- Mitral stenosis and left ventricular failure
- Bronchial adenoma
- Idiopathic pulmonary haemosiderosis
- Anticoagulation and blood dyscrasias

Differential diagnosis
Pointers to the significance of an episode of haemoptysis

Probably serious
- Middle-aged or elderly
- Spontaneous
- Previous or current smoker
- Recurrent
- Large amount

Probably not serious
- Young
- Recent infection
- Never smoked
- Single episode
- Small amount – if single episode

becomes yellow from the presence of leucocytes and this may turn to green by the action of the enzyme verdoperoxidase. Yellow or green sputum in asthma can be caused by the presence of eosinophils rather than infection. Questions on frequency are most useful in the diagnosis of chronic bronchitis, an epidemiological definition of this is 'sputum production on most days for 3 consecutive months for 2 successive years'. Sputum production is common in asthmatics and is occasionally the main complaint. The diagnosis of bronchiectasis is made on a story of daily sputum production stretching back to childhood.

Patients can often give an estimate of the amount of sputum they bring up each day, usually in terms of a cup or teaspoon and so on. Large amounts occur in bronchiectasis and lung abscess and in the rare bronchioloalveolar cell carcinoma.

Sticky 'rusty' sputum is characteristic of lobar pneumonia, and frothy sputum with streaks of blood is seen in pulmonary oedema.

Highly viscous sputum, sometimes with plugs, is characteristic of asthma and in some patients with chronic bronchitis. Small bronchial casts, like twigs, may be described by a patient with the condition of bronchopulmonary aspergillosis associated with asthma.

HAEMOPTYSIS

The coughing up of blood is often a sign of serious lung disease. Nevertheless, it is common in trivial respiratory infections. Like sputum production, it is essential to establish that it is coming from the lungs and not the nose or mouth or being vomited (haematemesis). Bleeding from the nose may run into the pharynx and be coughed out but usually the patient will also describe bleeding from the anterior nares. Bleeding in the mouth causes confusion, it is usually related to brushing the teeth (gingivitis).

The blood in haemoptysis is usually bright red at first, then followed by progressively smaller and darker amounts. This would be unusual in haematemesis.

All haemoptysis is potentially serious, although the most important is carcinoma of the bronchus. Repeated small haemoptyses every few days over a period of some weeks in a middle-aged smoker is virtually diagnostic of bronchial carcinoma.

Other serious causes are pulmonary embolism (sudden onset of pleuritic chest pain and dyspnoea followed by haemoptysis), tuberculosis (weight loss, fever, cough and sputum) and bronchiectasis (long history of sputum production and the haemoptysis associated with an exacerbation and increased sputum purulence). Blood-tinged sputum in pneumonia and pulmonary oedema has already been mentioned.

diagnosis is likely to be correct in a lifelong non-smoker. Patients seem to be generally accurate about their tobacco consumption contrasting sometimes with alcohol.

It is important not to appear censorious when enquiring about smoking. Tobacco is highly addictive and most patients would give up if only they could and are not being perverse when they continue despite evidence of lung damage. You should be aware that some patients claim to be nonsmokers when they only stopped last month, last week or even on the way to hospital! Ask nonsmokers 'have you smoked in the past?'. The risk of disease increases with the amount smoked. Cigarettes are the most dangerous; pipes and cigars are not free of risk. Risk declines steadily when smoking stops; it takes 10–20 years for the risk of lung cancer to equal that of lifelong nonsmokers.

Inhalation of another person's smoke at home or at work is increasingly recognised as a factor in lung disease. This is particularly true for asthma. Children in households with smokers have more respiratory infections.

Pets and hobbies

For many asthmatics, cats and dogs are common sources of allergen. The allergen may remain in the house long after the offending animal has been banished.

Exposure to racing pigeons, budgerigars, parrots and other caged birds can cause extrinsic allergic alveolitis. The cause is protein material derived from feathers and droppings. Acute symptoms are usually seen in pigeon fanciers who, a few hours after cleaning out their birds, develop cough, breathlessness and 'flu-like' symptoms. Recovery takes place over the next day or two unless there is re-exposure. Chronic symptoms are seen in budgerigar owners, presumably because they are exposed continuously to low doses of antigen. Their complaint is of progressive breathlessness.

Parrots and related species transmit the infectious agent of psittacosis, a cause of pneumonia. You may need to extend your enquires beyond the home because patients may be exposed to birds belonging to friends and relations.

Occupation

The question 'what work do you do?' is more important for respiratory disease than for any other. The nature of the job and not just the title is important because the latter may convey no meaning to you at all. The question is important in two ways. Respiratory disease may affect a patient's ability to perform a job but may also be the result of the occupation. Any job involving exposure to noxious agents of a respirable size is potentially damaging; the most obvious example is pneumoconiosis in coal miners.

Enquiry may need to be searching and, if occupational lung disease is suspected, then a full list of all jobs performed will need to be constructed. For example, in the case of asbestos there can be an interval of 30 years between exposure, say in shipyard work, and the development of asbestosis or mesothelioma. Some will deny working with asbestos but nevertheless were exposed when others were performing lagging (putting asbestos on pipes) or stripping (taking it off). Other occupations in which exposure may not be obvious, although real nonetheless, are building and demolition work, electrical repair work, railway engineering and gas mask and cement manufacture. Environmental exposure, including that of wives of asbestos workers, seems important occasionally.

The easiest way to diagnose pneumoconiosis is to ask the patient. Miners in the UK undergo regular chest radiography while working. If significant pneumoconiosis is diagnosed the patient will be told.

Occupational asthma

The list of causes of occupational asthma grows longer yearly. A good screening question to any asthmatic is: 'Does your work make any difference to your symptoms?'; follow this up with questions about improvement at weekends or on holiday. The latter is important because symptoms caused at work may not be manifest until the evening or night and sometimes changes take place over days or even weeks.

Common causes are isocyanates (paint hardeners and plastic manufacture) and colophony (soldering

Risk factors
Lung cancer

- Smoking
- Atmospheric pollution
- Asbestos exposure
- Radon exposure (natural and occupational)
- Work in gas and coke industry

Risk factors
Some occupational causes of lung disease

Occupation	Agent	Disease
Mining	Coal dust	Pneumoconiosis
Quarrying	Silica dust	Silicosis
Foundry work	Silica dust	Silicosis
Asbestos (Mining, heating, building, demolition)	Asbestos fibres	Asbestosis Mesothelioma Lung cancer
Farming	Actinomycetes	Alveolitis
Paint spraying	Isocyanates	Asthma
Plastics manufacture	Isocyanates	Asthma
Soldering	Colophony	Asthma

and electronics). The lack of an obvious culprit should not put you off the scent if the evidence is otherwise suggestive. Much detective work is necessary in individual cases.

Extrinsic allergic alveolitis

Extrinsic allergic alveolitis can be caused by occupation as well as birds. The best example is farmer's lung: the agent is the microorganism thermophilic actinomycetes contaminating stored damp hay. The story is of shortness of breath, cough and chills a few hours after forking out fodder for cattle in the winter. Other occupations with similar risks are mushroom workers, sugar workers (bagassosis: mouldy sugar cane), malt-workers and woodworkers, although the antigens vary in each case.

FAMILY HISTORY

The most common lung disease with a genetic basis is asthma, although the development of the disease in an individual is much more complicated. A family history of asthma and the related conditions of hay fever or eczema are often found but these diseases are so prevalent that enquiry beyond the immediate family is of little value. Other diseases that run in the family include cystic fibrosis and α_1-antitrypsin deficiency, a rare cause of emphysema.

Tuberculosis is usually passed on within families. In the UK, tuberculosis is common in Asian migrants, particularly in their first 10 years in the country, and in individuals who have revisited the subcontinent. Most of the increased incidence of the disease seen in recent years has occurred in conditions of poverty.

Enquiry into sexual habits will be necessary if the illness could be a manifestation of AIDS, remembering that this is now becoming more common in the heterosexual population, especially in individuals who have travelled abroad, particularly to Africa and Asia.

DRUG HISTORY

The most useful questions are those concerning past treatment. Successful use of bronchodilators and corticoids in airways obstruction will indicate asthma. Aspirin and sometimes other nonsteroidal anti-inflammatory drugs and β-adrenergic receptor blockers can make asthma worse, and angiotensin-converting enzyme inhibitors cause chronic dry cough. Steroid therapy predisposes to infections, including tuberculosis.

GENERAL EXAMINATION

Examination starts on first encounter. You should be able to continually pick up and store clues while talking and listening to the patient. As with all body systems, a good look at the patient as a whole will provide important evidence that will be missed in a rush to lay a stethoscope on the chest. Your findings should be divided into first impressions, then a more directed search for signs outside the chest likely to be helpful in lung disease and, finally, examination of the chest itself.

FIRST IMPRESSIONS

How breathless does the patient appear? Is it consistent with the story? If seen in the clinic or office, can the patient walk in comfortably and sit down or does the patient struggle to get in? Perhaps the patient is in a wheelchair; if so, is it because of breathing troubles or something else? Can the patient carry on a conversation with you or do they break up their sentences? How breathless is the patient when getting undressed? Details of breathing patterns are considered later but is the patient obviously distressed or quite comfortable? Is there stridor or wheeze? Is there cough, confirming or perhaps at variance with the history? Is there evidence of weight loss suggesting carcinoma or weight gain from steroid therapy?

Do not ignore clues around the patient. An air compressor by the bed will be used to deliver bronchodilator drugs. A packet of cigarettes in the pyjama jacket will have the opposite effect. In hospital you will be deprived of some of these features but not how the patient is positioned; does the patient have to sit up to breathe, confirming a history of orthopnoea. Is the patient receiving oxygen?

After extracting as much information as you can, position the patient comfortably on the bed or couch with enough pillows to support the chest at an angle of approximately 45° and begin the formal examination. This can conveniently start with the hands and a search for clubbing.

Clubbing

This refers to an increase in the soft tissues of the nail bed and the finger tip. The earliest stage is some softening of the nail bed which can be detected by rocking the nail from side to side on the nail bed (Fig. 5.25). This sign can be present to some extent in normal individuals but is exaggerated in the early stages of clubbing. Next, the soft tissue of the nail bed fills in the normal obtuse angle between the nail and the nail bed. This is usually approximately 160° but the area becomes flat, even convex in clubbing (Fig. 5.26). This is seen best by viewing the nail from the side against a white background, say the bedsheets. Not surprisingly, there can be considerable disagreement about the presence or absence of clubbing in the early stages. When normal nails are placed 'back to back' there is usually a diamond-shaped area between them. This is obliterated early in clubbing (Fig. 5.27).

In the next stage, the normal longtitudinal curvature of the nail increases. Some normal nails have a pronounced curve but in clubbing the increase in soft tissue in the nail beds needs to be present as well. In the final stage, the whole tip of the finger becomes rounded (a club) (Fig. 5.28). Clubbing less commonly affects the toes.

The pathogenesis of clubbing is unknown. There is increased vascularity and tissue fluid and this seems to be under neurogenic control because it can be abolished by vagotomy.

Clubbing is sometimes associated with hypertrophic pulmonary osteoarthropathy; this presents with pain in the joints, particularly the wrists, ankles and knees. The pain is not in the joint itself but over the shafts of the long bones adjacent to the joint. It is caused by subperiosteal new bone formation, which can be seen on a radiograph (Fig. 5.29). The condition is almost invariably associated with clubbing, although it can occur alone. Any cause of clubbing can also cause hypertrophic pulmonary osteoarthropathy; however, it is usually associated with a squamous carcinoma of the bronchus. The condition is often mistaken for arthritis, with consequent delay in diagnosis. Successful treatment of the cause will relieve clubbing and the pain of hypertrophic pulmonary osteoarthropathy. While searching for clubbing, note any nicotine staining of the fingers.

Cyanosis

Cyanosis, a bluish tinge to the skin and mucous membranes is seen when there is an increased amount of reduced haemoglobin in the blood (Fig. 5.30). Traditionally, it is thought to become visible when there is approximately 5 g/dl or more of reduced haemoglobin, corresponding to a saturation of approximately 85%; however, there is a good deal of interobserver variation. Severe anaemia and cyanosis cannot coexist otherwise most of the haemoglobin would be reduced. Conversely, in polycythaemia, in which there is an increase in red cell mass, there may be enough reduced haemoglobin to produce cyanosis, even though there is enough oxygenated haemoglobin to maintain a normal oxygen-carrying capacity.

Cyanosis can be divided into central and peripheral varieties. Central cyanosis is caused by disease of the heart or lungs and the blood leaving the left heart is blue. Peripheral cyanosis is caused by decreased circulation and increased extraction of oxygen in the peripheral tissues. Blood leaving the left heart is normal.

Central cyanosis

Although the whole patient may appear cyanosed, the best place to look is the mucous membranes of the lips and tongue (Fig. 5.31). Good natural light is best. Any severe disease of the heart and lungs will cause central cyanosis but the most common causes are severe airflow limitation, left ventricular failure and pulmonary fibrosis.

Peripheral cyanosis

Here, the peripheries, the fingers and the toes, are blue with normal mucous membranes. The usual cause is reduced circulation to the limbs, as seen in cold weather, Raynaud's phenomenon or peripheral vas-

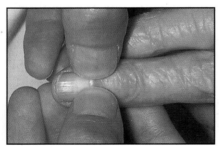

Fig. 5.25 Rocking the nail on the nail bed in clubbing.

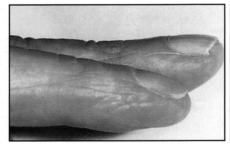

Fig. 5.26 Mild clubbing. The nail on the left shows obliteration of the angle at the nail fold compared with a normal nail on the right.

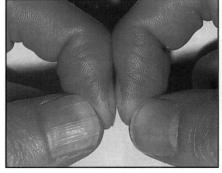

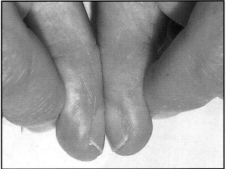

Fig. 5.27 Clubbing, showing how the diamond-shaped area formed between two normal nails (left) is obliterated (right).

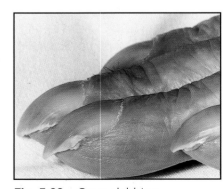

Fig. 5.28 Gross clubbing.

Differential diagnosis
Some common causes of clubbing

Pulmonary
- Bronchial carcinoma
- Chronic pulmonary sepsis
  - empyema
  - lung abscess
  - bronchiectasis
  - cystic fibrosis
- Cryptogenic fibrosing alveolitis
- Asbestosis

Cardiac
- Congenital cyanotic heart disease
- Bacterial endocarditis

Other
- Idiopathic/familial
- Cirrhosis
- Ulcerative colitis
- Coeliac disease
- Crohn's disease

cular disease. The peripheries are also usually cold. There may be an element of peripheral cyanosis in heart failure when the perfusion of the extremities is reduced.

Cyanosis can rarely be caused by the abnormal pigments methaemoglobin and sulphaemoglobin. Arterial oxygen tension is normal.

Tremors and carbon dioxide retention

The most common tremor in patients with respiratory disease is a fine finger tremor from stimulation of β-receptors in skeletal muscle by bronchodilator drugs. Carbon dioxide retention is seen in severe chronic airflow limitation. Clinically, it can be suspected by a flapping tremor (indistinguishable from that associated with hepatic failure), vasodilatation manifested by warm peripheries, bounding pulses, papilloedema and headache.

Pulse and blood pressure

Pulsus paradoxus is a drop in blood pressure on inspiration. A minor degree occurs normally. Major degrees occur in pericardial effusion and constrictive pericarditis but also in severe asthma. However, it probably adds nothing to other measures of severe asthma. For further discussion see Chapter 6.

Jugular venous pulse and cor pulmonale

The jugular venous pulse may be raised in cor pulmonale (right-sided heart failure due to lung disease). The common cause in the UK is chronic airflow limitation leading to hypoxia. The main mechanism is pulmonary vasoconstriction. Other signs are peripheral oedema (probably as much due to renal hypoxia as back pressure from the right heart), hepatomegaly and a left parasternal heave, indicating right ventricular hypertrophy. In severe cases, functional tricuspid regurgitation will lead to a pulsatile liver, large V waves in the jugular venous pulse and a systolic murmur in the tricuspid area (see Ch. 6). Sometimes

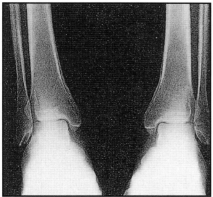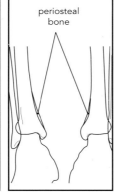

periosteal bone

Fig. 5.29 Hypertrophic pulmonary osteoarthropathy.

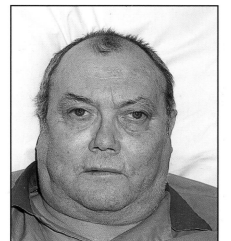

Fig. 5.30 Cyanosis in a patient with chronic airflow limitation.

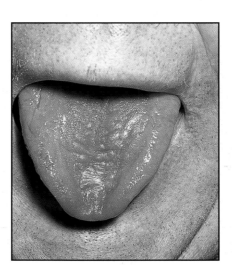

Fig. 5.31 Central cyanosis of the tongue.

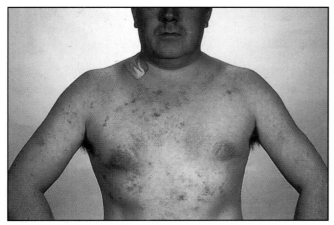

Fig. 5.32 Superior vena caval obstruction showing a swollen face and neck, dilated veins over the trunk and the site of a lymph node biopsy.

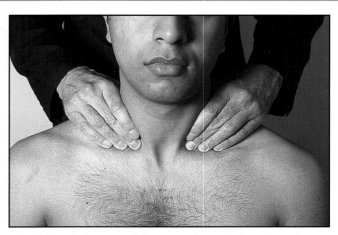

Fig. 5.33 Palpation of the supraclavicular lymph nodes from behind.

overinflation of the lungs will displace the liver downwards and also obscure the cardiac signs, leaving the jugular venous pulse as the only sign.

Superior vena cava obstruction is a common presentation of carcinoma of the bronchus but can rarely be caused by lymphoma, benign tumours and mediastinal fibrosis. The tumour compresses the superior vena cava near the point where it enters the right atrium. The resulting high pressure in the superior vena cava causes distension of the neck, fullness and oedema of the face, dilated collateral veins over the upper chest (Fig. 5.32) and chemosis or oedema of the conjunctiva. The internal jugular vein is, of course, distended but may be difficult to see because it does not pulsate (the 'dog-in-the-night-time' syndrome). The external jugular vein should be visible. The patient may have noticed that shirt collars have become tighter.

Lymphadenopathy

Lymph nodes may enlarge either because of generalised disease (e.g. lymphoma) or from local disease spreading through the lymphatics to the nodes. Both may be important in respiratory disease. Palpation of lymph nodes is considered in Chapter 2, so here the examination of only those lymph nodes draining the chest is considered.

Lymphatics from the lungs drain centrally to the hilum then up the paratracheal chain to the supraclavic-ular (scalene) or cervical nodes. Chest wall lymphatics, especially from the breasts, drain to the axillae. Lung disease, therefore, rarely involves the axillary nodes. Examination of the cervical chain can be carried out by palpation from the front of the patient. Supraclavicular lymphadenopathy is best detected from behind the patient by placing your fingers either side of the neck behind the tendon of the sternomastoid muscle. It helps if the neck is bent slightly forward (Fig. 5.33). Cervical nodes can be palpated this way too.

It is sometimes difficult to examine in the supraclavicular area because lymph nodes may be only slightly enlarged. If palpable, the nodes are usually the site of disease. Careful comparisons should be made between the two sides. If lymph nodes are enlarged then biopsy or aspiration may be a simple way to confirm a diagnosis. Beware of performing a cervical node biopsy too readily. Throat cancer can involve these nodes and painstaking block dissection is the correct treatment.

Respiratory diseases that involve these nodes are carcinoma, tuberculosis and sarcoidosis. Nodes containing metastatic carcinoma are hard and fixed. Tuberculous nodes, common in Asian patients in the

 Differential diagnosis
Common respiratory causes of supraclavicular lymphadenopathy

- Lung cancer
- Lymphoma
- Tuberculosis
- Sarcoidosis
- HIV infection

 Differential diagnosis
Erythema nodosum

Infections
- Streptococci
- Tuberculosis
- Systemic fungal infections
- Leprosy

Others
- Sarcoidosis
- Ulcerative colitis
- Crohn's disease
- Sulphonamides
- Oral contraceptive pill and pregnancy

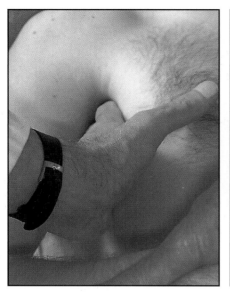

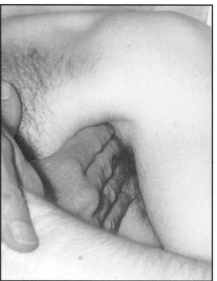

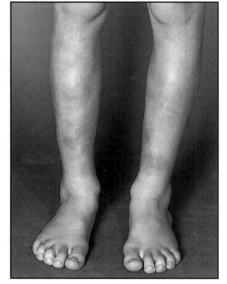

Fig. 5.34 Palpation of the axillary lymph nodes.

Fig. 5.35 Erythema nodosum, showing raised red lumps on the shins.

UK, are soft and matted and may have discharging sinuses. Healing and calcification leave small hard nodes.

Examination of the axillary nodes is shown in Figure 5.34. Abduct the patient's arm, place the fingers of your hand high up in the axilla, press the tips of the fingers against the chest wall, relax the patient's arm and draw your fingers downwards over the ribs to roll the nodes between your fingers and the ribs.

Skin

The early stages of sarcoidosis and primary tuberculosis are often accompanied by erythema nodosum (Fig. 5.35): painful red indurated areas usually on the shins; although occasionally more extensive, they fade through bruising. Severely affected patients may also have arthralgia. The most common cause of erythema nodosum in the UK is sarcoidosis. Sarcoidosis can also involve the skin, particularly old scars and tattoos, with nodules and plaques. Lupus pernio is a violaceous swelling of the nose from involvement by sarcoid granuloma.

Eyes

Horner's syndrome (miosis (contraction of the pupil), enophthalmos (backward displacement of the eyeball in the orbit), lack of sweating on the affected side of the face and ptosis (drooping of the upper eyelid) (see also Chapter 11)) is usually due to involvement of the sympathetic chain on the posterior chest wall by a bronchial carcinoma.

Sarcoidosis and tuberculosis can cause iridocyclitis. Miliary tuberculosis can produce tubercles visible on the retina by ophthalmoscopy. Papilloedema can be caused by carbon dioxide retention and cerebral metastases.

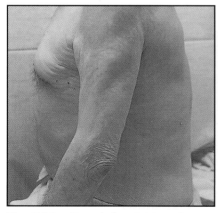

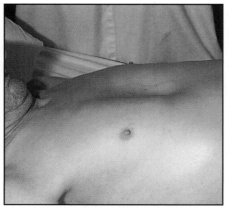

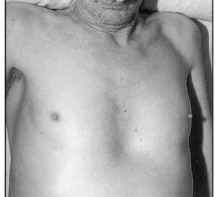

Fig. 5.36 'Barrel chest'. Note the increased anteroposterior diameter of the chest.

Fig. 5.37 Pectus excavatum, showing the depressed sternum.

EXAMINATION OF THE CHEST

You should follow the classical sequence of inspection, palpation, percussion and auscultation, not forgetting contemplation (Osler).

INSPECTION OF THE CHEST WALL

First look for any deformities of the chest wall. In 'barrel chest' the chest wall is held in hyperinflation (Fig. 5.36). In normal people the anteroposterior diameter of the chest is less than the lateral diameter but in hyperinflation the anteroposterior diameter may be greater than the lateral. The amount of trachea palpable above the suprasternal notch is reduced. The normal 'bucket handle' action of the ribs moving upwards and outwards, pivoting at the spinous processes and the costal cartilages, is converted into a 'pump handle' up and down motion. Barrel chest is seen in states of chronic airflow limitation, with the degree of deformity correlating with its severity.

In pectus excavatum ('funnel chest') (Fig. 5.37), the sternum is depressed: the condition is benign and needs no treatment but can produce unusual chest radiographic appearances, with the heart apparently enlarged and displaced to the left. In pectus carinatum ('pigeon chest'), the sternum and costal cartilages project outwards. It may be secondary to severe childhood asthma.

Examine the chest wall for any operative scars or the changes of thoracoplasty. This was an operation performed in the 1940s and 1950s for tuberculosis and designed to reduce the volume of the chest. It can produce marked distortion of the chest wall, more clearly seen from the back (Fig. 5.38).

Flattening of part of the chest can be due either to underlying lung disease (which usually has to be long-standing) or to scoliosis.

Kyphosis is forward curvature of the spine (Fig. 5.39) and scoliosis is a lateral curvature. Both, but scoliosis in particular, can lead to respiratory failure.

Air in the subcutaneous tissue is termed surgical emphysema, although it is as commonly associated with a spontaneous pneumothorax as trauma to the chest. The tissues of the upper chest and neck are swollen, sometimes grossly so (Michelin man), although the condition is not dangerous in itself. The tissues have a characteristic crackling sensation on palpation. In pneumothorax, the air probably tracks from ruptured alveoli, through the root of the lungs to the mediastinum, thence up into the neck. On auscultation of the precordium, you may hear a curious extra sound in time with the heart (mediastinal crunch) but this can occur in pneumothorax without pneumomediastinum. Mediastinal air may be visible on a radiograph.

BREATHING PATTERNS

A good deal can be learnt from simple observation of the chest wall movements. Note rate, depth and regularity. Does the chest move equally on the two sides? Does breathing appear distressing? Is it noisy?

Counting the respiratory rate is a traditional nursing observation, yet the precise rate is rarely of practical importance. You should note an increase in rate or depth. An increase in rate may occur in any severe lung disease and in fever. Patients with hyperventilation may breath both faster and more deeply, although the increase can be subtle and easily missed. Patients with acidosis from renal failure, diabetic ketoacidosis and aspirin overdosage will have deep sighing (Kussmaul) respirations as they try to excrete carbon dioxide. Acute massive pulmonary embolism gives a similar pattern.

Is the breathing regular? Cheyne–Stokes respiration is a waxing and waning of the respiratory depth over a minute or so from deep respirations to almost no breathing at all. It is thought to be caused by a failure

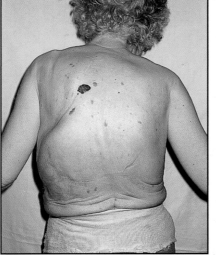

Fig. 5.38 Thoracoplasty with secondary changes in the spine.

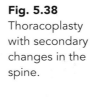

Fig. 5.39 Kyphosis.

of the central respiratory control to respond adequately to changes in carbon dioxide and is often seen in patients with terminal disease. Patients may seem unaware of the condition.

Is there any prolongation of expiration? The typical patient with airflow limitation has trouble breathing out. Inspiration may be brief, even hurried, but expiration is a prolonged laboured manoeuvre. Many of these patients breathe out through pursed lips as if they were whistling; this mechanism maintains a higher airway pressure and keeps open the distal airways to allow fuller although longer expiration.

Note if the chest expands unequally. If this is so and there is no structural abnormality of the chest or spine to account for it then air is probably not entering the lung so well on the affected side. The difference has to be marked to be appreciated. The causes will be considered under palpation. It is possible to measure overall expansion with a tape-measure (the result is of little value and certainly no substitute for measures of lung volume). Breathing mainly with the diaphragm suggests chest wall problems (e.g. pleural pain, ankylosing spondylitis). Breathing mainly with the rib cage suggests diaphragm paralysis, peritonitis or abdominal distension. Normally, as the diaphragm descends in inspiration the anterior abdominal wall will move outwards. If it moves inwards (abdominal paradox) then the diaphragm is probably paralysed. Similarly, in tetraplegia, when the chest wall muscles are paralysed, descent of the diaphragm produces indrawing of the chest wall (chest wall paradox).

Is the patient distressed by breathing? Can the patient carry on a normal conversation or does he or she have to break up sentences, even perhaps to single words at a time? Patients with severe respiratory distress use their accessory muscles of respiration. They fix the position of the shoulder girdle by pressing the hands on the nearest fixed object and throw back their heads. This gives a purchase for accessory muscles of respiration, mainly the sternomastoids.

Does the patient breathe more comfortably in certain positions? Can the patient lie flat or does he or she have to be propped up? Patients with pulmonary oedema and severe airflow limitation will be unable to lie down for long but then most patients with breathing difficulty are more comfortable sitting up. Is breathing audible? Wheeze is a prolonged expiratory noise often audible to the patient as well as the doctor and implies airflow limitation. Stridor is a harsh, chiefly inspiratory noise and implies obstruction in the central airways. This may be at laryngeal level when the voice is usually hoarse but otherwise implies tracheal or major bronchial obstruction. In children, croup and foreign bodies are the usual causes; in adults, carcinoma or extrinsic compression.

'Pink puffers' and 'blue bloaters'

The terms 'pink puffers' and 'blue bloaters' are applied to the overall appearances of some patients with chronic airflow limitation. They describe polar groups and most patients are in between. 'Blue boaters' (Fig. 5.40) are cyanosed from hypoxia and bloated from right-sided heart failure. Further investigation shows features of chronic obstructive bronchitis. Cough and sputum are common but breathlessness less so. Carbon dioxide retention is a feature. 'Pink puffers' (Fig. 5.41) are not cyanosed and are thin. Investigation shows features associated with emphysema. Cough and sputum are less common, but the patients are breathless. Carbon dioxide levels in the blood are normal or low.

PALPATION

Trachea and mediastinum

Start palpation by feeling for the position of the trachea. Do this from the front by placing two fingers either side of the trachea and judging whether the distances between it and the sterno-mastoid tendons are equal on the two sides (Fig. 5.42). An alternative is to

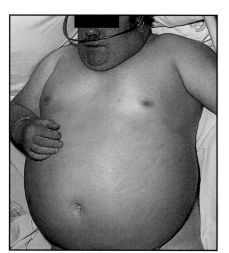

Fig. 5.40 A 'blue bloater' showing ascites from marked cor pulmonale.

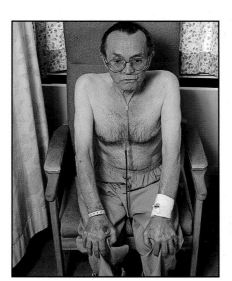

Fig. 5.41 'pink puffer'. Note the pursed-lip breathing.

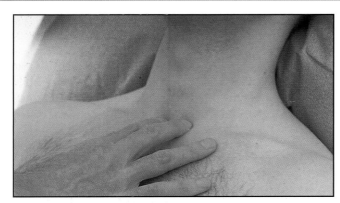

Fig. 5.42   Palpation of the trachea.

 Differential diagnosis
Mediastinal displacement

Away from the lesion
- Pneumothorax
- Effusion (large)

Towards the lesion
- Lung collapse from central airway obstruction
- Localised fibrosis

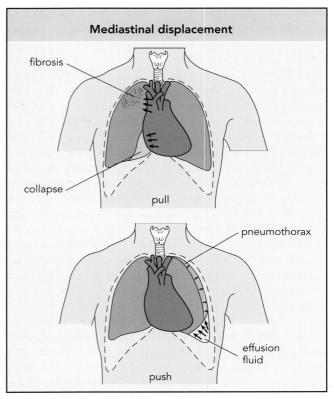

Fig. 5.43   Mediastinal displacement.

examine the patient from behind and hook your fingers round the tendons to meet the trachea. The trachea may be displaced by masses in the neck such as thyroid enlargement. Nonetheless, the trachea gives an indication about the position of the mediastinum, although often you will only be confident about tracheal displacement after you have seen the radiograph.

The position of the apex beat also gives information about the position of the mediastinum so long as the heart is not enlarged. The trachea moves with the upper part of the mediastinum, the apex beat with the lower. The mediastinum may be pushed or pulled to either side. Large effusions push the position of the apex beat but very large effusions are needed to displace the trachea. Pneumothorax pushes the mediastinum even though the lung collapses. This is because the pressure in the pleural space approaches or even exceeds atmospheric pressure, that is, increases. Lung collapse and fibrosis pull the mediastinum (Fig. 5.43). Tumour, especially the pleural tumour mesothelioma, may 'fix' the mediastinum so that it cannot move despite these changes.

Chest wall

If the patient complains of chest pain, then you should gently palpate the chest for local tenderness. If present, this usually indicates disease of bones, muscles or cartilage. As indicated earlier, one variety is called Tietze's syndrome, in which there is pain and swelling of one

or more of the upper costal cartilages, but much more commonly than this syndrome there is merely pain and tenderness of the cartilage but no swelling. Chest wall tenderness may also be present in pleurisy; point tenderness over a rib or cartilage is almost always due to benign local disease and the worried patient can be reassured.

A SYSTEMATIC APPROACH

From this point on, as with most parts of the physical examination, comparison is made between the two sides of the body as abnormality is likely to be confined to one side. Start from the front at the apex of the lung and work downwards, comparing each side immediately with the other. Remember that the heart will influence the result on the left. Do not forget the lateral sides and the axillae. Then sit the patient forwards and examine the back. Sometimes you will need an assistant to help a sick patient to lean forwards. When examining from the back, place the arms of the patient forwards in the lap. This will move the scapulae laterally and uncover more of the chest wall.

Vocal fremitus

This is performed by placing either the edge or the flat of your hand on the chest and asking the patient to say 'ninety-nine' or count 'one, two, three'. The vibrations produced by this manoeuvre are transmitted through the lung substance and are felt by the hand. The test is crude and the mechanism and the alterations in disease are the same as for vocal resonance.

Chest expansion

The purpose of this test is to determine if both sides of the chest move equally. Students often have difficulty with this examination. A good method is to put the fingers of both your hands as far round the chest as possible and then to bring the thumbs together in the midline but to keep the thumbs off the chest wall. The patient is then asked to take a deep breath in; the chest wall, by moving outwards, moves the fingers outwards and the thumbs are in turn distracted away from the midline (Fig. 5.44). The thumbs must be free: if they are also fixed to the chest wall they will not move. It is important to keep your fingers and thumbs in the same relationship to each other, for it is easy to move the thumb the way you think it ought to go. Examination can be performed on both the front and the back.

Expansion can be reduced on both sides equally. This is difficult to detect as there is no standard of comparison but is produced by severe airflow limitation, extensive generalised lung fibrosis and chest wall problems (e.g. ankylosing spondylitis).

Unilateral reduction implies that air cannot enter that side and is seen in pleural effusion, lung collapse, pneumothorax and pneumonia.

PERCUSSION

The purpose of percussion is to detect the resonance or hollowness of the chest. Use both hands, placing the fingers of one hand on the chest with the fingers separated and strike one of them with the terminal phalynx of the middle finger of the other hand (Fig. 5.45); it must be removed again immediately, like the clapper inside a bell, otherwise the resultant sound will be damped. The striking movement should be a flick of the wrist and the striking finger should be at right angles to the other finger. As well as hearing the percussion note, vibrations will be felt by your hand on the chest wall. Again, each side is compared with the equivalent area on the other from top to bottom. Do not forget the sides.

The finger on the chest should be parallel to the expected line of dullness (e.g. in an effusion, parallel to the floor). This will then produce a clearly defined change in note from normal to dull; a finger straddling the demarcation will not do this. It should be placed in the intercostal spaces. Do not percuss more heavily than is necessary: it gives no more information and can be distressing to patients. The apex of the lung can be

Differential diagnosis
Dullness to percussion

Moderate
- Consolidation
- Fibrosis
- Collapse

'Stony'
- Pleural fluid

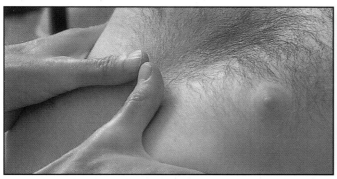
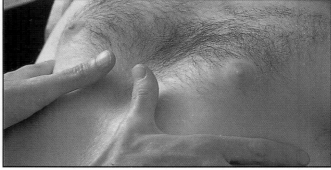

Fig. 5.44 Assessing chest expansion in expiration (left) and inspiration (right).

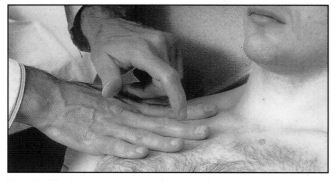

Fig. 5.45 Percussion over the anterior chest.

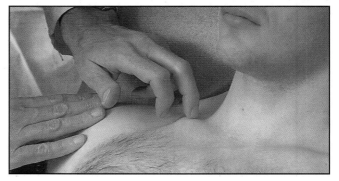

Fig. 5.46 Direct percussion of the clavicles for disease in the lung apices.

examined by tapping directly on the middle of the clavicle (Fig. 5.46). Remember that the lung extends much further down posteriorly than anteriorly (Fig. 5.4).

The degree of resonance depends on the thickness of the chest wall and on the amount of air in the structures underlying it. The possibilities are increased resonance, dullness and 'stony dullness'. Obese patients and individuals with thick chest walls show less resonance, yet it is equal on the two sides. In contrast, patients with overinflated lungs, particularly those with emphysema, have increased resonance; however, it is generalised and without a reference point is difficult to grade. It might be thought that air in the pleural space (pneumothorax) would increase resonance but the difference is often insufficient to identify from percussion alone which is the affected side.

Resonance is decreased moderately in consolidation and fibrosis of the lung and markedly if there is fluid of any kind between the lung and the chest wall, that is, stony dullness. A collapsed lobe can compress to a very small volume and compensatory overinflation of the other lobe fills the space. The percussion note may then be normal. A whole lung cannot collapse completely (unless there is also a pneumothorax) so the chest will be dull. Percussion can also be used to determine movement of the diaphragm because the level of dullness will descend as the patient breathes in (tidal

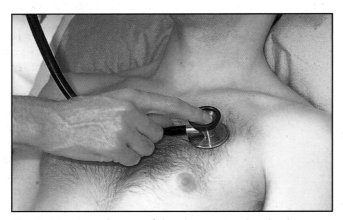

Fig. 5.47 Auscultation of the chest using the diaphragm.

percussion). Dullness is to be expected over the liver, which anteriorly reaches as high as the sixth costal cartilage, and over the heart. Resonance in these areas, again a subjective finding, implies increased air in the lungs and is common in overinflation and emphysema. Bilateral basal dullness is more usually due to failure or inability to take a deep breath, to obesity or to abdominal distension than to bilateral pleural effusions. The right diaphragm is normally higher than the left so expect a slightly higher level of dullness.

AUSCULTATION

Many doctors prefer to use the diaphragm of the stethoscope for auscultation of the chest (Fig. 5.47). In thin bony chests, the bell may give a more airtight fit and is less likely to trap hairs underneath, which produce a crackling sound.

Ask the patient to take deep breaths through the mouth, then listen in sequence over the chest as before. Start at the apices and compare each side with the other. Some patients fail to understand the instruction to breathe through the mouth but the sounds are much clearer if they do. To help them you may have to press gently on the jaw to open it. Some take enormous slow deep breaths that, although otherwise satisfactory, do prolong the examination. A quick demonstration of what you want will resolve any problems.

The breath sounds are produced in the large airways, transmitted through the airways and then attenuated by the distal lung structure through which they pass. The sounds you hear at the lung surface are therefore different from the sounds heard over the trachea and are modified further if there is anything obstructing the airways, lung tissue, pleura or chest wall. When reporting on auscultatory changes, you must distinguish between the breath sounds and the added sounds. Breath sounds are termed either vesicular or bronchial and the added sounds are divided into crackles, wheezes and rubs.

Vesicular breath sounds

This is the sound heard over normal lungs; it has a rustling quality and is heard on inspiration and the

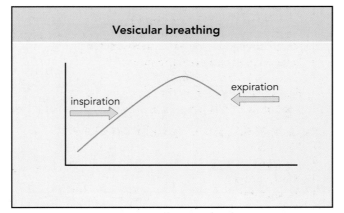

Fig. 5.48 Timing of vesicular breathing.

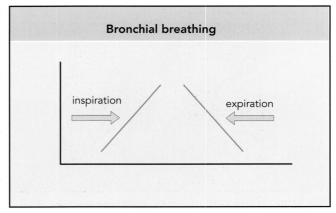

Fig. 5.49 Timing of bronchial breathing.

first part of expiration (Fig. 5.48). Reduction in vesicular breath sounds can be expected with airways obstruction as in asthma, emphysema or tumour. The so-called 'silent chest' is a sign of severe asthma: so little air enters the lung that no sound is produced. The breath sounds can be strikingly reduced in emphysema, particularly over a bulla. Generalised reduction in breath sounds also occurs with a thick chest wall or obesity.

Anything interspersed between the lung and the chest wall (air, fluid or pleural thickening) will reduce the breath sounds; this is likely to be unilateral and therefore more easily detected.

Avoid the term 'diminished air entry' when you mean diminished breath sounds. The two are not necessarily synonymous.

Bronchial breathing

Bronchial breathing causes much confusion because the essential feature of bronchial breathing, the quality of the sound, is difficult or impossible to put into words. Traditionally, it is described by its timing as occurring in both inspiration and expiration with a gap in between (Fig. 5.49). In this way it is contrasted with vesicular breathing. These features are undoubtedly true but lead to the confusion in the mind of the student that if anything is heard in middle or late expiration it must be bronchial breathing. Many normal people and individuals with airways obstruction have a prolonged expiratory component to the breath sounds (this is sometimes designated 'bronchovesicular' but this term increases the confusion rather than diminishing it). It is best to forget about the timing and concentrate on the essential feature, the quality of the sound. It can be mimicked to some extent by listening over the trachea with the stethoscope, although a better imitation can be obtained by putting the tip of your tongue on the roof of your mouth and breathing in and out through the open mouth.

Bronchial breathing is heard when sound generated in the central airways is transmitted more or less unchanged through the lung substance. This occurs when the lung substance itself is solid, as in consolidation, but the air passages remain open. Sound is conducted normally to the small airways but then, instead of being modified by air in the alveoli, the solid lung conducts the sound better to the lung surface and, hence, to the stethoscope. If the central airways are obstructed by say a carcinoma, then no transmission of sound will take place and no bronchial breathing will occur even though the lung may be solid. An exception is seen in the upper lobes. Here, if the bronchi to either lobe are blocked, sounds from the central airways can still be transmitted directly from the trachea through the solid lung to the chest wall (Fig. 5.50).

The main cause of bronchial breathing is consolidation, particularly from pneumonia, so much so that in the minds of most clinicians the three terms are synonymous. Lung abscess, if near the chest wall, can cause bronchial breathing, probably because of the consolidation around it. Dense fibrosis is an occasional cause. Breath sounds over an effusion will be diminished but bronchial breathing may be heard over its upper level, perhaps because the effusion compresses the lung.

Bronchial breathing is only heard over a collapsed lung if the airway is patent. This is rare as the collapse is usually caused by an obstructing carcinoma. Nevertheless, there is an exception with the upper lobes (see above).

Bronchial breathing has been divided into tubular, cavernous and amphoric but attempts to score points on ward rounds by using these terms are best left to others.

Vocal resonance

This is the auscultatory equivalent of vocal fremitus. Place the stethoscope on the chest and ask the patient to say 'ninety-nine'. Normally the sound produced is 'fuzzy' and seems to come from the chest piece of the stethoscope. The changes in disease should by now be predictable. The sound is increased in consolidation (better transmission through solid lung) and decreased

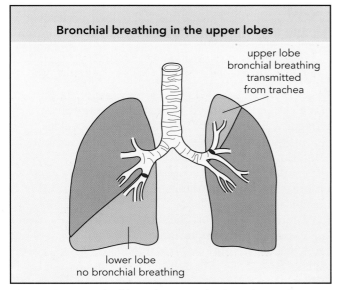

Bronchial breathing in the upper lobes

upper lobe bronchial breathing transmitted from trachea

lower lobe no bronchial breathing

Fig. 5.50 Bronchial breathing may be heard over the upper lobes even if the bronchus is blocked.

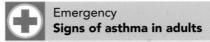

Emergency
Signs of asthma in adults

Signs of acute severe asthma in adults
- Unable to complete sentences
- Pulse >110 beats/min
- Respirations >25 breaths/min
- Peak flow <50% predicted or best

Signs of life-threatening asthma in adults
- Silent chest
- Cyanosis
- Bradycardia
- Exhaustion
- Peak flow <33% predicted or best

if there is air, fluid or pleural thickening between the lung and the chest wall. The changes of vocal fremitus are the same. Both tests are of little value in themselves, yet a refinement of vocal resonance can be very useful. Sometimes the increased transmission of sound is so marked that even when the patient whispers, the sound is still heard clearly over the affected lung (whispering pectoriloquy). When this is well developed there is a striking difference between the normal side, where the sound appears to come from the end of the stethoscope, and the abnormal side, where the syllables are much clearer and seem as if they are being whispered into your ear.

Bronchial breathing and whispering pectoriloquy often occur together. Consequently, if you are in doubt about the presence of bronchial breathing then whispering pectoriloquy may confirm it. Like bronchial breathing, whispering pectoriloquy is characteristic of consolidation but can also occur with lung abscess and above an effusion.

Added sounds

There are three types of added sounds: wheezes, crackles and pleural rubs. Much confusion has been generated in the past by other terms such as rhonchi, which are equivalent to wheezes, and crepitations and rales, which are equivalent to crackles. Further subdivision is often attempted but is of very limited value.

Wheezes

These are prolonged musical sounds largely occurring on expiration, sometimes on inspiration, and are due to localised narrowing within the bronchial tree. They are caused by the vibration of the walls of a bronchus near to its point of closure. Most patients with wheeze have many, each coming from a single, narrowed area. As the lung gets smaller on expiration, so the airways get smaller too; each narrowed airway reaches a critical phase when it produces a wheeze then ceases to do so. Thus, during expiration, numerous narrowings produce numerous wheezes in sequence and together. A single wheeze can occur and may then suggest a single narrowing, often caused by a carcinoma or foreign body (fixed wheeze).

Wheezes are typical of airway narrowing from any cause. Asthma and chronic bronchitis are the most common and the narrowing is caused by a combination of smooth muscle contraction, inflammatory changes in the walls and increased bronchial secretions. Sometimes patients with these conditions have few or no wheezes. If so, ask the patient to take a deep breath and then to blow out hard. This may produce a marked wheeze. Occasionally, wheezing is heard in pulmonary oedema, presumably because of bronchial wall oedema.

The term bronchospasm suggests narrowing caused only by smooth muscle contraction and should be avoided as the bronchial narrowing is usually multifactorial.

Differential diagnosis
Crackles

- Left ventricular failure
- Fibrosing alveolitis
- Extrinsic allergic alveolitis
- Pneumonia
- Bronchiectasis
- Chronic bronchitis
- Asbestosis

Wheeze-like breath sounds can disappear in severe asthma and emphysema because of low rates of airflow. The amount of wheeze is not a good indicator of the degree of airways obstruction. Peak expiratory flow measurement is much better.

Stridor

Stridor may be heard better without a stethoscope by putting your ear close to the patient's mouth and asking the patient to breathe in and out. As indicated earlier, it is a sign of large airway narrowing in the larynx, trachea or main bronchi.

Crackles

In a sense the term crackles is self-explanatory. Problems arise because of various descriptions that are often added, such as coarse, medium, fine, wet or dry. These add little to our understanding; nonetheless, it is possible to distinguish two main types. The first occurs when there is fluid in the larger bronchi and a coarse bubbling sound can be heard that clears or alters as the secretions causing the sound are shifted on coughing or deep breathing.

The sound of other 'fine' crackles can be imitated by rolling the hairs of your temple together between your fingers. They occur in inspiration and are high-pitched, explosive sounds. The mechanism of their production is thought to be as follows. Many conditions lead to premature closure of the small airways at the end of expiration. During the succeeding inspiration, these units can only be reopened by overcoming the surface tension that keeps them closed. When they eventually 'pop open' crackles are produced. During inspiration, larger bronchi will open before smaller ones so crackles from chronic bronchitis and bronchiectasis tend to occur early. Conditions that largely involve the alveoli, such as left ventricular failure, fibrosis and pneumonia, tend to produce crackles later on inspiration. This distinction is of clinical value.

Note whether the crackles are localised. This would be expected in pneumonia and mild cases of bronchiectasis. Pulmonary oedema and fibrosing alveolitis typically affect both lung bases equally.

Normal people, especially smokers, may have a few basal crackles; these often clear with a few deep breaths.

Pleural rub

This is caused by the inflamed surfaces of the pleura rubbing together. The sound has been likened to new leather when it is bent or, more vividly, to the creaking noises made in a sailing ship heeling to the wind, which you may have experienced from films if not in reality. Some idea of the quality of the sound can be obtained by placing one hand over the ear and rubbing the back of that hand with the fingers of the other. Pleural rubs are usually heard on both inspiration and expiration. At first you may think that you are moving the stethoscope on the chest. Sometimes coarse crackles can sound like rubs; a cough will shift the former. If there is any pain, ask the patient to point to the site of the pain, this often localises the rub too. Rubs are heard in all varieties of pleural inflammation, such as in pneumonia and pulmonary embolism. Any effusion will separate the pleura and the rub may well go but sometimes remain above the effusion.

COMMON PATTERNS OF ABNORMALITY

This section summarises what has been said before but from the perspective of the disease process. The diagnosis itself will need the integration of the history and any other information. Those considered are consolidation, pleural fluid, pneumothorax, chronic airflow limitation, lung or lobar collapse and fibrosis. Not all the signs are present in every case and often there is more than one disease process at a time. The radiograph often illustrates the anatomical nature of the process, so examples are shown.

CONSOLIDATION

Consolidation is a confusing term as it means different things to different specialists. To a radiologist it means an alveolar-filling process with no presumption about aetiology. To a pathologist it means a heavy airless lung and to a clinician it means bronchial breathing that is usually equated with pneumonia. To use pneumonia as an example, the affected lung or lobe is the same size or very slightly larger than normal lung.

Differential diagnosis
Some causes of pneumonia

- *Streptococcus pneumoniae*
- *Mycoplasma pneumoniae*
- *Haemophilus influenzae*
- Influenza virus
- *Legionella pneumophila*
- Psittacosis
- Q fever
- Chemical (for example, aspiration of vomit)
- Radiation

Differential diagnosis
Some causes of pleural fluid

Transudates
- Congestive cardiac failure
- Cirrhosis
- Nephrotic syndrome

Exudates
- Tumours – primary, secondary and lymphomas
- Pneumonia
- Tuberculosis
- Rheumatoid arthritis and other connective tissue disorders
- Pulmonary embolism and infarction

Blood
- Trauma
- Pulmonary embolism
- Tumours

Pus
- Pneumonia
- Trauma

Lymph
- Tumours, especially lymphoma

The alveoli are full of exudate, yet the air passages are open. The pleura are inflamed. The differential diagnosis box lists some causes. Note that not all are infections.

Inspection of the chest may show diminished movement on the affected side, palpation shows no shift of the mediastinum but expansion is reduced, vocal fremitus may be increased, percussion note will be moderately impaired, breath sounds will be bronchial over the affected area with whispering pectoriloquy and there may be a pleural rub. Early and late in the disease process there may also be crackles and these may be the only auscultatory change in mild cases. In lobar pneumonia, the changes are localised to a lobe, which means that the signs are detected either anteriorly or posteriorly but not usually both. More widespread changes suggest 'bronchopneumonia', a complication of chronic bronchitis, or 'atypical pneumonia' caused by viruses, mycoplasma and other organisms. Radiology may show an 'air bronchogram': air in the bronchi outlined by fluid in the alveoli (Fig. 5.51).

PLEURAL FLUID

Whether this be from an increase in pleural transudate, pleural exudate from inflammation, blood, pus or lymph, the signs are the same. A large amount of fluid is needed to displace the heart and an even larger amount, filling most of the hemithorax, to displace the trachea. The displacement is away from the fluid. Expansion is diminished on the affected side, vocal fremitus is reduced, percussion note is markedly

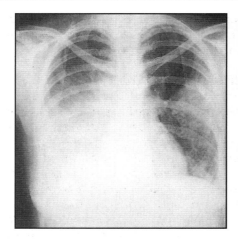

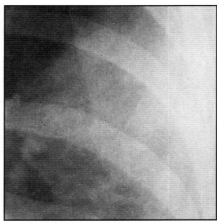

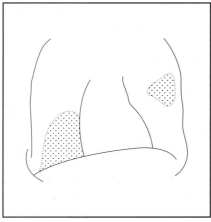

Mediastinum central
Expansion ↓
Percussion note ↓
Breath sounds bronchial
Whispering pectoriloquy
Crackles
Pleural rub

Fig. 5.51 Consolidation (unusual because it affects both lungs). Enlarged view showing air bronchogram.

> **Risk factors**
> **Some causes of pneumothorax**
>
> • No cause found
> • Apical blebs
> • Chronic bronchitis and emphysema
> • Staphylococcal pneumonia
> • Asthma
> • Tuberculosis
> • Cystic fibrosis
> • Trauma

reduced, 'stony dullness', and breath sounds are absent or markedly reduced. Bronchial breathing and a rub may be heard at the upper level of the effusion. An effusion, if large enough, is detected both anteriorly and posteriorly (Figs 5.52, 5.53)

PNEUMOTHORAX

The pressure in the pleural space is normally negative with respect to atmospheric pressure. In a pneumothorax, the affected side is at a higher pressure, that is, less negative. This pressure tends to displace the mediastinum to the opposite side, and if there is a flap valve effect producing a tension pneumothorax this can be extreme and dangerous. The affected side moves less well, vocal fremitus is reduced and the percussion note is normal. The expected increased resonance can be difficult to detect and it is the conjunction of diminished breath sounds with a normal percussion note that distinguishes it from other causes of diminished breath sounds when there is also dullness to percus-

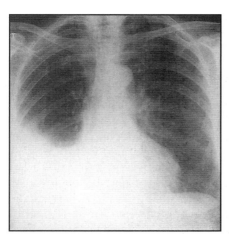

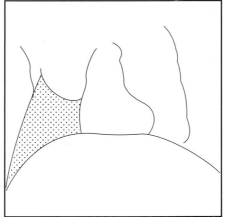

Mediastinum usually central
Expansion ↓
Percussion ↓
Breath sounds ↓
Sometimes bronchial breathing
    or a pleural rub at upper level

Fig. 5.52 Small effusion.

Emergency
Bedside assessment of acute respiratory failure

- Bedside diagnosis of acute respiratory failure difficult but
- Look first for respiratory rate, cyanosis, respiratory distress, use of accessory respiratory muscles, ankle swelling
- Consider upper airways obstruction (e.g. anaphylactic shock, laryngeal tumour, foreign body, obstructive sleep apnoea)
  - look for swelling of lips and tongue, stridor, hoarse voice, snoring
- Consider central airways obstruction (e.g. tumour)
  - look for stridor, unilateral reduced breath sounds
- Consider generalised airway narrowing (e.g. asthma, COPD)
  - look for flapping tremor, wheeze, prolonged expiration, silent chest
- Consider parenchymal lung disease (e.g. pneumonia, pulmonary oedema, alveolitis)
  - look for crackles, bronchial breathing
- Consider pleural problems (e.g. effusion, pneumothorax)
  - look for displaced trachea, dullness with silence, resonance with silence
- Consider chest wall problems (e.g. ankylosing spondylosis, neurological disease)
  - look for scoliosis, upper limb weakness, poor chest wall movement, poor diaphragm movement, muscle fasciculations.

Further analysis depends crucially on vital capacity, chest radiograph, arterial blood gases, oxygen saturation

sion. Vocal resonance is reduced and there are no added sounds (Fig. 5.54). Some causes of pneumothorax are given in the risk factors box.

CHRONIC AIRFLOW LIMITATION

This term covers the entities of chronic obstructive bronchitis, emphysema and asthma, which are not always readily distinguishable from each other. There may be hyperinflation of the chest, pursed lip breathing and use of accessory muscles of respiration. Expansion may well be reduced but usually equally so. The mediastinum is not displaced. Vocal fremitus is normal, percussion is usually normal but there may be increased resonance and reduced hepatic and cardiac dullness. Breath sounds are vesicular and sometimes reduced, presumably from low flow rates; the added sounds are wheezes and often crackles. The radiograph is usually normal but sometimes shows overinflation with low flat diaphragms (Fig. 5.55).

LUNG AND LOBAR COLLAPSE

The usual cause is a central bronchial carcinoma, although a foreign body has the same effect. If the lung or lobe is not ventilated, the air within it is absorbed by the blood and the lung collapses. If the whole lung is involved, then the degree of collapse is limited by the capacity of the chest to shrink, but if a lobe is involved, then the other lobe can fill the space and the affected lung may come to occupy only a very small area. Lung collapse can also follow infection: tuberculosis and bronchiectasis are good examples. Here the airways remain open.

The findings on examination depend on whether the whole lung or only one lobe is involved. There is diminished movement on the affected side, with the mediastinum deviating to that side. The percussion note is markedly reduced if the whole lung is involved but can be difficult or impossible to detect if only a lobe is involved and has shrunk to a small space. Breath sounds are diminished but remain vesicular in lobar collapse and may be absent if the whole lung is

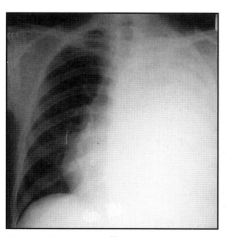

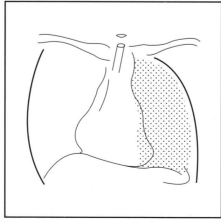

Mediastinum displaced
Expansion ↓
Percussion ↓
Breath sounds ↓

Fig. 5.53 Large effusion with mediastinal displacement.

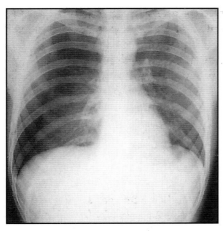
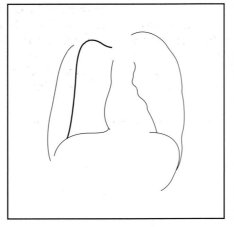

Fig. 5.54   Pneumothorax on right.

Mediastinum sometimes
   displaced
Expansion ↓
Percussion normal or ↑
Breath sounds ↓
No added sounds

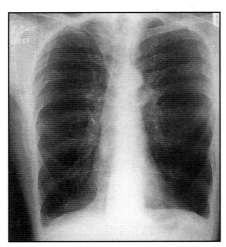
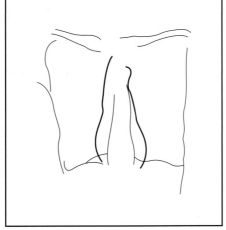

Fig. 5.55   Chronic airflow limitation.

Hyperinflation
Mediastinum central
Hepatic and cardiac dullness ↓
Vesicular breath sounds
Wheezes and crackles
Radiograph often normal but
   here shows overinflation
   and low flat diaphragms

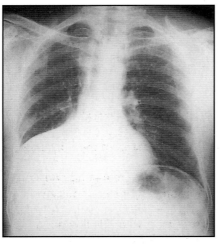
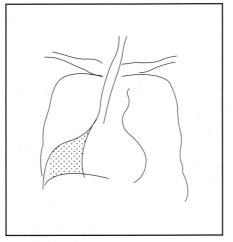

Fig. 5.56   Right middle and lower lobe collapse.

Mediastinum displaced
Expansion reduced
Percussion normal or ↓
Breath sounds vesicular
   but ↓ or sometimes
   bronchial

involved. Vocal resonance is decreased. As already indicated, bronchial breathing, increased vocal resonance and whispering pectoriloquy can be heard in upper lobe collapse because of direct transmission of sound from the trachea. Bronchial breathing is also heard in collapse of other lobes if (unusually) the airways remain patent (Fig. 5.56). Crackles and wheeze may be present if the cause is damage from an old infection.

LUNG FIBROSIS

This may be the end result of many lung conditions and minor degrees are undetectable clinically. Localised changes produce similar signs to lung collapse. Generalised disease is best illustrated by cryptogenic fibrosing alveolitis. The lungs are stiff, expansion may be reduced, but equally, and the mediastinum is central. Vocal fremitus is normal, percussion note is normal or slightly reduced, breath sounds are vesicular, although occasionally bronchial, yet there are marked crackles, initially confined to the bases but later extending up the chest (Fig. 5.57).

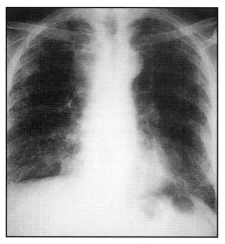
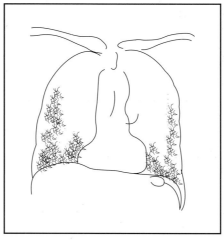

Mediastinum central
Expansion equally ↓
Percussion normal or ↓
Breath sounds vesicular
   (occasionally bronchial)
Crackles

Fig. 5.57 Cryptogenic fibrosing alveolitis.

Examination of elderly people
Respiratory examination

- Be aware of multiple problems
- Occupational history still valid
  - mesothelioma occurs long after exposure
  - pneumoconiosis changes persist for life
- Not all breathless elderly patients have chronic obstructive pulmonary disease
- Respiratory and cardiac disease often coexist
- Right ventricular failure as a consequence of lung disease is difficult to distinguish from congestive cardiac failure
- Disability may be multifactorial

Review
Framework for the routine examination of the respiratory system

1. While taking the history, watch for respiratory distress, particularly while talking. Note any clues from the patient's surroundings
2. Look at the hands for clubbing, cyanosis and evidence of carbon dioxide retention
3. Look at the mucous membranes for central cyanosis
4. Check the jugular venous pulse for evidence of cor pulmonale
5. Palpate for supraclavicular lymph nodes
6. Inspect the chest wall for deformities and inequalities
7. Note the pattern of breathing
8. Palpate the trachea for any displacement
9. Palpate the front of the chest for vocal fremitus and for right ventricular hypertrophy
10. Assess expansion of the chest from the front and note any inequalities
11. Percuss the front of the chest comparing one side with the other and noting any areas of dullness; include the axillae
12. Auscultate the chest similarly and decide on the presence and nature of the breath sounds
13. Test for vocal resonance and, where appropriate, whispering pectoriloquy
14. Note any added sounds
15. Repeat last six steps on the back of the chest
16. If appropriate, measure the peak flow rate

6.
The Heart and Cardiovascular System

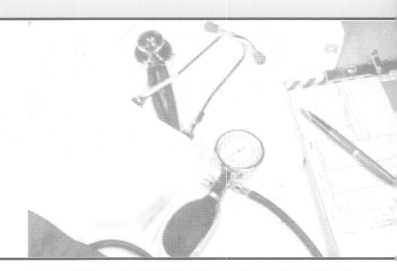

The cardiovascular system is fundamental to the functioning of almost every other organ system. Despite the availability of many sophisticated imaging techniques which will be discussed later, the fundamental simplicity and accessibility of the structure and function of the heart and vascular system make its physical examination both important and extremely rewarding.

STRUCTURE AND FUNCTION

The adult heart (Fig. 6.1) consists of two pumps working in series. The 'right heart', comprising the right atrium, tricuspid valve, right ventricle, pulmonary valve and pulmonary artery, is a low pressure pump receiving blood from the systemic veins and pumping it to the

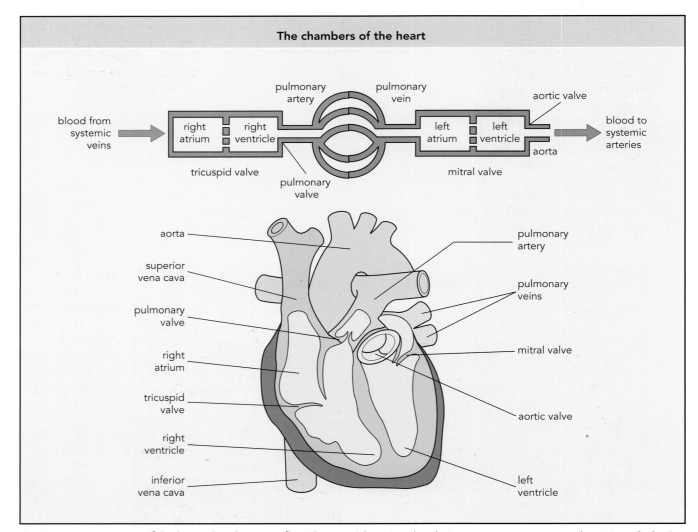

Fig. 6.1 Arrangement of the heart chambers as a flow diagram (above) and in their approximate anatomical positions (below).

lungs. The left heart, comprising the left atrium, mitral valve, left ventricle, aortic valve and aorta, is a high pressure pump receiving blood from the lungs and pumping it round the body. In the early embryo, the heart forms as a simple tube down the midline of the body. As the embryo grows, the tube elongates more rapidly than the tissues around it and thus develops a loop and a twist. It also becomes divided into left and right chambers by the growth of a partition or septum down the middle. In the ninth week of gestation, the fetal heart rotates in a clockwise direction until the right ventricle comes to rest anteriorly behind the sternum. Most of the left ventricle comes to lie posteriorly, apart from a small portion of left ventricular muscle which forms the left heart border when seen from the front and the extreme tip or apex of the heart (Fig. 6.2). The way the heart is situated within the chest cavity is also well demonstrated on the computerised tomographic scan of the chest shown in Figure 6.3. Note that the heart lies obliquely in the chest and that its long axis, the planes of the interatrial and interventricular septum, and the planes of the various valves, are not aligned with any of the conventional anatomical planes. The chambers of the heart can be examined after death by injecting wax or plastic and dissolving away the muscle (Fig. 6.4). They can also be examined during life by injecting radio-opaque contrast medium through catheters placed in the various chambers of the heart and taking cine radiographs. By tilting the X-ray tube and image detector appropriately, it is possible to obtain detailed pictures of the full extent of the ventricular cavities (Fig. 6.5).

HEART MUSCLE

Ventricles

Heart muscle or myocardium is a special type of muscle that is extremely resistant to fatigue. As a result of the higher pressures that it normally generates, the wall of the left ventricle is much thicker than the wall of the right ventricle. In a section taken through both ventricles, left ventricular myocardium, including the intraventricular septum, has a roughly circular outline

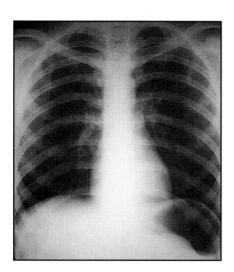

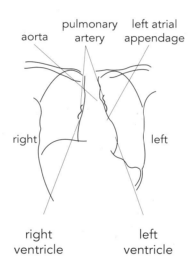

Fig. 6.2 Most of the anterior surface of the heart is formed by the right ventricle and pulmonary artery. The tip of the left ventricle and the left atrial appendage also appear on the left border of the heart.

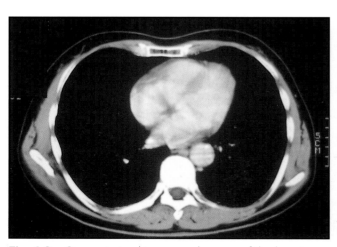

Fig. 6.3 Computerised tomography scan of the heart showing the position of the heart within the chest cavity. Viewed from below.

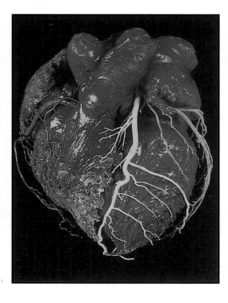

Fig. 6.4 A 'corrosion cast' of the chambers of the heart, made by filling the chambers with wax or plastic and dissolving away the muscle.

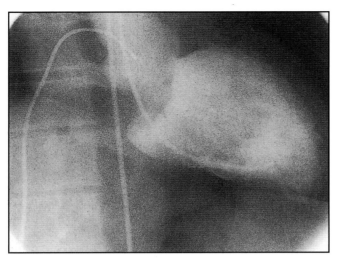

Fig. 6.5 Left ventricular cine-angiogram made by injecting radio-opaque contrast medium into the heart through a catheter passed via the femoral artery and aorta. The X-ray tube and image intensifier are tilted into the 'right anterior oblique' position to outline the full extent of the left ventricle.

with the right ventricle appearing to be wrapped around one side of it (Fig. 6.6). The muscle fibres of the heart are arranged in a complicated spiral arrangement so that when they contract (systole) not only is blood forced out of the ventricles but the heart also elongates and rotates on the fixed base provided by the attachment of the major blood vessels. It is this movement that is felt as the beating of the heart by a hand placed on the chest. The heart normally lies in its own serous cavity, the pericardium, which allows it to move without friction. Apart from moving with each heart beat, the position of the pericardium and the heart can be altered by the phase of respiration or by rolling from one side to the other.

Atria

The atria of the heart are also muscular but are much thinner walled than the ventricles (Fig. 6.7). They contract a fraction of a second before the ventricles and, in doing so, they assist in the filling of the ventricles, particularly when there is a need for increased cardiac output. Patients in whom, as a result of disease, the atria are paralysed or are beating out of synchrony with the ventricles are usually comfortable at rest but may become short of breath on exercise.

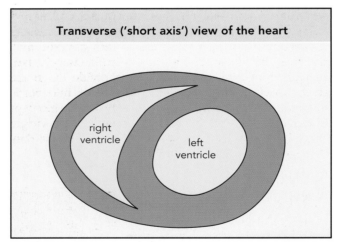

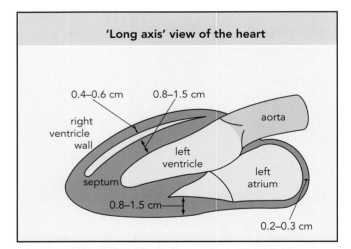

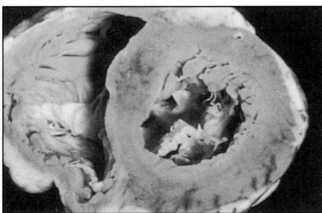

Fig. 6.6 'Short axis' view of the heart. In the short axis or transverse section, the thinner (low pressure) right ventricle is 'wrapped around' the left ventricle.

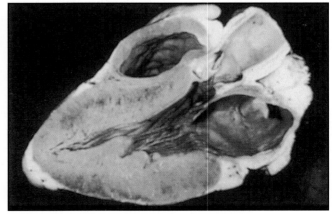

Fig. 6.7 Relative thickness of muscle in different parts of the heart.

CARDIAC HYPERTROPHY AND DILATATION

Like any muscle, cardiac muscle responds to an increased workload by growth. The heart responds in different ways to pressure load and volume load. Pressure load is caused by an increased resistance to ejection of blood from the heart. The response to pressure load is cardiac hypertrophy, initially without dilatation of the chamber involved. For example, in aortic stenosis, the left ventricular wall becomes excessively thickened but the left ventricular cavity remains of normal size. Eventually, when the pressure load is extreme or growth of the heart muscle has outstripped its blood supply, failure of the muscle occurs and the cavity begins to enlarge.

The heart responds to a volume load, for example, a leaking mitral or aortic valve, an arteriovenous fistula or left-to-right shunt, by both hypertrophy of the myocardium and dilatation of the chamber involved. This is to accompany the increased stroke volume that is required to deal with the volume load. The chest radiograph shows cardiac enlargement (Fig. 6.8) and this is also found on echocardiography. Both hypertrophy and dilatation produce characteristic electrocardiographic changes and it is possible to identify the cardiac chamber involved from the electrocardiographic appearances.

HEART VALVES

There are four heart valves. They fall anatomically and functionally into two groups: the inflow or atrioventricular valves and the outflow or 'semilunar' valves. The tricuspid and mitral valves separate right atrium and right ventricle and left atrium and left ventricle, respectively. Both develop from the endocardial cushions of the embryonic heart and are composed of thin flexible leaflets that are prevented from prolapsing back into the atrium when the ventricle contracts by being attached by

 Differential diagnosis
Increased pressure load (afterload) on the heart

Right ventricular pressure load
- Pulmonary valve stenosis
- Increased pulmonary vascular resistance
  - chronic hypoxia
  - chronic lung disease
  - secondary to left heart failure
  - Eisenmenger's syndrome
  - primary pulmonary hypertension

Left ventricular pressure load
- Aortic valve stenosis
- Subaortic stenosis
- Supravalvar aortic stenosis
  - discrete membrane
  - hypertrophic obstructive cardiomyopathy
- Coarctation of the aorta
- Systemic hypertension

chordae tendineae to specialised portions of ventricular muscle, the papillary muscles (Fig. 6.9). The hydrodynamic efficiency of the mitral and tricuspid valves is very high. Their pliable edges smooth out eddies and turbulence in blood flow and allow the rapid transfer of blood from atrium to ventricle with a very small pressure differential. The aortic and pulmonary valves develop from two spiral ridges that divide the single great vessel leaving the embryonic heart into aortic and pulmonary trunks. Each normally has three cusps whose arrangement reflects their embryonic origin (Fig. 6.10). As each cusp is shaped like a half moon, they are sometimes called the semilunar valves.

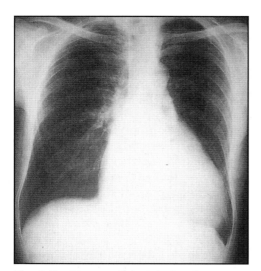

Fig. 6.8 Chest radiograph showing cardiac enlargement in response to a volume load chronic mitral regurgitation. (Compare with Fig. 6.2.)

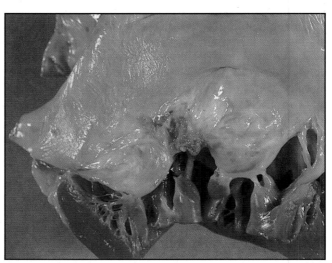

Fig. 6.9 Postmortem specimen showing attachment of valve cusps to papillary muscles by chordae tendineae.

caused by the cyclical depolarisation and repolarisation of the heart cells. Electrical potentials are picked up by electrodes that are attached to the skin. The points at which the electrodes are attached and the conventional ways in which they are connected enable the ECG to 'look at' the heart from a series of different directions (Fig. 6.14). The cycle of electrical changes during a single heart beat is termed an ECG complex. Different parts of the ECG complex reflect the activation of different parts of the heart. The P wave indicates atrial activity and the QRS complex indicates ventricular activity (Fig. 6.15).

In patients suspected of intermittent arrhythmias, the ECG may be displayed as a continuous monitor trace (Fig. 6.16). In patients outside hospital, the ECG can be recorded continuously on magnetic tape for periods of 24–48 h and then played back to analyse any rhythm disturbances. This process is sometimes called 'Holter mon-

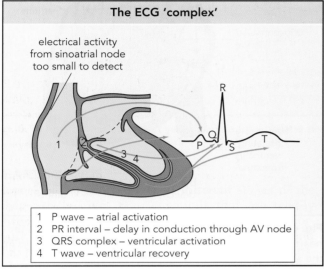

The ECG 'complex'

electrical activity from sinoatrial node too small to detect

1   P wave – atrial activation
2   PR interval – delay in conduction through AV node
3   QRS complex – ventricular activation
4   T wave – ventricular recovery

Fig. 6.15   Different parts of an ECG 'complex'.

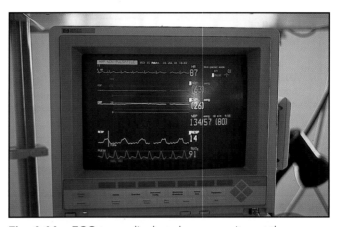

Fig. 6.16   ECG trace displayed on a monitor at the nursing station or bedside.

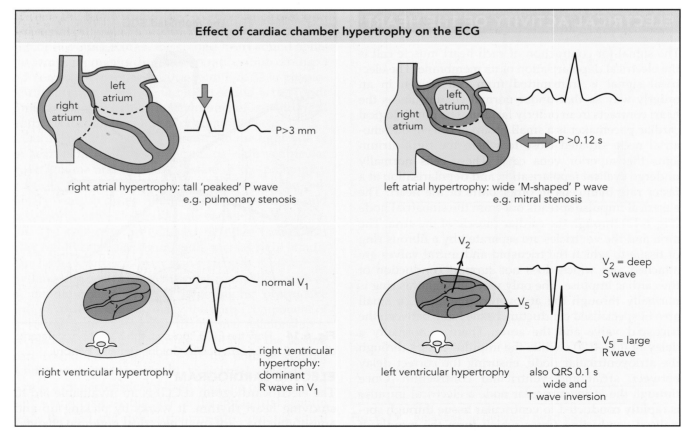

Effect of cardiac chamber hypertrophy on the ECG

right atrial hypertrophy: tall 'peaked' P wave
e.g. pulmonary stenosis

P>3 mm

left atrial hypertrophy: wide 'M-shaped' P wave
e.g. mitral stenosis

P >0.12 s

right ventricular hypertrophy

normal V$_1$

right ventricular hypertrophy: dominant R wave in V$_1$

left ventricular hypertrophy

V$_2$ = deep S wave

V$_5$ = large R wave

also QRS 0.1 s wide and T wave inversion

Fig. 6.17   Electrocardiographic changes can be used to identify hypertrophy of the cardiac chambers.

itoring'. The ECG can be used to detect hypertrophy of the different chambers of the heart (Fig. 6.17), abnormal rhythms or cardiac damage.

CARDIAC ARRHYTHMIAS

Abnormalities of heart rhythm can be divided into those in which the heart goes too slowly (bradycardia) and those in which the rate is abnormally rapid (tachycardia). Physiologically, heart rate can vary in a normal young adult from 40 beats/min during sleep to 180 beats/minute or more during vigorous exercise. The physiological control of heart rate is due to a balance between sympathetic nervous activity, which speeds the heart rate, and vagal activity, which slows it down.

BRADYCARDIA

Bradycardia may be caused by drugs, particularly β-adrenoceptor blocking drugs ('beta blockers'); it may also be a physiological finding in young athletes with a high vagal tone. Extreme bradycardia may be caused by heart block where there is failure of conduction of the electrical impulse, usually as it passes through the atrioventricular node or bundle of His (Fig. 6.18).

TACHYCARDIA

Ectopic beats

As all heart muscle and not just the sinoatrial node retains the capacity for spontaneous depolarisation, it is not uncommon to find an 'ectopic focus' of electrical activity which can initiate extra beats out of time with the normal cardiac cycle. These extra beats or extrasys-

> **Dx** Differential diagnosis
> **Autonomic effects on the heart**
>
> **Vagal tone (slows the heart)**
> Increased in children, athletes
> - Stimulated by: carotid baroreceptors, pain, trauma (via hypothalamus) ventricular stretch receptors (fainting reflex)
> - Excessive in: malignant vasovagal syncope carotid sinus syncope
> - Blocked by: atropine
>
> **Sympathetic tone (speeds up the heart)**
> - Increased by: fear, pain, hypovolaemia, heart failure, physical activity
> - Decreased: during sleep
> - Blocked by: β-adrenoceptor blocker

toles may be generated in the atrium or in the ventricle. In otherwise healthy people, extrasystoles are usually benign and harmless. Nevertheless, they may act as markers for metabolic damage and, consequently, excessive irritability of the heart muscle (e.g. after myocardial infarction or during a viral infection of the heart) (Fig. 6.19).

Sustained tachycardia

A persistent tachycardia may be caused by several ectopic beats occurring in sequence (e.g. as the manifestation of a particularly irritable ectopic focus). This is called a 'focal tachycardia'.

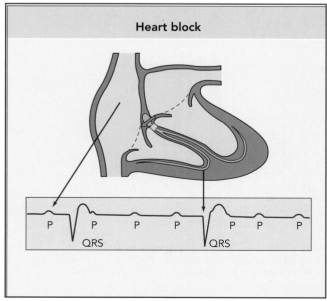

Fig. 6.18 Heart block is one cause of bradycardia; there is failure of conduction of the electrical impulses from atrium to ventricle.

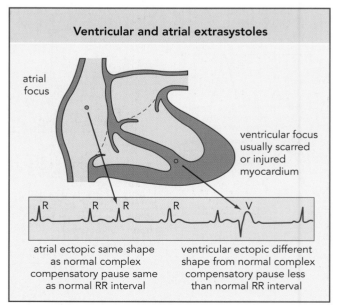

Fig. 6.19 Extrasystoles are caused by an ectopic focus of electrical activity.

A more common mechanism for sustained tachycardia, however, is the phenomenon of re-entry (Fig. 6.20). The basic principle of a re-entry tachycardia is that there are two alternative pathways for the conduction of the electrical impulse; these pathways differ both in their speed of conduction and in their refractory period. Under normal conditions, the cardiac impulse will be conducted by both pathways but an exceptionally early beat may find one pathway still refractory to conduction and therefore the impulse will be conducted down the other one alone. However, by the time it reaches the end of this pathway, the other pathway will have recovered and be able to conduct the impulse in the reverse direction. This sets up the possibility of a 'circus movement' or oscillation and the re-entry circuit can act as a focus for generating a tachycardia. This tachycardia may continue until one of the pathways fatigues and cannot conduct fast enough to maintain

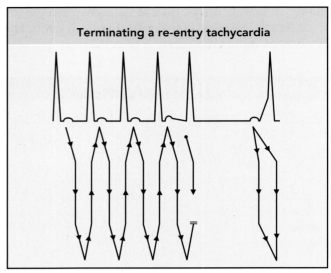

Terminating a re-entry tachycardia

Fig. 6.21 A critically timed extra stimulus can terminate a re-entry tachycardia by making both pathways refractory.

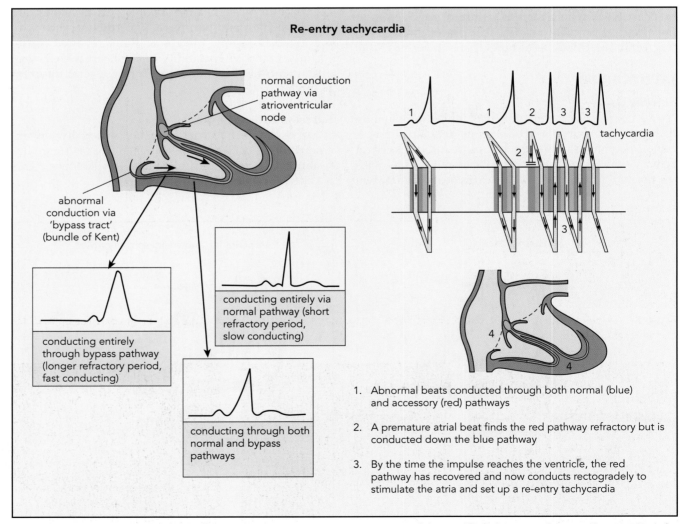

Re-entry tachycardia

normal conduction pathway via atrioventricular node

abnormal conduction via 'bypass tract' (bundle of Kent)

conducting entirely through bypass pathway (longer refractory period, fast conducting)

conducting entirely via normal pathway (short refractory period, slow conducting)

conducting through both normal and bypass pathways

tachycardia

1. Abnormal beats conducted through both normal (blue) and accessory (red) pathways

2. A premature atrial beat finds the red pathway refractory but is conducted down the blue pathway

3. By the time the impulse reaches the ventricle, the red pathway has recovered and now conducts rectogradely to stimulate the atria and set up a re-entry tachycardia

Fig. 6.20 Mechanism of a re-entry tachycardia, based on the 'paradigm' of the Wolff–Parkinson–White syndrome. The left hand diagram shows the ECG pattern produced when conduction is all along the bypass pathway, when it is all along the normal pathway and when it is along both simultaneously.

the circuit or until the process is interrupted by an electrical stimulus which breaks the circuit and re-establishes normal conduction (Fig. 6.21).

Fibrillation

The most extreme form of arrhythmia occurs when the coordinated conduction of impulses between cells completely breaks down and individual cells contract haphazardly. This process is termed fibrillation. Atrial fibrillation is common but not particularly hazardous because the atrioventricular node acts as a filter, preventing the ventricles from being stimulated at too rapid a rate. Ventricular fibrillation is, however, rapidly lethal because the ventricles are unable to pump any blood into the circulation. The only effective treatment for ventricular fibrillation is to pass a large electric current through the heart (defibrillation). This transiently wipes out all electrical activity and allows the whole system to reset (Fig. 6.22).

BLOOD SUPPLY TO THE HEART

Heart muscle needs a supply of blood to support both its basal metabolic needs and the increased oxygen requirements of exercise. The blood supply must be capable of increasing to meet the heart's demands during exercise because heart muscle, unlike skeletal muscle, can only work aerobically. The arterial blood supply to the heart is provided by the right and left coronary arteries. The right coronary artery supplies mainly the right ventricle and the inferior surface of the left ventricle. The left coronary artery divides soon after its origin into the left anterior descending coronary artery, which supplies the interventricular septum, the anterior surface and the apex of the left ventricle, and the circumflex coronary artery which supplies the lateral part of the left ventricle (Fig. 6.23).

In common with other arteries in the body, coronary arteries are prone to atheroma and this in turn may

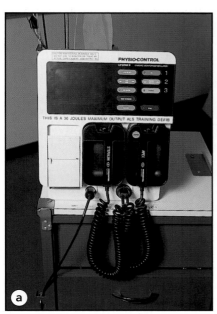

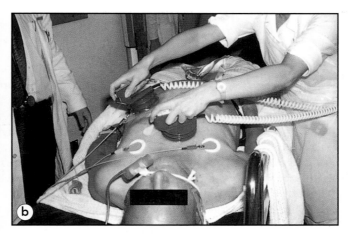

Fig. 6.22 A defibrillator (a). An electrical charge is built up within the machine and discharged through paddles applied to the patient's chest (b).

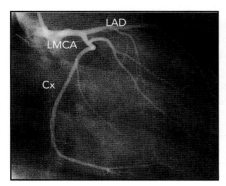

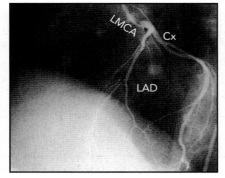

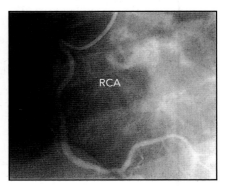

Fig. 6.23 Cine-angiograms to show (left and middle) the left coronary artery and (right) the right coronary artery (RCA). (Cx, left circumflex artery; LAD, left anterior descending artery; LMCA, left main coronary artery).

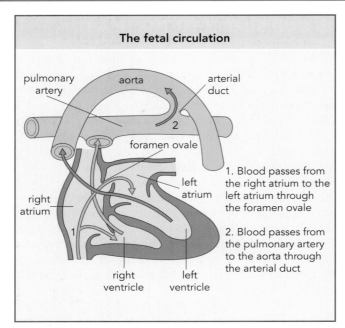

Fig. 6.24   In the fetal circulation, oxygenated blood from the umbilical vein bypasses the liver through the ductus venosus; a portion is shunted from the right to left atrium through the foramen ovale and a further portion passes through the arterial duct.

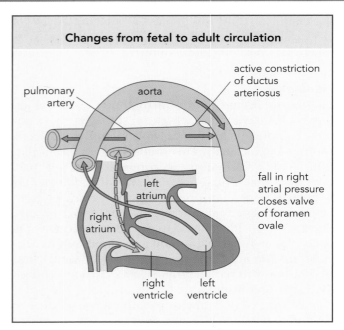

Fig. 6.25   Changes that occur in the fetal circulation at birth. The ductus arteriosus constricts and the fall in right arterial pressure as the lungs expand closes the foramen ovale.

lead to thrombosis, which causes coronary artery obstruction. The clinical features of coronary thrombosis and the myocardial infarction that may result are described later.

INTRACARDIAC SHUNTING

In the fetus, the lungs do not participate in respiratory gas exchange (this is done by the placenta) and the unexpanded lungs offer a high resistance to blood flow. Both sides of the fetal heart work to pump a mixture of deoxygenated blood from the systemic veins and oxygenated blood from the placenta into the aorta and thus to the rest of the body. Blood collecting in the right atrium may pass either through the tricuspid valve into the right ventricle or through the foramen ovale (a hole in the intra-atrial septum) into the left atrium. Blood that enters the right ventricle is pumped into the pulmonary artery, with only a small proportion of it entering the lungs. The remainder passes via the ductus arteriosus into the aorta (Fig. 6.24).

After birth, the vascular resistance of the lungs falls rapidly as they are inflated with air. This causes a fall in right atrial pressure and a rise in left atrial pressure, thus closing the valve-like foramen ovale. At the same time, the ductus arteriosus constricts and closes (Fig. 6.25). This normally separates the work of the right and left sides of the heart and causes them to work in series rather than in parallel. However, abnormalities in the process of transition from fetal to adult circulation, or anatomical defects in the partitions or 'septa' dividing the right and left sides of the heart, may lead to short-circuits or 'shunts'.

Left to right shunt

A congenital or acquired defect in the interatrial septum or the interventricular septum or the failure of closure of the ductus arteriosus without other associated abnormality will produce a left to right shunt. Blood follows the path of least resistance from the high pressure left-sided chamber to the lower pressure right-sided chamber. The result is that, instead of the left and the right sides of the heart having exactly identical outputs, the right side of the heart has to cope not only with its normal output but also with the extra load of blood transferred from the left. A two-to-one shunt means that the output at the right side of the heart is twice that of the left side of the heart. Eventually, the increased workload on the right side of the heart may lead to heart failure or, alternatively, the excessively high blood flow through the lungs may lead to damage to the lung blood vessel and the development of pulmonary hypertension. Examples of left to right shunts are shown in Figure 6.26.

Right to left shunt

If a septal defect or persistent ductus arteriosus is combined with another lesion that raises the pressure on the right side of the heart then, instead of blood flowing from the left-sided chamber to the right-sided chamber, it will flow in the opposite direction, from the right side of the heart to the left. The most common example of congenital heart disease causing a right to left shunt is Fallot's tetralogy (Fig. 6.27) which is physiologically equivalent to a ventricular septal defect plus pulmonary valve stenosis. A right to left shunt can sometimes occur

Examples of left to right shunts: atrial septal defect

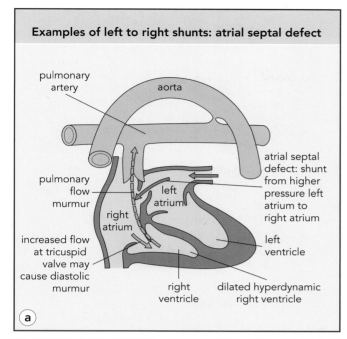

(a)

Left to right shunt: ventricular septal defect

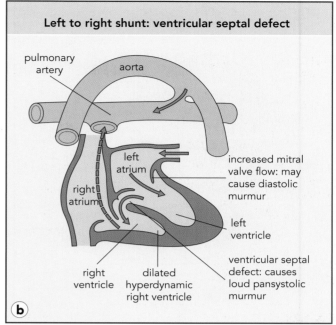

(b)

Left to right shunt: persistent ductus arteriosus

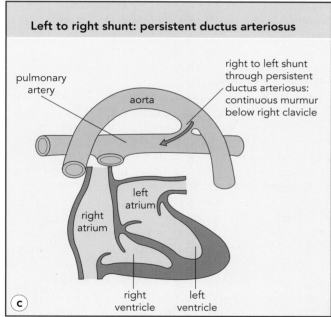

(c)

Fig. 6.26 (a) Left to right shunt atrial septal defect. Blood passes from the left to right atrium. The overall result is an increase in pulmonary blood flow. (b) Left to right shunt: ventricular septal defect. Blood passes from the high pressure left ventricle to the lower pressure right ventricle. (c) Left to right shunt: persistent ductus arteriosus. Blood passes from the high pressure aorta to the lower pressure pulmonary artery.

patient a higher concentration of oxygen to breathe will not make any difference.

Features of long-term adaptation to a reduction in systemic arterial oxygen saturation that are seen in patients with right to left shunts include finger clubbing (Fig. 6.29), polycythaemia (increased production of red blood cells) and acne (particularly in adolescent children).

ARTERIAL SYSTEM

when pulmonary vascular damage in a patient with a severe left to right shunt causes the resistance offered by the pulmonary arteries to rise, thus leading to increased pressure on the right side of the heart and a reversal of the shunt. This is called Eisenmenger's syndrome (Fig. 6.28).

The striking clinical feature about patients with right to left shunts is that they are centrally cyanosed. This cyanosis is due to the admixture of desaturated venous blood with saturated blood coming from the pulmonary vein. It differs from cyanosis that is caused by lung disease or to pulmonary oedema, in that it is not corrected by giving the patient oxygen to breathe because the blood leaving the pulmonary veins is already fully saturated with oxygen, so giving the

The arterial system exists to distribute oxygenated blood from the heart to the tissues and organs of the body. Where arteries pass close to the surface of the body or can be compressed against the bony skeleton they can be felt as 'pulses' (Fig. 6.30). During each cardiac cycle, the left ventricle ejects blood into the aorta and initiates a pulse wave that is transmitted to the periphery. It is important to remember that the pulse wave travels to the periphery much more rapidly than the actual flow of blood. An intra-arterial recording of pressure against time indicates the shape of the pulse wave, which approximates to that which would be felt by a finger on the arterial wall (Fig. 6.31). The shape of the arterial pulse wave depends on many factors (see differential diagnosis box).

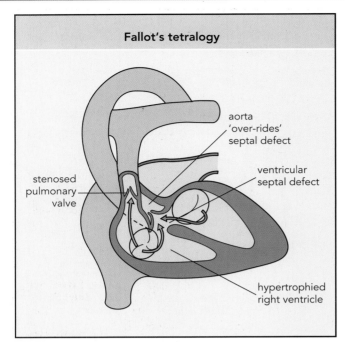

Fallot's tetralogy

aorta 'over-rides' septal defect

ventricular septal defect

stenosed pulmonary valve

hypertrophied right ventricle

Fig. 6.27 Fallot's tetralogy is the most common 'congenital' cause of a right to left shunt. (The 'tetralogy' comprises pulmonary stenosis, ventricular septal defect, over-riding aorta and right ventricular hypertrophy.) (Note that cyanosis sometimes develops several weeks after birth because dynamic hypertrophy of muscle in the right ventricular outflow tract worsens the obstruction.)

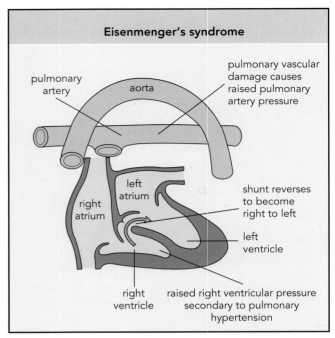

Eisenmenger's syndrome

pulmonary artery

aorta

pulmonary vascular damage causes raised pulmonary artery pressure

left atrium

right atrium

shunt reverses to become right to left

left ventricle

right ventricle

raised right ventricular pressure secondary to pulmonary hypertension

Fig. 6.28 Eisenmenger's syndrome is caused by a secondary rise in pulmonary vascular resistance as a consequence of pulmonary damage from increased blood flow initially due to a left to right shunt. (In some children, the pulmonary vasculature may never develop normally in the presence of such a shunt.)

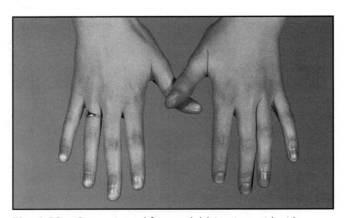

Fig. 6.29 Cyanosis and finger clubbing in a girl with Eisenmenger's syndrome.

The most important way in which individual organs can adjust their blood supply according to their metabolic needs is by decreasing or increasing the resistance of the arterioles (very small arteries 200–300 μm in diameter) that supply them. Thus, the act of eating food considerably reduces vascular resistance in the gut and increases gut blood flow. Similarly, exercising skeletal muscle strikingly reduces its vascular resistance, thereby increasing local blood flow. Alteration of blood flow to the skin is one of the important mechanisms whereby the body loses or conserves heat. The arteriolar resistance in the skin and the gut is also under the control of the sympathetic nervous

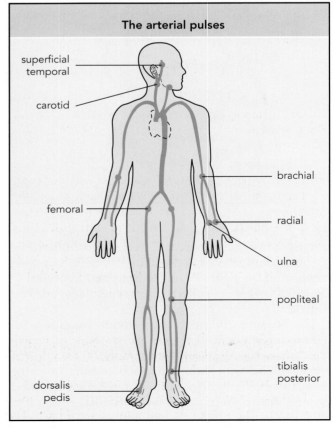

The arterial pulses

superficial temporal

carotid

brachial

femoral

radial

ulna

popliteal

tibialis posterior

dorsalis pedis

Fig. 6.30 Some of the points at which arterial pulsation can be felt. (Note the similarity to first-aiders' 'pressure points'.)

Differential diagnosis
Factors that affect the shape of the pulse

- Velocity of cardiac ejection
- Stroke volume (decreased with tachycardia, heart failure)
- Peripheral resistance (low peripheral resistance leads to 'collapsing' pulse)
- Left ventricular outflow obstruction ('slow rising' pulse in aortic stenosis)
- Elasticity of peripheral vessels (inelastic vessels, e.g. in elderly people, may 'sharpen' pulse waves)
- Reflection of pulse waves from the periphery

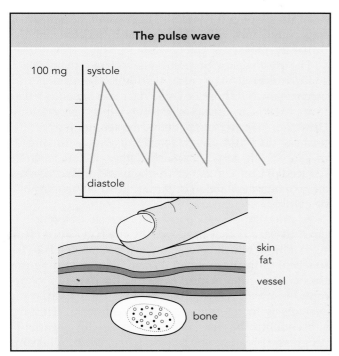

Fig. 6.31   Relationship between the pulse and the arterial waveform.

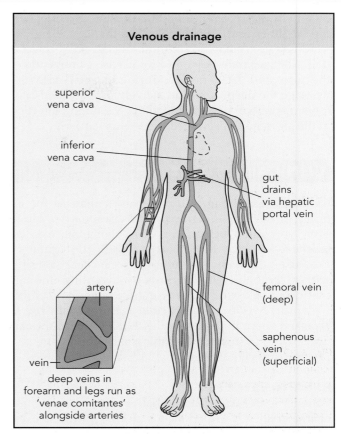

Fig. 6.32   Principal veins of the body.

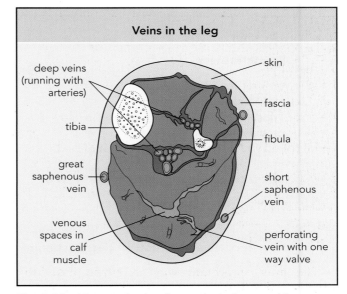

Fig. 6.33   Veins in the leg form a 'muscle pump' in conjunction with the calf muscles. Muscle contraction forces blood from superficial to deep veins, and from periphery to centre.

system as part of the general body response to 'fright, fight or flight'. Sympathetic nervous system stimulation causes arteriolar constriction and as a result tends to raise the blood pressure. The most important blood vessels for the control of peripheral vascular resistance are the small muscular arteries and arterioles; larger blood vessels such as the femoral, carotid or radial arteries simply act as conduits and play little or no role in the control of blood pressure.

VENOUS SYSTEM

The principal veins of the body are shown in Figure 6.32. Systemic veins collect blood from the tissues and return it to the right atrium of the heart. The venous return from the gut is a special case because it is collected by the hepatic portal vein and carried first of all to the liver. The venous system operates at a much lower pressure than the arterial system. Veins draining the chest and abdomen drain passively into the vena cava, either directly or via the azygos vein. In the upright position, venous drainage from the head and neck is assisted by gravity. Passive venous drainage alone is inadequate for the limbs and, in particular, for the legs. Here, the venous system is divided into superficial and deep veins (Fig. 6.33) separated by one-way valves. Contraction of the arm and leg muscles during normal activities massage the deep veins and actively propel blood back towards the heart. Flow of blood in the wrong direction in the leg veins is prevented by venous valves.

CLINICAL HISTORY

Carefully taking the history greatly enhances the efficacy of the subsequent physical examination. However, you must beware of what the great medical teacher, Maurice Pappworth, called the crime of Procrustes, namely, making your physical signs fit with a preconceived diagnosis by inventing findings that do not exist or suppressing findings that conflict with your hypothesis. Particular features that need to be asked about in the history with relevance to the cardiovascular system are breathlessness, chest pain, palpitation and claudication.

BREATHLESSNESS

Patients with heart disease that causes breathlessness characteristically experience it during physical exertion (exertional dyspnoea) and sometimes when they lie flat in bed (positional dyspnoea or orthopnoea). There is evidence that orthopnoea is caused by stimulation of

Questions to ask
Breathlessness

- Do you ever feel short of breath?
- Does this happen on exertion?
- How much can you do before getting breathless?
- Do you ever wake up gasping for breath?
- If so, do you have to sit up or get out of bed?
- How many pillows do you sleep on?
- Do you cough or wheeze when you are short of breath?

Symptoms and signs
New York Heart Association classification of heart failure

Grade	
I	No symptoms at rest, dyspnoea only on vigorous exertion
II	No symptoms at rest, dyspnoea on moderate exertion
III	May be mild symptoms at rest, dyspnoea on mild exertion, severe dyspnoea on moderate exertion
IV	Significant dyspnoea at rest, severe dyspnoea even on very mild exertion. Patient often bed bound

Differential diagnosis
Dyspnoea

- Heart failure
- Ischaemic heart disease (atypical angina)
- Pulmonary embolism
- Lung disease
- Severe anaemia

fine nerve endings in the lungs as a consequence of a rise in pulmonary capillary pressure, which is caused by a redistribution of fluid between peripheral tissues and the lungs when the patient lies flat. Sometimes, the patient awakes from sleep extremely breathless and has to sit up gasping for breath. This is often accompanied by a cough and white frothy sputum (paroxysmal nocturnal dyspnoea).

The mechanism of exercise-associated dyspnoea is controversial. It may partly be due to the same sort of mechanism as orthopnoea, with increased venous return from exercising muscles raising left atrial pressure. However, in exercising patients, the sensation of breathlessness does not always correlate well with directly measured left atrial pressure. Other factors such as reduced oxygen content of arterial blood and some alteration of muscle function in chronic heart failure may also be involved.

A popular classification of exercise tolerance in heart disease is that proposed by the New York Heart Association, which is used widely in clinical trials. For practical purposes, when taking and recording the history, it is often helpful to record the patient's symptoms as much as possible in their own words and perhaps with reference to local landmarks. This can subsequently be very useful in assessing a patient's progress. Breathlessness associated with wheezing may sometimes be due to heart disease but should raise the suspicion of obstructive airways disease.

Patients who feel that they suddenly have to take a deep breath unrelated to any physical exertion, who find themselves sighing excessively or who have a constant feeling of not being able to get enough breath in are not describing common features of heart disease. These may, however, be features of anxiety.

It can sometimes be difficult to decide whether a patient's breathlessness is caused by heart or lung disease. Paroxysmal nocturnal dyspnoea or orthopnoea point towards heart disease and wheezing as a

Differential diagnosis
Chest pain on exertion

- Angina caused by coronary atheroma
- Aortic stenosis
- Hypertrophic cardiomyopathy
- 'Anginal syndrome with normal coronary arteries'

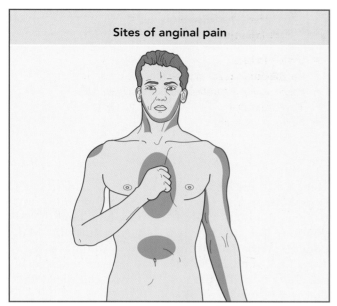

Sites of anginal pain

Fig. 6.34 Characteristic distribution of anginal pain.

prominent feature to lung disease but the distinction can often only be made after the clinical examination.

CHEST PAIN

Chest pain caused by myocardial ischaemia

Over 50% of patients presenting to cardiology clinics in the UK do so with the predominant symptom of chest pain. The most common type of chest pain associated with heart disease is called angina pectoris and is caused by an imbalance between the actual blood supply to a portion of heart muscle and the blood supply that this muscle needs for normal metabolism. Most patients with angina have a narrowing or stenosis in one or more coronary arteries and the pain is precipitated when the metabolic needs of the heart are increased by physical or emotional exertion. Less often, angina is a symptom of aortic stenosis or hypertrophic cardiomyopathy. The characteristic features of anginal pain are listed in the summary box and its distribution is illustrated in Figure 6.34. The single most characteristic feature of angina is chest pain that comes on during

Symptoms and signs
Anginal pain

- Brought on by physical or emotional exertion
- Relieved by rest
- Usually crushing, squeezing or constricting in nature
- Usually retrosternal (Fig. 6.34)
- Often worse after food or in cold winds
- Often relieved by nitrates

exertion and that goes away again as soon as or very shortly after the exertion stops. It is usually described as a crushing, squeezing or constricting pain (the Greek word from which it is derived means choking).

Pain that is similar in nature to angina but comes on at rest may be caused by unstable angina or myocardial infarction. The pain of myocardial infarction is severe, persistent and often accompanied by nausea and a feeling of impending death ('angor animi').

Pericarditis

Pericarditis is an inflammation of the pericardium, the serous sac that surrounds the heart. It may be a complication of myocardial infarction or it may result from a viral or bacterial infection. Another important cause is uraemia. The patient characteristically complains of pain that is usually described as a constant soreness behind the breast bone and that often gets much worse if the patient takes a deep breath. Unlike the pain of angina or myocardial infarction, pericarditic pain is related to movement (e.g. turning over in bed) but not to physical exertion. It sometimes radiates to the tip of the left shoulder.

Musculoskeletal chest pain

Pain arising in the chest wall or thoracic spine is often mistaken for cardiac pain. Characteristically, it tends to be an aching pain, the onset of which may relate to a particular twist or movement: the pain persists at rest. There is often localised tenderness, particularly over the costal cartilages. A variant of musculoskeletal pain

Questions to ask
Angina

- Do you get pain in your chest on exertion, (e.g. climbing stairs)?
- Whereabouts in the chest do you feel it?
- Is it worse in cold weather?
- Is it worse if you exercise after a big meal?
- Is it bad enough to stop you from exercising?
- Does it go away when you rest?
- Do you ever get similar pain if you get excited or upset?

Differential diagnosis
Chest pain at rest

- Myocardial infarction
- Unstable angina
- Dissecting aortic aneurysm
- Oesophageal pain
- Pericarditis
- Pleuritic pain
- Musculoskeletal pain
- Herpes zoster (shingles)

is the precordial catch syndrome, in which the patient describes a sudden, sharp needle-like jabbing pain in the precordium. The pain is short lasting but may recur; the prognosis is benign.

Dissecting aortic aneurysm

Dissecting aneurysm of the thoracic aorta causes a rare but characteristic form of chest pain that usually starts as a 'tearing' sensation, often felt most between the shoulder blades or in the back. The pain is usually severe and persistent and may be mistaken for the pain of myocardial infarction.

Other chest pains

Other chest pains that may masquerade as cardiac pain include the pain of pleurisy, of an acute pneumothorax or of shingles.

Palpitation

Palpitation is defined as abnormal awareness of the heart beat. This may be because the heart is beating abnormally fast or irregularly as the result of an arrhythmia or because the cardiac impulse is more forceful, perhaps as a result of excessive vasodilatation. It is important to find out which of these the patient means. It is often helpful to ask the patient to tap out the heart rhythm on the table. In patients with extrasystoles, it is often not the extra beat itself which the patient perceives but the one following it, which is characterised by a longer than usual pause and an excessively forceful beat. The patient may say that their heart jumps or that it feels that it is about to stop. Ask about the circumstances when the patient feels the palpitation. Ectopic beats are often more apparent when the background heart rate is slow (e.g. when the patient lies down to rest); whereas paroxysmal tachycardias are often precipitated by exercise or by particular movements (e.g. stooping down to open a drawer or reaching to remove something from a high shelf).

The need to treat an arrhythmia is often determined by the haemodynamic effects it is having. Find out whether the arrhythmia is simply a transient incon-

Differential diagnosis
Palpitation

- Extrasystoles
- Paroxysmal atrial fibrillation
- Paroxysmal supraventricular tachycardia
- Thyrotoxicosis
- Perimenopausal

venience to the patient or whether the patient has to stop working and lie down. Some arrhythmias cause patients to lose consciousness. Ask how long the palpitations last and whether they stop abruptly. Many patients with paroxysmal tachycardia have learnt some trick such as the Valsalva maneouvre (forceably breathing out with the nose and the mouth held shut) that will terminate an attack.

In some patients, palpitation is precipitated by certain foods, in particular, tea, coffee, wine and chocolates. You should also ask carefully about any medication, particular decongestants and 'cold cures' which often contain sympathomimetic drugs.

Syncope (fainting, blackouts)

Syncope is defined as loss of consciousness resulting from a transient failure of blood supply to the brain. The main differential diagnosis is from epilepsy. Note that any patient may have convulsions if the blood supply to the brain is interrupted for long enough. The common causes of syncope are simple fainting (vasovagal syncope), its variants such as micturition syncope, postural hypotension, vertebrobasilar insufficiency and cardiac arrhythmias, particularly intermittent heart block. Simple fainting is caused by a vagally mediated heart slowing combined with sudden reflex vasodilatation. It is usually caused by a combination of diminished venous return (e.g. standing still on a hot parade ground or in an operating theatre), coupled with increased sympathic drive (excitement, fear, disgust). Micturition syncope characteristically occurs at night in middle-aged or elderly men with a degree of prostatic obstruc-

Questions to ask
Palpitation

- Please could you tap out on the table the rate you think your heart goes at during an attack?
- Is the heart beat regular or irregular?
- Is there anything that sets attacks off?
- Can you do anything to stop an attack?
- What do you do when you have an attack?
- Are there any foods that seem to make symptoms worse?
- What medicines are you taking?

Questions to ask
Syncope

(Wherever possible history should be taken from a family member or observer as well as the patient.)

- What were the exact circumstances of the blackout?
- Did you have any warning of the attack?
- How quickly did you recover?
- Did you go pale or red during or after the attack?
- Are you taking any medication?

tion, in which the fall in venous return is caused by straining to empty the bladder and the sympathic stimulation by the anticipation of the consequences of not doing so.

In fainting, loss of consciousness is seldom abrupt; the patient looks pale or 'green' both before and immediately afterwards. Rapid relief is provided by elevating the legs. In contrast, syncope caused by heart block is often sudden, unheralded and complete. The patient looks pale while collapsed, recovery (which is often equally sudden) may be heralded by a pink flush. Vertebrobasilar insufficiency is common in elderly patients: there may be restricted neck movement and active or passive movements of the neck may precipitate symptoms. Postural hypotension is more common in elderly people and may be exacerbated by antihypotensive medication. Important clinical questions in taking the history are highlighted in the question box.

Claudication

Claudication is derived from a Latin word meaning limping. Intermittent claudication is the name given to a condition in which the patient experiences pain in one or both legs on walking which eases up when the patient rests. Just as angina is the usual initial symptom of atheromatous disease affecting the coronary arteries, so intermittent claudication is usually the earliest symptom of narrowing in the arteries supplying the legs. The pain is usually an aching pain felt in the calf, thigh or buttocks. Intermittent claudication is more common in men and much more common in smokers than in nonsmokers. More advanced symptoms of peripheral arterial disease are discussed in the section on peripheral vascular disease.

OCCUPATIONAL AND FAMILY HISTORY

A family history is very important in evaluating patients with heart disease because many cardiac diseases involve an underlying genetic predisposition (e.g. towards hyperlipidaemia). Sometimes it is more helpful to ask whether specific family members are still alive or about the circumstances of their death because the significance of this may not be apparent to the patient. For example, early death from stroke may indicate a family susceptibility to hypertension. The patient's occupation may be very relevant to the significance of the disease: coronary artery disease or arrhythmias may be incompatible with a continuing career as an airline pilot or truck driver.

Do not forget to enquire specifically about smoking, alcohol intake and any medication the patient may be taking.

Questions to ask
Family history

- Is there any heart disease in the family?
- Are your parents still alive?
- Did they live to a good age?
- Do you know what they died from?
- Have you any brothers or sisters?
- Do any of them have a heart problem?

CLINICAL EXAMINATION OF THE CARDIOVASCULAR SYSTEM

There are three interlinking facets to the examination of the cardiovascular system. First, the student will wish to establish an examination routine that will ensure that all important aspects of the cardiovascular system are examined smoothly and efficiently and that nothing important is forgotten. Second, he or she will wish to concentrate on certain specific points to confirm or to refute a working diagnosis based on the clinical history. Third, it will frequently happen that routine clinical examination will disclose an unexpected abnormality, such as a heart murmur, whose differential diagnosis must then be considered.

A FRAMEWORK FOR THE ROUTINE PHYSICAL EXAMINATION OF THE CARDIOVASCULAR SYSTEM

The author's schedule for the routine examination of the cardiovascular system can be seen in the review box. It is not the only possible schedule, nor necessarily the best one, and it is constantly being modified in the light of increasing experience. It will, however, serve as a framework for discussion.

HANDS IN HEART DISEASE

The temperature of the hands gives a guide to the extent of peripheral vasodilatation. Patients in heart failure are usually vasoconstricted and their hands feel cold and sometimes sweaty from increased adrenaline secretion. The fingernails may show splinter haemorrhages (Fig. 6.35) in subacute infective endocarditis and finger clubbing in endocarditis or cyanotic congenital heart disease.

FEELING THE PERIPHERAL PULSES

The right radial pulse is usually best felt with the fingers of the examiner's left hand (Fig. 6.36). It is used to assess heart rate and rhythm. As the radial pulse is a relatively long way from the heart, it is not a good pulse from which to attempt to assess pulse character.

Review
Framework for routine examination of the cardiovascular system

1. While taking the history, watch the patient's face for features of anxiety, distress, breathlessness or features of specific diseases
2. Take the patient's hand and assess warmth, sweating and peripheral cyanosis; examine the nails for clubbing or splinter haemorrhages
3. Palpate the radial pulse and assess the rate and rhythm
4. Locate and palpate the brachial pulse and assess its character. Measure the blood pressure. If there is any suspicion of a problem with the aortic arch, compare pulses in both arms
5. With the patient lying supine at 45°, assess the jugular venous pressure and the jugular venous pulse form
6. Take an opportunity for a closer look at the face, the conjunctivae, the tongue and the inside of the mouth
7. Palpate the carotid pulse and assess its character
8. With the patient's chest exposed, inspect the precordium and assess the breathing pattern

and the presence of any abnormal pulsation
9. Palpate the precordium, locate the apex beat and assess its character. Assess the feel of the rest of the precordium and the presence of any abnormal vibrations or thrills
10. Listen with the stethoscope and assess heart sounds and murmurs. If appropriate, listen over the carotid artery for radiating murmurs or bruits
11. Percuss and auscultate the chest both front and back looking for pleural effusions. Listen for crepitations at the lung bases
12. Lie the patient flat and palpate the abdomen, feeling in particular for the liver and any dilatation of the abdominal aorta
13. Assess the femoral pulses and the popliteal and foot pulses. Look for ankle or sacral oedema
14. If appropriate, assess the patient's exercise tolerance by taking the patient for a short walk
15. Test the urine

If there is any suspicion of an abnormality in the aortic arch or of some abnormality in the brachial artery on either side, it may be helpful to feel both radial pulses and compare their volume and timing simultaneously. In patients with suspected coarctation of the aorta, it is helpful simultaneously to feel the radial and the femoral pulse. In the presence of coarctation not only is the volume of the femoral pulse diminished but it is also appreciably delayed compared with the radial pulse (Fig. 6.37).

Brachial pulse
The best way to feel the patient's right brachial pulse is to use the thumb of the right hand, applied to the front of the elbow just medial to the biceps tendon with the fingers cupped round the back of the elbow (Fig. 6.38). Students are sometimes taught never to use the thumb for feeling a pulse because pulsation in the examiner's own thumb may lead to mistakes in the detection of very faint peripheral pulses in patients with peripheral arterial disease. However, in most patients we are not actu-

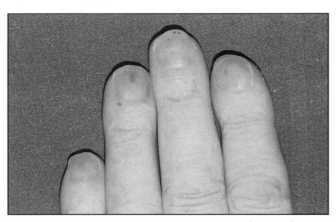

Fig. 6.35 Splinter haemorrhage in the ring finger of a man with infective endocarditis. There is an older, fading 'splinter' under the nail of the index finger. Splinter haemorrhages are often smaller and darker than this.

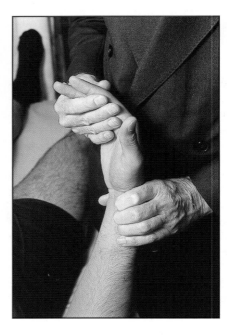

Fig. 6.36
Feeling the right radial pulse.

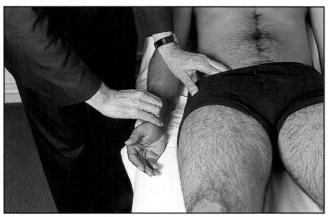

Fig. 6.37   Simultaneous palpation of the radial and femoral pulses: a delayed femoral pulse is a feature of aortic coarctation.

Pulse character		
Name	**Feels like**	**Associated with**
Normal		—
Slow rising		Aortic stenosis
Bisferiens ('two peaks')		Mild aortic stenosis plus reflux
Collapsing		Aortic reflux Persistent ductus arteriosus
No pulse		Occluded bronchial or axillary artery

Fig. 6.39   Different pulse waveforms are associated with different cardiac or vascular abnormalities.

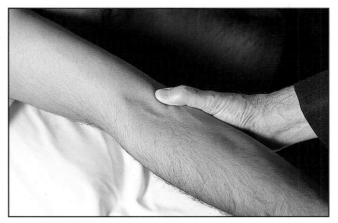

Fig. 6.38   Using the thumb to assess the character of the brachial pulse. The artery lies just medial to the tendinous insertion of the biceps muscle and deep to the fascial insertion of this muscle. It was called the 'grâce à dieu' (thanks be to God) fascia by medieval barber surgeons because it saved them from fatally damaging the artery when blood letting at the elbow!

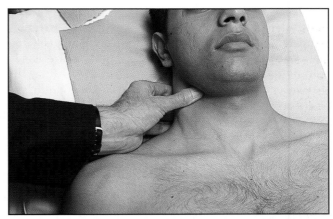

Fig. 6.40   Palpation of the carotid artery using the thumb.

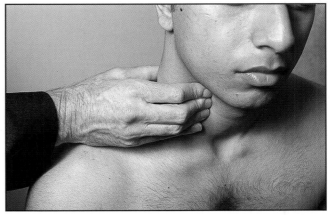

Fig. 6.41   Palpation of the carotid artery by different means.

ally concerned with whether or not the brachial pulse is present but with its character (Fig. 6.39) and here the extreme kinaesthetic sensitivity of the examiner's thumb compared with the other fingers is a distinct advantage.

Carotid pulse

The carotid pulse is even closer to the heart than the brachial pulse and therefore even better for assessing pulse character as a reflection of the way the left ventricle is working. The best way to feel the patient's right carotid artery is to locate the tip of the examiner's left thumb against the patient's larynx and then gently but firmly press directly backwards so that the carotid artery is felt against the precervical muscles (Fig. 6.40). Alternatively, the carotid pulse can be felt from behind by curling the fingers around the side of the neck (Fig. 6.41).

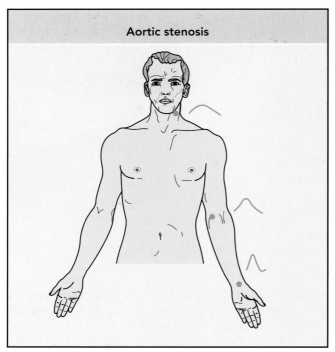

Fig. 6.42 Pulse wave changes in aortic stenosis.

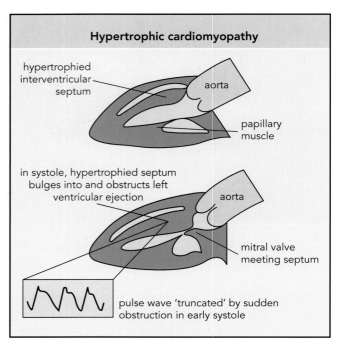

Fig. 6.43 Hypertrophic cardiomyopathy. A 'jerky' carotid pulse may result from dynamic left ventricular outflow obstruction.

In severe aortic stenosis, there is characteristically a slow rising carotid pulse, often with a palpable shudder. If the carotid pulse is difficult to feel in a patient whose radial and brachial pulses are easily felt, the cause may be aortic stenosis because the pulse form becomes more 'normal' the nearer the periphery it is felt (Fig. 6.42). Another sign best appreciated at the carotid is the jerky pulse of hypertrophic cardiomyopathy. This starts normally and then suddenly peters out as the contracting left ventricular outflow tract obstructs ejection (Fig. 6.43).

Femoral pulse

The femoral pulse is almost as valuable as the carotid pulse in assessing cardiac performance. It is more likely to be weak or absent in patients with disease of the aorta or iliac arteries. It is best examined, with the patient unclothed and lying flat, by placing the thumb or finger directly above the superior pubic ramus and midway between the pubic tubercle and anterior superior iliac spine (Fig. 6.44).

Methods for assessing the popliteal and foot pulses are given here for completeness but their main use lies in assessing peripheral arterial disease (see section on peripheral vascular disease).

Popliteal pulse

The popliteal pulse lies deep within the popliteal fossa but is readily felt by compressing it against the posterior surface of the distal end of the femur. The patient

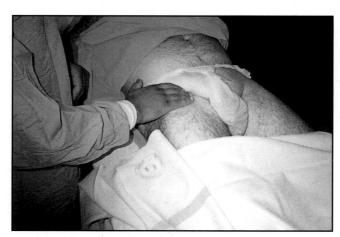

Fig. 6.44 Palpation of the femoral artery.

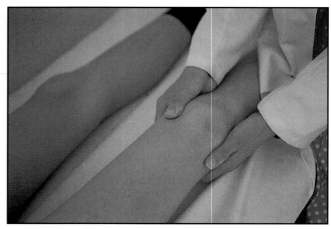

Fig. 6.45 Palpation of the popliteal artery.

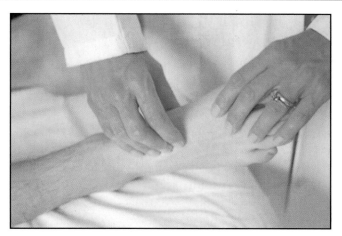

Fig. 6.46   Palpation of the dorsalis pedis pulse.

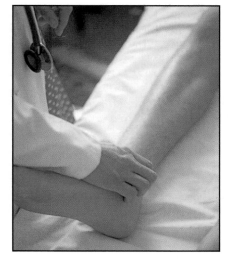

Fig. 6.47
Palpation of the tibialis posterior pulse.

lies flat with the knee slightly flexed. The fingers of one hand are used to press the tips of the fingers of the other hand into the popliteal fossa to feel the popliteal artery against the back of the knee joint (Fig. 6.45). Palpating the popliteal artery is mainly useful in evaluating patients with peripheral vascular disease, particularly patients presenting with intermittent claudication.

Dorsalis pedis and tibialis posterior pulses

Palpation of these pulses is mainly used for assessing peripheral vascular disease, although they can sometimes be used for monitoring pulse rate and rhythm during anaesthesia or recovery. The dorsalis pedis pulse is felt with the fingers aligned along the dorsum of the foot lateral to the extensor hallucis longus tendon (Fig. 6.46); the tibialis posterior pulse is felt with the fingers cupped round the ankle just posterior to the medial malleolus (Fig. 6.47).

MEASURING BLOOD PRESSURE

The most convenient way of measuring blood pressure in the clinic is with a stethoscope and sphygmomanometer. The sphygmomanometer is placed around the upper arm (Fig. 6.48) and air is pumped into the cuff. As the pressure in the sphygmomanometer cuff increases above the systolic pressure in the brachial artery, the artery is compressed and the radial pulse becomes impalpable. As the pressure in the cuff is gradually lowered, blood can force its way past the obstruction for part of the cardiac cycle, creating sounds that can be heard with a stethoscope placed over the brachial artery at the elbow. These sounds are called the Korotkoff sounds after the Russian physician who first described them. As pressure in the cuff is lowered, the Korotkoff sounds become louder and more ringing in nature and then suddenly become muffled. Very shortly afterwards, the sounds usually disappear altogether. It is this

point of disappearance of the Korotkoff sounds (sometimes called phase 5) that is now used to define diastolic pressure for clinical and epidemiological purposes. In fact, it is the point of muffling of the sounds (phase 4) that corresponds most closely to the diastolic pressure, as measured by an indwelling arterial cannula, but phase 5 readings have proved to be more reproducible among different observers. The generation of the Korotkoff sounds is shown diagrammatically in Figure 6.49.

To measure the blood pressure reliably in the clinic, all clothing must be removed from the arm and the sphygmomanometer cuff smoothly applied. The patient's arm should be supported at heart level by an arm rest or by the examiner. It is good practice to check the systolic pressure roughly by palpation of the radial artery before applying the stethoscope. This is because in some patients with very high blood pressure the Korotkoff sounds may disappear and then reappear again as cuff pressure is lowered, a phenomenon called the auscultatory gap. For accurate measurement, pressure in the cuff should be

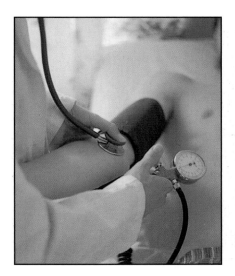

Fig. 6.48
Measuring blood pressure using a sphygmomanometer and stethoscope. The sphygmomanometer cuff is smoothly applied around the unclothed upper arm and the examiner supports the patient's arm at 'heart height'.

reduced slowly, ideally at about 1 mmHg/s. Mercury manometers must be upright and not tilted. Aneroid manometers invariably become inaccurate with time and can be regularly recalibrated against mercury manometers; however, mercury manometers are being phased out. Most people consciously or unconsciously round off the blood pressure reading to the nearest 5–10 mmHg. This is frowned on by purists. If really accurate results are needed for research purposes, it is best to use a random zero sphygmomanometer in which the operator presses levers to indicate when he or she thinks systolic and diastolic pressures have been reached and then opens the back of the instrument to read the results off a concealed scale.

Patients with very high blood pressure often have other evidence of hypertensive disease in the form of retinal changes, left ventricular hypertrophy and proteinuria. In patients without these features, it is important not to make a definitive diagnosis of hypertension on the basis of a single casual blood pressure recording. Repeated blood pressure measurements will nearly always show some tendency to revert towards normal. Some patients have high blood pressure when measured in a hospital clinic, yet measurements in their own home or by continuous blood pressure monitoring show a more normal pattern. The definition of what constitutes higher blood pressure has long been a subject for controversy. In any given population, the distribution of systolic and diastolic blood pressures is continuous. In Western populations, there is a ten-

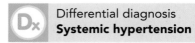

Differential diagnosis
Systemic hypertension

- Primary 'essential' hypertension
- Secondary: Aortic coarctation
- Hormonal: Congenital
                        – adrenal hyperplasia
                        – 11-hydroxylase deficiency
                      Acquired
                        – phaeochromocytoma
                        – Conn's syndrome
                        – Cushing's syndrome
- Renal: Polycystic kidneys
                Renal artery stenosis
                Acute glomerulonephritis
                Chronic renal disease
- Drug-related: Steroids
                        Contraceptive pill
                        Nonsteroidal anti-inflammatory
                            drugs
                        Ciclosporin

dency for both systolic and diastolic pressures to increase with age, although this does not necessarily apply to other populations, particularly peoples in whom there is a low salt intake. Most authorities would accept a phase 5 diastolic pressure of over 100 mmHg on repeated measurement as defining a hypertensive population. A diastolic pressure of greater than 120 mmHg and evidence of end organ damage would define patients with severe hyper-

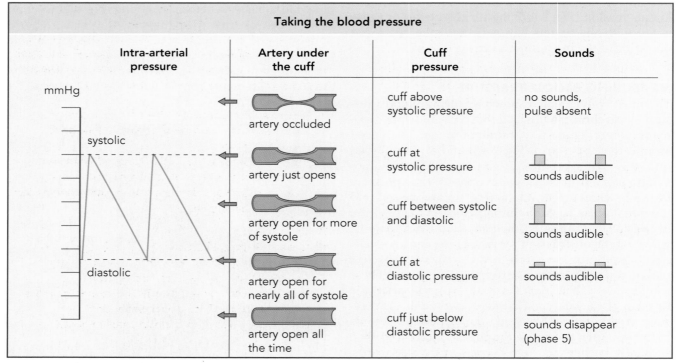

	Taking the blood pressure		
Intra-arterial pressure	**Artery under the cuff**	**Cuff pressure**	**Sounds**
mmHg	artery occluded	cuff above systolic pressure	no sounds, pulse absent
systolic	artery just opens	cuff at systolic pressure	sounds audible
	artery open for more of systole	cuff between systolic and diastolic	sounds audible
diastolic	artery open for nearly all of systole	cuff at diastolic pressure	sounds audible
	artery open all the time	cuff just below diastolic pressure	sounds disappear (phase 5)

Fig. 6.49   The relationship between cuff pressure, Korotkoff sounds and arterial pressure.

Symptoms and signs
Important points about measuring blood pressure

- Remove all clothing from arm
- Support arm comfortably at heart level
- Use correct size of cuff: wide cuff for obese arms, paediatric cuff for children
- Check systolic pressure by palpitation
- Release pressure no faster than 1 mmHg/s
- Take phase 5 (disappearance of sounds) as diastolic pressure
- Check aneroid manometers regularly against mercury manometer
- If using a mercury manometer, it must be absolutely upright

Differential diagnosis
Hypotension

Impaired cardiac output
- Myocardial infarction
- Pericardial tamponade
- Massive pulmonary embolism
- Acute valve incompetence

Hypovolaemia
- Haemorrhage
- Diabetic precoma
- Dehydration from diarrhoea or vomiting

Excessive vasodilatation
- Anaphylaxis
- Gram-negative septicaemia
- Drugs
- Autonomic failure

tension. Important points about the measurement of blood pressure are summarised in the symptoms and signs box.

The converse of hypertension is hypotension or low blood pressure. Although a systolic blood pressure of less than 100 mmHg is part of the definition of shock, hypotension is usually defined by its consequences (e.g. impaired cerebral or renal function) rather than by some arbitrary pressure level. Some patients have postural hypotension, which most commonly manifests itself as dizziness when the patient attempts to stand upright. The diagnosis is made by measuring the blood pressure with the patient lying and standing.

Emergency
Severe hypotension (shock)

Emergency medical assessment of the patient with severe hypotension (shock)
1. History (from patient, relatives or attendants)
- Has there been any trauma, haemorrhage or substance abuse?
- Has onset been sudden or gradual (over hours or days, e.g. diabetic ketoacidosis, dysentery)?
- Has there been any pain (i) in the chest (myocardial infarction, dissecting aneurysm) or (ii) elsewhere (e.g. headache in meningococcal septicaemia)?
- Is there any other relevant history (e.g. bed rest, airline travel in massive pulmonary embolism)?

2. Clinical examination
- Before starting the examination, check that the patient's airway is safe and, if possible, attach an ECG monitor
- Check whether the patient is more comfortable sitting up (think of pulmonary oedema) or lying flat (think of hypovolaemia or pulmonary embolism)
- Remove external clothes and conduct a quick but thorough examination for signs of trauma or haemorrhage if appropriate. Usually the skin in shock is pale and cold but if it is warm or red think of septicaemia or allergy
- Assess the pulse. Normally it would be fast (100–120 beats/min) in shock, if very slow think of heart block, if more rapid consider an arrhythmia

- Quickly assess the major pulses (carotid, femorals). If asymmetrical, think of dissecting aortic aneurysm
- Try and assess the jugular venous pressure. A very high jugular venous pressure suggests pulmonary embolism or cardiac tamponade
- Check that the trachea is central and that air entry can be heard on both sides of the chest (if not, think of tension pneumothorax). If there are widespread crackles in the lungs, think of pulmonary oedema
- Listen to the front of the chest for murmurs or abnormal heart sounds (often very difficult if the heart rate is rapid)
- Gently palpate the abdomen for tenderness or pulsation (think of ruptured aortic aneurysm)
- If appropriate consider rectal or vaginal examination for hidden haemorrhage

3. Investigation
- As soon as possible record an ECG (diagnosis of myocardial infarction, arrhythmia, pulmonary embolism) and take a chest radiograph (and if appropriate other radiographs, for example, in the case of trauma). Consider emergency echocardiography if diagnosis is still in doubt

EVALUATION OF THE JUGULAR VENOUS PULSE

The evaluation of the jugular venous pulse is a key factor in assessing the performance of the 'input' side of the heart. The internal jugular vein is in direct communication, without intervening valves, with the superior vena cava and the right atrium. The normal pressure in the right atrium is equivalent to that exerted by a column of blood 10–12 cm tall. Therefore, when the patient is standing or sitting upright, the internal jugular vein is collapsed, and when the patient is lying flat, it is completely filled. If the patient lies supine at approximately 45°, the point at which jugular venous pulsation becomes

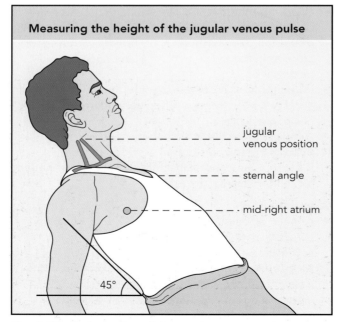

Fig. 6.50 Assessing the jugular venous pressure. With the patient lying supine at 45°, jugular pulsation is normally just visible above the clavicle.

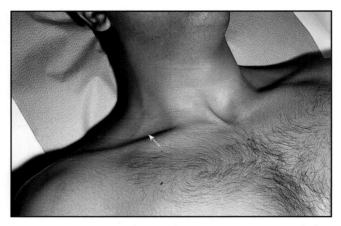

Measuring the height of the jugular venous pulse

jugular venous position

sternal angle

mid-right atrium

45°

Fig. 6.51 Relationship of the jugular venous pulsation, right atrium and manubriosternal angle.

visible is usually just above the clavicle; this is the position usually chosen for examination of the jugular venous pulse (Fig. 6.50). It is best if the patient rests his or her head comfortably against a pillow, with the neck slightly flexed and looking straight ahead. It is important not to tense the sternomastoid muscles because the internal jugular vein lies directly beneath them. Reliable ways of telling the jugular venous pulse from the carotid arterial pulse are listed in the differential diagnosis box. It is sometimes said that jugular venous pulsation can be obliterated by gentle pressure with the finger and that the jugular pulse is never palpable but these two statements are incorrect, particularly in the presence of tricuspid regurgitation.

Once the jugular venous pulse has been identified, the examiner must try to assess, first, the mean height of pulsation above right atrial level and, second, the waveform of jugular venous pulsation. As it is not actually possible to see or feel the right atrium, it is usual to express the height of jugular venous pulsation above the manubriosternal angle (Fig. 6.51). The height of the manubriosternal angle above the mid-right atrium is approximately constant irrespective of whether the patient is lying, sitting or standing. A normal jugular venous pressure is less than 4 cm above the manubriosternal angle.

In patients with a very high jugular venous pressure (e.g. individuals with pericardial tamponade or constrictive pericarditis), the internal jugular vein may be completely filled with the patient lying at 45°

 Differential diagnosis
Distinction between jugular venous and carotid pulses

Venous
- Most rapid movement inward
- Two peaks per cycle (in sinus rhythm)
- Affected by compressing abdomen
- May displace earlobes (if venous pressure raised)

Arterial
- Most rapid movement outward
- One peak per cycle
- Not affected by compressing abdomen
- Never displaces earlobes

 Differential diagnosis
Raised jugular venous pressure

- Congestive or right-sided heart failure
- Tricuspid reflux
- Pericardial tamponade
- Pulmonary embolism
- Iatrogenic fluid overload
- Superior vena cava obstruction

and it is necessary to sit the patient bolt upright to see the top of the pulsation. As a quick rule of thumb, if jugular venous pulsation is visible above the clavicle with the patient sitting bolt upright, then the jugular venous pressure must be raised.

Even sitting the patient upright is sometimes not adequate to assess a very high venous pressure. A rough estimate can sometimes be made in these patients by raising the hand until the veins on the back of the hand collapse and by assessing the difference in height between the hand and the right atrium or sternal angle.

Examples of different jugular pressure waveforms are shown in Figure 6.52. In practice, by far the most common and most important abnormal waveform to recognise is that of tricuspid regurgitation, which is characterised by large systolic waves that are often palpable and cannot be obliterated by pressing with a finger. By far the most common cause of a raised jugular venous pressure is congestive heart failure, in which the raised venous pressure reflects the right ventricular failure component. A raised but nonpulsatile jugular venous pressure should bring to mind the possibility of superior vena cava obstruction.

PALPATION OF THE PRECORDIUM

Palpate the precordium by laying the flat of the hand and the outstretched fingers on the chest wall to the left of the sternum (Fig. 6.53). You are literally trying to feel how the heart is working. The first thing to do

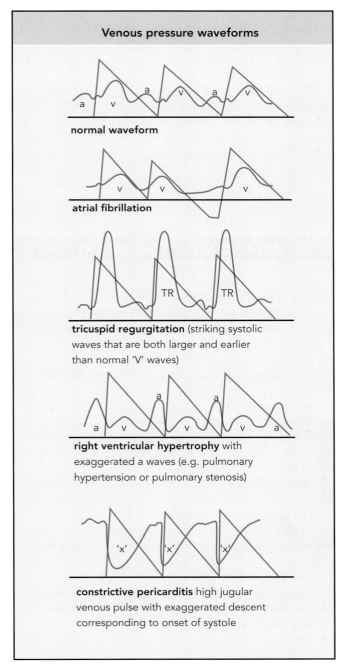

Venous pressure waveforms

normal waveform

atrial fibrillation

tricuspid regurgitation (striking systolic waves that are both larger and earlier than normal 'V' waves)

right ventricular hypertrophy with exaggerated a waves (e.g. pulmonary hypertension or pulmonary stenosis)

constrictive pericarditis high jugular venous pulse with exaggerated descent corresponding to onset of systole

Fig. 6.52 Examples of different jugular pressure waveforms.

 Differential diagnosis
Causes and characteristics of raised jugular venous pressure

Common
- Congestive heart failure
- Tricuspid regurgitation
- Normal wave pattern usually preserved
- Large 'V' waves

Less common
- Pericardial tamponade
- Massive pulmonary embolism
- Grossly elevated venous pressure, wave pattern difficult to assess because patient becomes hypotensive when sitting upright

Rare
- Superior caval obstruction
- Constrictive pericarditis
- Tricuspid stenosis

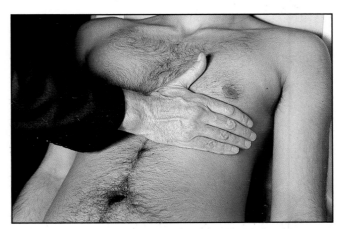

Fig. 6.53 Palpating the precordium. For locating the apex beat, the patient should lie flat on the back but to assess the quality of the impulses the patient should be rolled onto the left side.

is to locate the 'apex beat'. This is the furthest outward and downward point at which pulsation is easily palpable. Its site is usually expressed in terms of fixed landmarks such as the intercostal spaces, the clavicle and the axilla. The normal adult apex beat with the patient lying supine at 45° is in the fifth or sixth left intercostal space, in the midclavicular line. Remember that the heart has some mobility within the chest, so if you roll the patient onto, for example, the left side, the apex beat will move further outwards. Sometimes, particularly in an obese individual or one with an emphysematous chest, you will actually need to roll the patient onto their left side in order to feel cardiac pulsation properly. Do not attempt, however, to describe the position of the apex beat in these patients.

Just as important as the position of the apex beat is the quality of the impulse that you feel (Fig. 6.54). The quality of the normal apex beat and the range that this encompasses must be learnt by experience. A forceful apex beat usually indicates increased cardiac output (e.g. in a patient with a fever or after exercise). A diffuse poorly localised apex beat is commonly found after damage to the ventricular muscle, either by myocardial infarction or as a result of cardiomyopathy. This diffuse impulse can often be seen as well as felt by inspecting the precordium. The

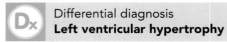

Differential diagnosis
Left ventricular hypertrophy

- Hypertension
- Aortic stenosis
- Hypertrophic cardiomyopathy

character of the cardiac impulse in left ventricular hypertrophy is very distinctive, being a sustained and forceful heave rather than a short sharp impulse. In mitral stenosis, the cardiac apex is often described as tapping. To some extent, this is caused by displacement of the left ventricle nearer to the examining hand by an enlarged left atrium and, partly, due to a loud first heart sound which is palpable as well as audible. Right ventricular hypertrophy or dilatation is felt as a heave close to the left sternal border.

While palpating the heart, the examining hand will sometimes detect a vibration or 'thrill'. Thrills are really 'palpable murmurs' and are always accompanied by an easily heard murmur on auscultation. A diastolic thrill (which feels very like the sensation of stroking a purring cat) may sometimes be felt in patients with mitral stenosis. Systolic thrills may accompany aortic stenosis, ventricular septal defect or mitral reflux.

AUSCULTATION OF THE HEART

Cardiac auscultation is easier with a good quality stethoscope. The stethoscope was originally introduced into medical practice by the French physician Laennec at the beginning of the nineteenth century. In its original form it consisted of a wooden cylinder with a small hole drilled from end to end. In addition to introducing a decorous distance between the head of the physician and the chest of the patient, the stethoscope has two principal functions. First, it transmits sounds from the chest of the patient and helps to exclude extraneous noise and, second, it selectively emphasises sounds of certain frequencies, enabling the examiner to concentrate on them.

An indiscriminate amplification of the sound coming from the chest, as would be produced by a sensitive high fidelity microphone, actually produces a signal that is very hard for the human ear to interpret. A modern stethoscope consists of two ear pieces connected by tubing to a chest piece which usually has both diaphragm and bell attachments. The ear pieces should be angled forwards to match the direction of the examiner's external auditory meati. They should fit snugly but comfortably. The tubing should not be too long (cardiologists seldom wear their stethoscopes round their collars). The bell and diaphragm chest pieces selectively emphasise sounds of different frequencies. The bell is central for listening to low-pitched sounds such as the mid-diastolic

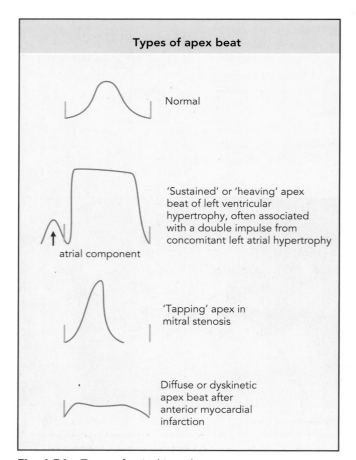

Types of apex beat

Normal

'Sustained' or 'heaving' apex beat of left ventricular hypertrophy, often associated with a double impulse from concomitant left atrial hypertrophy

atrial component

'Tapping' apex in mitral stenosis

Diffuse or dyskinetic apex beat after anterior myocardial infarction

Fig. 6.54   Types of apical impulse.

murmur of mitral stenosis or the third heart sound of cardiac failure. In contrast, the diaphragm filters out low-pitched sounds and, therefore, emphasises high-pitched ones. The diaphragm is best for analysing the second heart sound, for ejection and mid-systolic clicks and for the soft but high-pitched early diastolic murmur of aortic regurgitation.

It is worthwhile buying a good stethoscope, taking care of it and making use of every opportunity to appreciate the normal range of heart and chest sounds, both at rest and after exertion.

When auscultating the heart, you should as a minimum listen at the apex, at the base (the part of the heart between the apex and the sternum) and in the aortic and pulmonary areas to the right and left of the sternum, respectively (Fig. 6.55). Obviously, if anything abnormal is found, the stethoscope should be moved around until the abnormality is heard most clearly. It is good practice to relate the auscultatory findings to the cardiac cycle by simultaneously palpating the carotid artery while listening to the heart (Fig. 6.56).

It is helpful when learning, or when confronted with a difficult problem, to analyse your oscillatory findings under three headings, namely, first and second heart sounds, murmurs and any additional heart sounds. In practice, as you gain experience, particular auscultatory patterns will be recognised as a whole, just as one recognises speech.

HEART SOUNDS

First and second heart sounds

The mechanism of the first and second heart sounds and the mechanism and physiology of splitting the second heart sound have already been described. The first heart sound can usually be heard easily with both the bell and the diaphragm but the diaphragm is invaluable for analysing the second heart sound, with the stethoscope usually best placed at the midleft sternal edge. It is usual to record the heart sounds in a shorthand notation which derives from the records made by phonocardiography (Fig. 6.57).

Factors that may cause a change in the intensity of the heart sounds are shown in the differential diagnosis box. The most common causes of a loud first heart sound are an increased cardiac output or mitral stenosis. The most common causes of an abnormally quiet first heart sound are reduced cardiac output

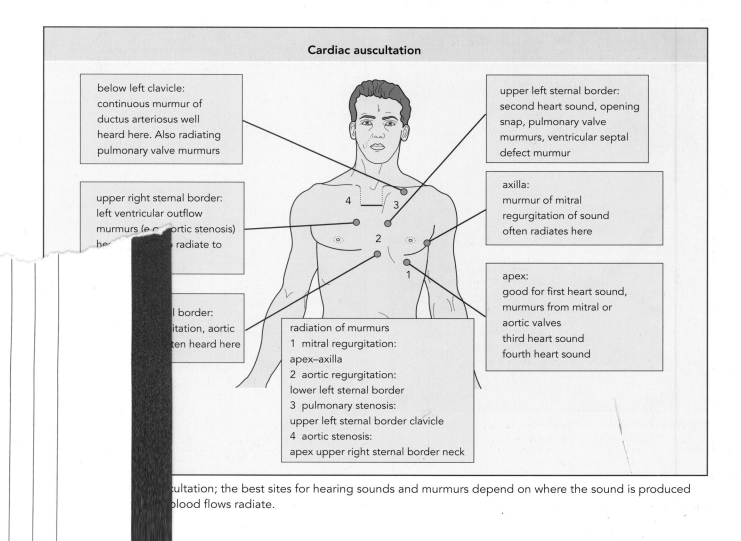

Cardiac auscultation

below left clavicle: continuous murmur of ductus arteriosus well heard here. Also radiating pulmonary valve murmurs

upper right sternal border: left ventricular outflow murmurs (e.g. aortic stenosis) he... radiate to

...l border:
...itation, aortic
...ten heard here

upper left sternal border: second heart sound, opening snap, pulmonary valve murmurs, ventricular septal defect murmur

axilla: murmur of mitral regurgitation of sound often radiates here

apex: good for first heart sound, murmurs from mitral or aortic valves third heart sound fourth heart sound

radiation of murmurs
1 mitral regurgitation: apex–axilla
2 aortic regurgitation: lower left sternal border
3 pulmonary stenosis: upper left sternal border clavicle
4 aortic stenosis: apex upper right sternal border neck

...ultation; the best sites for hearing sounds and murmurs depend on where the sound is produced
...blood flows radiate.

Differential diagnosis
Factors that may influence the intensity of the heart sounds

Loud first sound
- Hyperdynamic circulation (fever, exercise)
- Mitral stenosis
- Atrial myxoma (rare)

Soft first sound
- Low cardiac output (rest, heart failure)
- Tachycardia
- Severe mitral reflux (caused by destruction of valve)

Variable intensity of first sound
- Atrial fibrillation
- Complete heart block

Loud aortic component of second sound
- Systemic hypertension
- Dilated aortic root

Soft aortic component of second sound
- Calcific aortic stenosis

Loud pulmonary component of second sound
- Pulmonary hypertension

and either a thick chest wall or emphysema. A loud ringing second heart sound may be a feature of systemic hypertension or occasionally of pulmonary hypertension.

Third and fourth heart sounds

These are abnormal heart sounds that are heard in addition to the normal sounds in patients with certain specific conditions. The third heart sound is a low-pitched, thudding sound that occurs in diastole and coincides with the end of the rapid phase of ventricular filling. It occurs in two distinct sets of circumstances, one of which is physiological, the other pathological. A physiological third heart sound occurs in young fit adults under circumstances of increased cardiac output (e.g. in athletes, in the presence of a fever or during pregnancy). It is of no pathological significance. A pathological third heart sound is usually a marker for severe impairment of left ventricular function. It can be heard in dilated cardiomyopathy, after acute myocardial infarction or (in this case, coming from the right ventricle) in acute massive pulmonary embolism. In patients with a pathological third heart sound, there is nearly always a tachycardia and the first and second heart sounds are relatively quiet. The cadence of first,

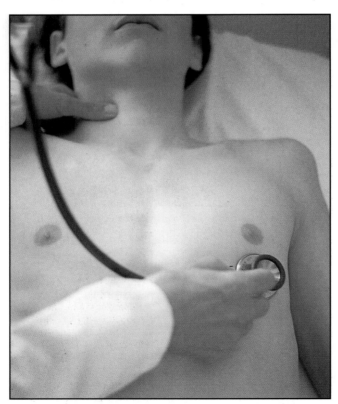

Fig. 6.56 Simultaneously listening to the heart sounds and timing them against the carotid pulse.

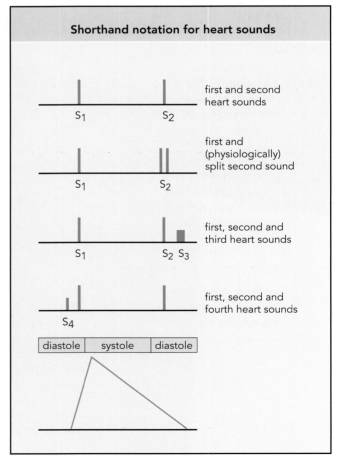

Fig. 6.57 Shorthand notation (derived from phonocardiography) for recording the heart sounds.

...rt sounds therefore sounds ...-boom, da-da-boom' and has ... a gallop rhythm. (The doctor ..., Phillippe Potain, served in ...so presumably knew a gallop

...d is an extra heart sound that ...ontraction. It is usually best ...e left atrium is hypertrophied ... of systemic hypertension or ...yopathy). It is not, however, ...s. A fourth sound sounds a little ...b-dup' (Fig. 6.58).

...unds

...is a high-pitched ringing sound ... very shortly after the first heart ... is a feature of aortic or pulmonary valve stenosis, in which it is probably caused by the sudden opening of the deformed valve. Sometimes, patients with a dilated pulmonary artery or an ascending aorta may have an ejection click without a stenotic valve.

Opening snap This is a diastolic sound heard in mitral stenosis and associated with the tensing of the diaphragm formed by the stenosed mitral valve. It is best heard to the left of the sternum and sounds rather like the second part of a widely split second heart sound.

Mid-systolic clicks These are usually associated with mitral valve prolapse and are caused by the tensing of the long and redundant chordae tendineae of these

valves. The clicks may or may not be associated with a late systolic murmur (Figs 6.60, 6.61).

Sounds from artificial heart valves The ball, disc or poppet in an artificial heart valve usually makes a noise both when it opens and when the valve closes. The closing sound is usually louder than the opening sound. Thus, an aortic prosthesis will have a soft opening click just after the first heart sound and a loud closing click which contributes to the second heart sound. Conversely, a mitral valve will give a soft opening click in a similar position to the opening snap of mitral stenosis and a loud closing click which contributes to the first heart sound.

Murmurs

Murmurs are more or less musical sounds occurring at specific points in the cardiac cycle and resulting from turbulent blood flow. The important points in analysing a murmur are where it occurs in the cardiac cycle, what it sounds like, where it is best heard, where it radiates to and what happens in manoeuvres like deep breathing.

Systolic murmurs Systolic murmurs are due to one of three things: leakage of blood through a structure

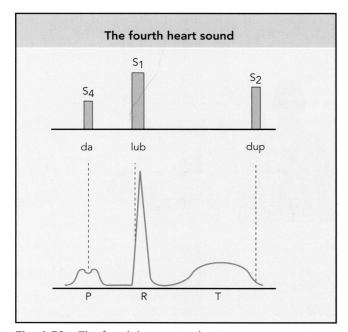

Fig. 6.58 The fourth heart sound.

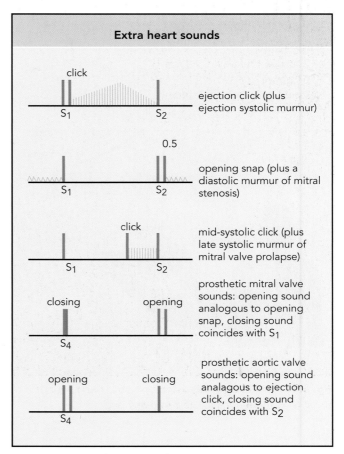

Fig. 6.59 Extra heart sounds.

that is normally closed during systole (mitral or tricuspid valves or the interventricular septum) blood flow through a valve normally open in systole but which has become abnormally narrowed

(e.g. aortic or pulmonary stenosis) or increased blood flow through a normal valve (a flow murmur).

Murmurs that are due to leakage of blood through an incompetent mitral or tricuspid valve or a ventricular septal defect are usually of similar intensity throughout the length of systole. They are called pansystolic or holosystolic murmurs (Fig. 6.60). Occasionally, a valve is competent at the start of systole but starts to leak half way through. This is common in patients with mitral valve prolapse. The result is a murmur that starts in mid- or late systole

Symptoms and signs
Grading the intensity of murmurs

- Grade 1 – just audible with a good stethoscope in a quiet room
- Grade 2 – quiet but readily audible with a stethoscope
- Grade 3 – easily heard with a stethoscope
- Grade 4 – a loud, obvious murmur
- Grade 5 – very loud, heard not only over the precordium but elsewhere in the body

Differential diagnosis
Systolic murmurs

Ejection systolic
- Innocent systolic murmur
- Aortic stenosis
- Pulmonary stenosis
- Hypertrophic cardiomyopathy
- Flow murmurs
  - atrial septal defect
  - fever
  - athlete's heart

Pansystolic
- Tricuspid reflux
- Mitral reflux
- Ventricular septal defect

Differential diagnosis
Sites of radiation of murmurs

Cause	'Primary site'	Radiation
Tricuspid regurgitation	Lower left sternal edge	Lower right sternal edge, liver
Pulmonary stenosis	Upper left sternal edge	Towards left clavicle, beneath left scapula
Mitral regurgitation	Apex	Left axilla, beneath left scapula
Aortic regurgitation	Left sternal edge	Down left sternal edge towards apex
Aortic stenosis	Apex	Towards upper right sternal edge, over carotids
Ventricular septal defect	Left sternal edge	All over pericardium
Mitral stenosis	Apex	Does not radiate

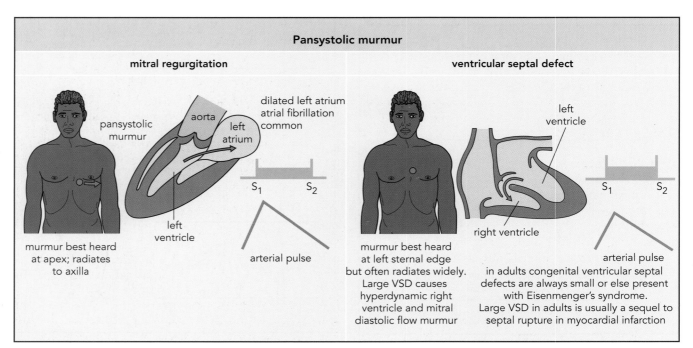

Pansystolic murmur

mitral regurgitation

pansystolic murmur

aorta

left atrium

dilated left atrium
atrial fibrillation common

left ventricle

S_1 S_2

arterial pulse

murmur best heard at apex; radiates to axilla

ventricular septal defect

left ventricle

right ventricle

S_1 S_2

arterial pulse

murmur best heard at left sternal edge but often radiates widely. Large VSD causes hyperdynamic right ventricle and mitral diastolic flow murmur

in adults congenital ventricular septal defects are always small or else present with Eisenmenger's syndrome. Large VSD in adults is usually a sequel to septal rupture in myocardial infarction

Fig. 6.60 Pansystolic (holosystolic) murmurs: mitral regurgitation (left), ventricular septal defect (right).

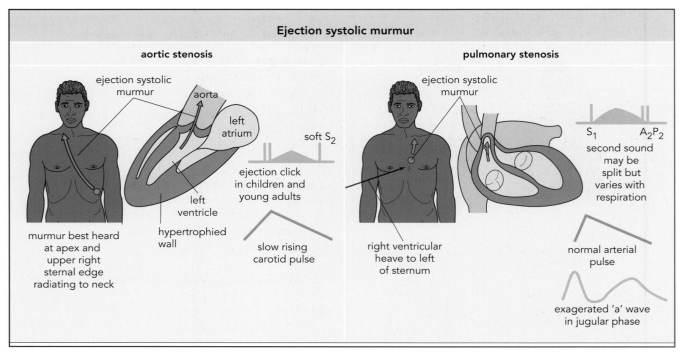

Fig. 6.61   Ejection systolic murmurs: aortic stenosis and pulmonary stenosis.

and is called a mid-systolic or late systolic murmur, respectively (Fig. 6.59).

Murmurs that are due to blood being forced through a narrow aortic or pulmonary valve or to increased blood flow through a normal aortic or pulmonary valve tend to start quietly at the beginning of systole, rise to a crescendo in midsystole and then become quiet again towards the end of systole. Such murmurs are called ejection systolic murmurs (Fig. 6.61).

Innocent murmurs   Innocent murmurs are murmurs that are not associated with any major structural abnormality in the heart nor with any haemodynamic disturbance. They are common in children and young adults. They have the following characteristics: always systolic and always quiet (less than grade 3); usually best heard at the left sternal edge; no associated ventricular hypertrophy; and normal heart sounds, pulses, chest radiograph and ECG.

Diastolic murmurs   Diastolic murmurs can be divided into early diastolic murmurs and mid-diastolic murmurs. An early diastolic murmur is nearly always caused by incompetence of either the aortic or the pulmonary valve. It is maximal at the beginning of diastole when aortic or pulmonary pressure is highest and rapidly becomes quieter (decrescendo) as pressure in the great vessel falls. The sound of an aortic diastolic murmur has aptly been described as like a whispered letter 'r' (Fig. 6.62).

A mid-diastolic murmur is usually caused by either blood flow through a narrowed mitral or tricuspid valve or, occasionally, to increased blood flow through

one of these valves (e.g. in children with atrial septal defect). The characteristic murmur of mitral stenosis is a low-pitched, rumbling murmur heard throughout diastole (Fig. 6.63). Sometimes, in patients in sinus rhythm, it gets louder just before the onset of systole as a result of atrial contraction increasing blood flow through the narrowed valve. Sometimes patients with aortic reflux have a mid-diastolic murmur. This is

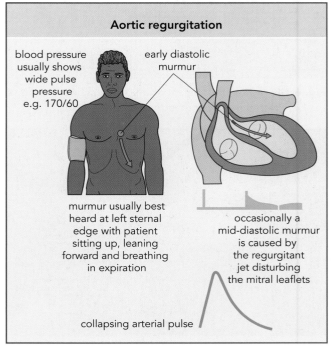

Fig. 6.62   Aortic regurgitation as an example of an early diastolic murmur.

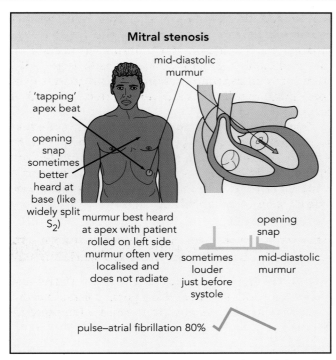

Mitral stenosis

mid-diastolic murmur

'tapping' apex beat

opening snap sometimes better heard at base (like widely split S₂)

murmur best heard at apex with patient rolled on left side murmur often very localised and does not radiate

sometimes louder just before systole

opening snap

mid-diastolic murmur

pulse–atrial fibrillation 80%

Fig. 6.63   Mitral stenosis as an example of a mid-diastolic murmur.

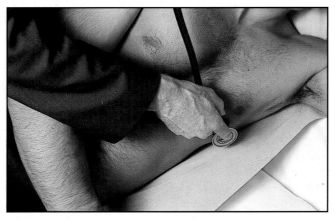

Fig. 6.64   Mitral diastolic murmurs are best heard using the bell, with the patient rolled onto the left side.

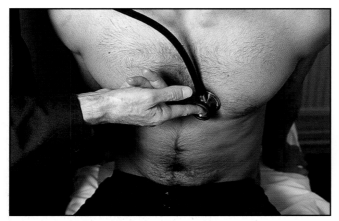

Fig. 6.65   Aortic diastolic murmurs may be heard more easily if the patient sits up, leans forward and holds the breath in expiration.

Differential diagnosis
Behaviour of murmurs in respiration

Louder immediately on inspiration
- Pulmonary stenosis
- Pulmonary valve flow murmurs

Quieter immediately on inspiration (may become louder later)
- Mitral regurgitation
- Aortic stenosis

Louder during Valsalva manoeuvre
- Hypertrophic obstructive cardiomyopathy
- The murmur of mitral prolapse may become louder or softer during inspiration

caused by the regurgitant blood from the incompetent aortic valve setting up a vibration of the anterior leaflet of the mitral valve (Austin Flint murmur).

Murmurs tend to be heard best over the site of the lesion that is causing them and in the direction of the turbulent bloodstream that is producing the sound. It is sometimes possible to make murmurs easier to hear by putting the patient into special positions. The murmur of mitral stenosis is best heard if the patient is rolled onto his or her left side and the stethoscope bell applied to the cardiac apex (Fig. 6.64). The murmur of aortic reflux is sometimes best heard if the patient is made to sit up, lean forward and breathe out fully while the stethoscope is applied at the left side of the lower part of the sternum (Fig. 6.65).

The behaviour of murmurs during respiration sometimes gives a clue to their nature. Systolic murmurs arising at the pulmonary valve (i.e. pulmonary stenosis flow murmurs) tend to get louder during inspiration and quieter during expiration. Conversely, murmurs arising on the left side of the heart tend to get quieter during inspiration. Making the patient perform a Valsalva maneuvre (forceful expiration against a closed glottis) makes most murmurs quieter, for cardiac output is diminished, whereas the murmur of hypertrophic obstructive cardiomyopathy (an ejection systolic murmur arising from the left ventricular outlet tract) tends to get louder as the degree of obstruction increases. The murmur of mitral stenosis is often easier to hear if the patient is made to exercise before listening for it.

CARDIOVASCULAR SYSTEM AND CHEST EXAMINATION

The most important feature to look for in a patient with cardiac disease is the presence of crackles at the lung bases. These occur during inspiration and are an early sign of pulmonary oedema. In mild heart failure, crackles are confined to the lung bases but in severe failure they may be heard all over the chest. Patients with severe heart failure and peripheral oedema may also develop pleural effusions. Examination of the chest is discussed in detail in Chapter 5.

CARDIOVASCULAR SYSTEM AND ABDOMINAL EXAMINATION

Abdominal examination (see Ch. 7) also plays an important part in the examination of patients with suspected cardiovascular disease. The principal points to check for are the presence of ascites, an enlarged or pulsatile liver, an aortic aneurysm and, particularly in patients with high blood pressure, the presence of enlarged kidneys or a renal artery bruit.

The liver is a very vascular organ and will enlarge in response to any rise in right atrial pressure. Sometimes, particularly if the enlargement is rapid, this leads to acute discomfort in the right upper quadrant of the abdomen. The liver edge is characteristically firm and even. In patients with tricuspid reflux, there is a marked hepatic pulsation in time with the regurgitation waves in the jugular venous pulse and with the arterial pulse.

In severe heart failure, the spleen may also become passively enlarged. However, this is less common and less prominent than hepatic enlargement. Enlargement of the spleen in its role as part of the immune system is seen in subacute bacterial endocarditis.

Aneurysm of the abdominal aorta is common, particularly in men over the age of 60 years. It is important to detect because early elective surgery carries a much lower mortality than emergency surgery. The characteristic finding on examination is pulsation at about the level of the umbilicus. It is easy to feel the normal aorta at this level, yet the characteristic features of an aneurysm are that it is enlarged in comparison with a normal aorta and that the pulsation it generates is expansile (Fig. 6.66). Abdominal ultrasound examination is a good way of confirming the diagnosis of aortic aneurysm and of measuring its size.

Enlarged kidneys caused by polycystic disease sometimes present as hypertension, even heart failure. Another cause of hypertension is renal artery stenosis. In this condition, it is sometimes possible to hear a murmur or bruit with the stethoscope applied to one side or other of the umbilicus.

PERIPHERAL VASCULAR SYSTEM

Assess the skin temperature in the feet and feel and record the popliteal and dorsalis pedis pulses. Look for varicose veins and venous ulcers and for the presence of oedema.

OEDEMA
Oedema is the collection of an abnormal amount of tissue fluid. This fluid accumulates in the extracellular spaces between cells and leads to local swelling. Tissue fluid is normally in dynamic equilibrium with plasma, so that the amount of fluid escaping from blood vessels is normally exactly balanced by the quantity of fluid being returned to the blood vessels in addition to that which is drained away by the lymphatic vessels (Fig. 6.67). Heart failure is an important cause of oedema. The oedema of heart failure is largely the result of increased venous pressure but factors such as a slightly reduced plasma albumin concentration and abnormal capillary permeability may also play a role.

The oedema of heart failure can be divided into pulmonary oedema and peripheral oedema. Peripheral oedema is usually a feature of right-sided heart failure or congestive heart failure. It character-

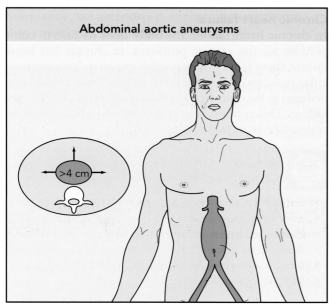

Fig. 6.66 Abdominal aortic aneurysm is felt as an 'expansile swelling' in the abdomen.

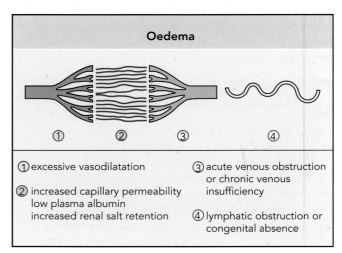

① excessive vasodilatation
② increased capillary permeability low plasma albumin increased renal salt retention
③ acute venous obstruction or chronic venous insufficiency
④ lymphatic obstruction or congenital absence

Fig. 6.67 The factors contributing to oedema formation.

Symptoms and signs
Hyperlipidaemia

Common
- Corneal arcus (nonspecific in patients over 50 years old)
  Xanthelasma (nonspecific in patients over 50 years old)
- Tendon xanthomas (mainly in familial hypercholesterolaemia)

Less common
- Palmar xanthomas
- Eruptive xanthomas
- Ejection systolic murmur (familial hypercholesterolaemia)
- Lipaemia retinalis

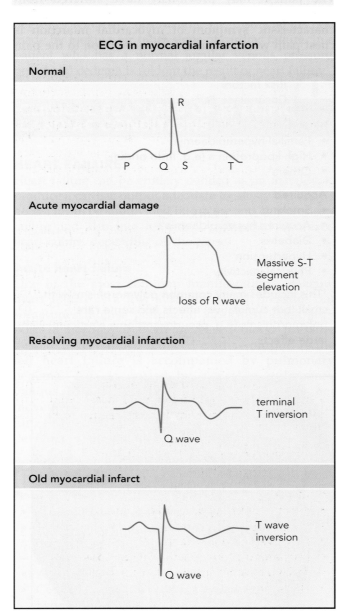

Fig. 6.72 ECG showing features of acute myocardial infarction.

Symptoms and signs
Acute myocardial infarction

Symptoms
- Severe pain
- Pain persists despite rest

Physical signs
- Signs of sympathetic activation (pallor, sweating)
- Narrow pulse pressures
- May be extrasystoles
- May be added (third) heart sound

of angina but is usually much more severe and persists even when the patient rests. In a small proportion of patients, particularly elderly people and individuals with diabetes mellitus, myocardial infarction can be relatively painless.

On physical examination, there is nearly always marked evidence of sympathetic nervous system activation, the blood pressure tends to be low with a narrow pulse pressure, there may be a third heart sound and there are frequently ventricular extrasystoles. The diagnosis of myocardial infarction is usually confirmed by electrocardiography (Fig. 6.72) and by characteristic changes in the plasma level of cardiac enzymes.

The main risk in the early stages of acute myocardial infarction is of ventricular fibrillation. This requires constant observation of the patient and treatment if necessary with a defibrillator. Later complications include arrhythmias, cardiac rupture and, occasionally, the development of ventricular septal defect or mitral reflux.

Chronic heart failure due to ischaemic heart disease has the clinical features of any other form of chronic heart failure but diagnosis is usually made on the basis of the history.

PERIPHERAL VASCULAR DISEASE

This can be considered under two headings: disease of the peripheral arterial system and disease of the peripheral venous system. Peripheral arterial disease is mainly to do with acute or chronic impairment of the blood supply to a limb. This may result from atheromatous narrowing of the artery, from thrombosis or much more rarely from embolism from the heart.

Acute arterial obstruction presents with a cold, white, painful, pulseless limb. The site of obstruction is usually obvious from examining the pulses but confirmation by ultrasound or by angiography before surgery is generally necessary. It is important to check pulses in the other limbs as well, even if they are not obviously ischaemic. Embolism to multiple sites may be the first clue to a cardiac disease such as atrial myxoma.

Chronic arterial insufficiency is much more common in the lower limb and usually presents as intermittent claudication. The patient is aware of pain, in the leg, the thigh or the buttock, which comes on with walking and goes away when stopping to rest. Examination of the leg reveals weak or absent foot, knee and sometimes femoral pulses. There may be a murmur or bruit over the femoral artery because of turbulence due to narrowing upstream in the internal or external iliac arteries. As the disease progresses, pain comes on with progressively less exertion until finally the patient experiences pain at rest. Pain is often worse at night. Patients with severe chronic arterial insufficiency in the legs often gain partial relief by hanging their leg over the side of the bed outside the bedclothes. Paradoxically, this often makes perfusion of the foot worse. The skin tends to become discoloured and shiny, and hair is lost from the foot. Infection, which often starts with a small injury such as one derived from paring the toenails, spreads rapidly. Eventually, gangrene may affect the toes and foot (Fig. 6.73).

Patients with diabetes mellitus are particularly susceptible to peripheral arterial disease. As diabetes affects both large and small blood vessels and also the intercellular matrix of the tissues, peripheral tissue damage tends to be more severe than would be expected from the large vessel pulses alone. The position is made worse by diabetic neuropathy, which means that patients may sustain injuries giving rise to infection without noticing much discomfort until the infection is well established.

The main aids to clinical diagnosis in peripheral arterial disease are ultrasound examination, which can detect both vessel diameter and blood flow, and angiography.

DISEASES OF THE PERIPHERAL VEINS

The principal diseases of the peripheral veins are varicose veins, thrombophlebitis and deep venous thrombosis.

Varicose veins

Varicose veins are excessively dilated superficial leg veins. They usually result from defects in the 'muscle pump' system that normally pumps venous blood from the legs via the deep veins against the force of gravity. In adopting an upright posture, the human race has considerably increased the difficulty of securing adequate venous drainage from the legs. The two major causes of varicose veins are defective valves in the 'perforating veins' which connect the deep and superficial venous systems in the calf and defective valves in the upper part of the long saphenous vein where it joins the femoral vein at the thigh. Commonly, the problem is initiated by incompetent valves in the perforating veins and saphenofemoral incompetence is secondary to the resulting dilatation of the superficial venous system.

Varicose veins are always most apparent when the patient is standing upright and empty completely when the legs are raised above heart level. By elevating the legs to empty the veins and then watching the veins fill as the leg is lowered, it is often possible to see the sites of incompetent perforating veins and to control them by local finger pressure. If the saphenofemoral junction is incompetent, it may be necessary first to prevent blood flowing back from the femoral vein by tying a tourniquet around the upper thigh. Identification of the site of perforating veins is an important step in treating varicose veins by injecting a sclerosant solution around incompetent perforators. Very advanced varicose veins may still need to be treated by ligating and stripping the long (and sometimes the short) saphenous vein. The importance of the long saphenous vein as a conduit in coronary bypass surgery makes it important to preserve this vessel if possible.

Chronic venous insufficiency

Failure or inadequacy of the 'muscle pump' mechanism may also lead to chronic oedema of the legs and feet, with or without obvious varicose veins. This is more common in elderly, obese and sedentary patients and tends to become self-perpetuating because the legs are often painful to walk on. The oedema is often relatively firm and pits only reluctantly on pressure; it is usually least apparent in the morning and gets worse as the day goes on. The condition is distinguished from heart failure because the jugular venous pressure is normal. Sometimes chronic venous insufficiency is associated with obstruction of the inferior vena cava but in this case

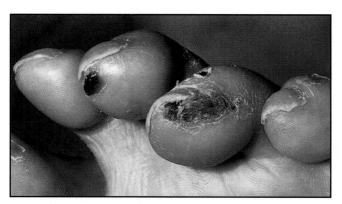

Fig. 6.73 Gangrene of toes in peripheral vascular disease.

 Risk factors
Varicose veins

- Obesity
- Stasis from sitting or standing (position)
- Pregnancy
- Pelvic venous obstruction
- Damage to deep veins from thrombosis
- Trauma to short or long saphenous vein
- Hereditary

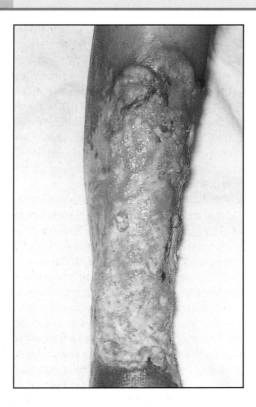

Fig. 6.74
Severe varicose ulceration of the leg.

there are usually grossly distended veins on the abdominal wall.

Varicose ulceration and eczema

Chronic venous insufficiency results in a rise in tissue pressure in the skin and subcutaneous tissues which can interfere with adequate nutrient blood flow. This may lead to skin necrosis and ulceration, most commonly at the ankle just above the malleoli. The skin is often dusky and indurated. Scarring as part of the healing process tends to impair the microcirculation further and the condition may become self-perpetuating (Fig. 6.74).

Thrombophlebitis

Superficial thrombophlebitis is inflammation and thrombosis of a superficial vein. This commonly results either from local trauma or from an intravenous infusion but may occur spontaneously. There is local pain, redness and tenderness over the course of the vein. The condition is usually benign and self-limiting but septic thrombophlebitis from a drip site infection can lead to septicaemia.

Deep vein thrombosis

Thrombosis of the deep veins in the calf or pelvis usually occurs as a result of a combination of damage to the endothelial lining of the veins, with stasis of the blood within them as a consequence of physical inactivity. Until measures were taken to prevent it by encouraging early mobilisation and using low dosage heparin, it was a common complication of any form of major surgery. In some patients, deep vein thrombosis occurs in the absence of any obvious external cause; it is important

that these patients should be investigated for abnormalities of the blood clotting and fibrinolytic systems.

The characteristic clinical features of deep vein thrombosis in the leg are pain, swelling and occasionally redness. The pain is a deep aching pain which is worse on activity but persists at rest. Sometimes it is absent. The leg may be swollen (compare it with the other one) and there is often dilatation of the superficial veins and a warm skin as a result of blood flow diversion from the deep to the superficial veins. Pain in the calf can sometimes be produced by dorsiflexing the foot but as this can sometimes cause a detachment thrombus in the form of an embolism it is not recommended. If pain and swelling are mainly below the knee, then it is likely that the thrombosis is in the calf veins. If, however, the swelling and tenderness extend to the thigh or the groin, then the thrombosis may involve the femoral or iliac veins: this is potentially more serious because thromboembolism from these sites is frequently massive.

The main differential diagnosis of deep vein thrombosis in legs is from spontaneous rupture of the gastrocnemius muscle and rupture of an arthritic Baker's cyst from the knee joint. The diagnosis of deep vein thrombosis needs to be confirmed with either ultrasound scanning or phlebography. It is important to remember that deep vein thrombosis, particularly in elderly people, may be accompanied by very few clinical signs and often goes unnoticed until it presents as pulmonary embolism.

The intact endothelium in the veins of the body normally prevents thrombus formation and any small quantity of thrombus that does form is dealt with by the body's own thrombolytic mechanisms. If extensive thrombi do form in veins, one may become detached and travel through the great veins to the heart, where it may either lodge in the right ventricle or in the pulmonary artery. Clinically, pulmonary embolism may present in three ways: pulmonary infarction, acute massive pulmonary embolus and chronic thromboembolic pulmonary hypertension.

Acute pulmonary infarction

This is usually the consequence of a relatively small pulmonary embolus that lodges in a branch of the pulmonary artery. As a result of spasm and reduced air entry, a wedge-shaped section of the lung downstream

 Differential diagnosis
Deep vein thrombosis

Pain and swelling in the leg may be caused by:
- deep vein thrombosis
- ruptured head of gastrocnemius muscle
- ruptured osteoarthritic cyst (Baker's cyst) of knee joint
- anterior compartment syndrome (skin splints)

of the block becomes necrotic. This induces pleural inflammation over the infarct and the resulting pleurisy causes pain. The clinical presentation is with the relatively sudden onset of pleuritic chest pain. The patient may be moderately breathless but is seldom hypotensive. Arterial blood gas measurements often show marked hypoxaemia, but the partial pressure of carbon dioxide is normal. The chest radiograph may show a wedge-shaped opacity based on the pleura. A perfusion lung scan often shows other perfusion defects besides that causing the infarct. It is important to look for other evidence of deep vein thrombosis, both by clinical examination and by phlebography, because the pulmonary infarction may be a warning of a possible massive pulmonary embolus later on.

Acute massive pulmonary embolism

This is most common in postoperative patients. The patient suddenly becomes extremely short of breath, severely hypotensive and may not be able to sit upright. There is often an urge to evacuate the bowels. The jugular veins are markedly distended and the liver may also be enlarged. Heart sounds are usually quiet because of the reduced cardiac output. Nonetheless, there may be a third sound best heard to the left of the sternum. The chest radiograph is usually unhelpful but the ECG shows characteristic features of acute right ventricular strain. Echocardiography shows a dilated, poorly contracting, right ventricle and a small underfilled left ventricle. Definitive diagnosis is by pulmonary angiography.

Chronic pulmonary hypertension

Chronic thromboembolic pulmonary hypertension is a result of multiple pulmonary emboli over a period of time. The clinical features are those of chronic pulmonary hypertension. The causal diagnosis can sometimes be made on the basis of recurrent history of deep vein thrombosis but sometimes has to be made on the basis of pulmonary angiography or lung biopsy.

INFECTIVE ENDOCARDITIS

Infective endocarditis is an infection of the endocardial lining of the heart. There are three principal clinical types: acute endocarditis, subacute endocarditis and postoperative endocarditis.

Acute endocarditis

Acute endocarditis is the result of infection of a normal or abnormal heart with a virulent organism such as *Staphylococcus aureus* or *Streptococcus pneumoniae*. The infection usually involves one of the heart valves but may involve the endocardium next to a defect such as a ventricular septal defect. The infection may cause destruction of valve tissue, abscess formation or the formation of large vegetations which are composed of masses of bacteria, platelets and thrombin. The patient is nearly always severely ill with a fever and marked systemic symptoms. One of the characteristic clinical findings is that heart murmurs develop or change rapidly as the destructive process goes on. There may also be systemic emboli as portions of vegetation break off and are carried away by the bloodstream. There may be finger clubbing and splinter haemorrhages but often they do not have time to develop, so rapid is the course of the disease.

Subacute endocarditis

Subacute endocarditis may result either from infection of a diseased heart valve or septal defect with an indolent organism, such as *Streptococcus sanguis*, or from the partial treatment of acute endocarditis with inadequate doses of antibiotics. The time course of the illness is much more insidious. Patients present with unexplained fever, excessive tiredness, depressive symptoms or with the consequences of valve destruction or systemic embolisation. There is nearly always a heart murmur: the combination of fever and a heart murmur should always lead to suspicion of endocarditis. As in acute endocarditis, the murmurs may change but this is usually over a time course of days or weeks rather than hours. Finger clubbing and splinter haemorrhages are common. In neglected cases there may be anaemia and a brown pigmentation of the skin. There is often splenomegaly. There may be localised subconjunctival haemorrhages, tender swellings (Osler's nodes) in the finger pulps and haemorrhagic spots (Roth spots) in the retina. All these are features of a systemic vasculitis.

Postoperative endocarditis

Postoperative endocarditis occurs in patients who have had open heart surgery and may involve artificial heart valves or other implanted material. The most common organism is a coagulase-negative staphylococcus. The clinical features may resemble those of acute or subacute endocarditis.

MYOCARDITIS

Myocarditis is an inflammatory infection of heart muscle, usually the result of a virus infection. Clinically, this may present with heart failure or an arrhythmia. There may be cardiac dilatation, a third heart sound or a systolic murmur from 'functional' mitral incompetence resulting from dilatation of the ventricle.

CARDIOMYOPATHY

Cardiomyopathy is a general term meaning 'heart muscle disease'. Clinically, cardiomyopathy can be classified into hypertrophic, dilated and restrictive types.

Hypertrophic cardiomyopathy

Hypertrophic cardiomyopathy is characterised by excessive cardiac muscle hypertrophy in the absence of a stimulus such as hypertension. The hypertrophy may be 'asymmetrical', that is, it specifically affects the

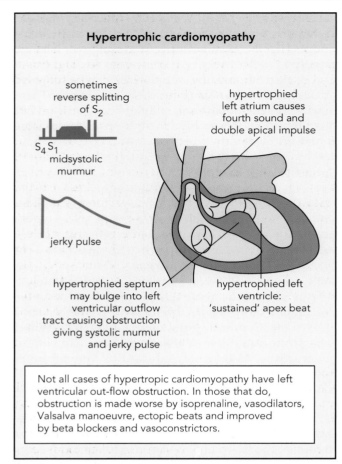

Hypertrophic cardiomyopathy

sometimes reverse splitting of S₂

$S_4 S_1$ midsystolic murmur

jerky pulse

hypertrophied left atrium causes fourth sound and double apical impulse

hypertrophied septum may bulge into left ventricular outflow tract causing obstruction giving systolic murmur and jerky pulse

hypertrophied left ventricle: 'sustained' apex beat

Not all cases of hypertropic cardiomyopathy have left ventricular out-flow obstruction. In those that do, obstruction is made worse by isoprenaline, vasodilators, Valsalva manoeuvre, ectopic beats and improved by beta blockers and vasoconstrictors.

Fig. 6.75   Findings in hypertrophic cardiomyopathy.

interventricular septum, which bulges into the left ventricular outflow tract and causes obstruction to blood flow. This variant is called hypertrophic obstructive cardiomyopathy; some patients with this condition die suddenly, often when engaged in sport or exercise. The clinical features of hypertrophic obstructive cardiomyopathy are summarised in Figure 6.75.

Dilated cardiomyopathy
Dilated cardiomyopathy is characterised by a global impairment of left ventricular function, leading to progressive dilatation of the ventricles. The basic cause is unknown but similar patterns can be reproduced in association with excessive alcohol intake or systemic diseases (e.g. sarcoidois). Clinical presentation is usually with heart failure. There is a displaced apex beat, a gallop rhythm and possibly secondary mitral or tricuspid regurgitation.

Restrictive cardiomyopathy
This is a rare condition in Western countries. The clinical presentation mimics constrictive pericarditis.

ACUTE RHEUMATIC FEVER
Acute rheumatic fever is a consequence of an auto-immune response to heart tissue precipitated by exposure to certain strains of streptococcus. It is now very uncommon in Western countries, although its long-term consequences are still seen as an important cause of chronic valvular heart disease. Clinically, acute rheumatic fever presents in children or young adults either with an acute, migratory (i.e. flitting from joint to joint) polyarthritis or with chorea.

Cardiac involvement is usually signalled by the development of a murmur: either a pansystolic murmur of mitral regurgitation or a soft mid-diastolic murmur that resembles that of mitral stenosis. The latter is called a Carey Coombs murmur and is probably caused by oedema of the mitral valve cusps and by small platelet vegetations. There is commonly a skin rash, which again is often fleeting and variable. Rheumatic nodules are not seen in all cases but are virtually pathognomonic; they consist of firm subcutaneous nodules, often on the extensor surfaces of knees and elbows.

PERICARDIAL DISEASE
The heart normally contracts within a smooth, closely fitting serous cavity: the pericardium. The principal pericardial diseases are acute pericarditis, pericardial effusion and chronic constrictive pericarditis.

Acute pericarditis
The symptoms of acute pericarditis have already been discussed under chest pain. The most characteristic physical finding is the pericardial rub. This is often mistaken for a murmur but it usually has a distinct scratchy quality. In patients in sinus rhythm, there are often three components to the pericardial rub, corresponding to atrial contraction, ventricular contraction and ventricular relaxation. Pericardial rubs are often best heard if the patient is made to sit up, lean forward and breathe out fully (similar to the position for hearing aortic diastolic murmurs). It is characteristic of a pericardial rub in that it comes and goes over a period of a few hours. Patients with acute pericarditis are often pyrexic and may feel systemically unwell.

Pericardial effusion
Normally, there is only just sufficient fluid in the pericardial cavity to lubricate the heart in its movements. An excess of accumulation of pericardial fluid is called a pericardial effusion.

The clinical features of a pericardial effusion depend both on the amount of fluid and the speed with which it accumulates. A large amount of fluid or the very rapid accumulation of fluid causes compression of the heart, particularly the right ventricle, and can cause a substantial reduction in cardiac output. This is cardiac tamponade and is a medical emergency. The patient is often very ill, hypotensive and peripherally constricted. There may be pulsus paradoxus: a variation in pulse volume with respiration (Fig. 6.76). The jugular venous pressure is very high but this may be hard to see because the patient may be too hypotensive to sit upright. Even a small amount of fluid, if it accumulates rapidly, can cause cardiac tamponade, meaning that signs such as cardiac enlargement on a chest radiograph or an increased area of dullness to percussion in the front of the chest are unreliable in diagnosing cardiac tamponade. The best way of confirming the diagnosis is by bedside echocardiography, which can be followed immediately by pericardiocentesis.

If fluid accumulates slowly in the pericardium over days or weeks, then it is often accommodated by stretching of the pericardium rather than cardiac tamponade. The chronic pericardial effusion may be picked up by accident or (more commonly) it presents as chronic predominantly right-sided cardiac failure, often with very marked peripheral oedema and perhaps ascites. There may or may not be a pericardial rub. There is often an enlarged area of dullness on percussion to the left of the sternum. The jugular venous pressure is usually markedly elevated. There may be a paradoxical pulse but it is often less prominent than in acute cardiac tamponade. Chest radiography shows cardiac enlargement. Again, echocardiography is the simplest investigation to confirm the diagnosis.

Chronic constrictive pericarditis

Chronic as opposed to acute inflammation of the pericardium may lead to a thickened fibrotic pericardial membrane that, as a long-term result of scarring, constricts and compresses the heart. Worldwide, the most common cause of this is chronic tuberculous pericarditis but it may also follow acute viral pericarditis or cardiac surgery.

The clinical features of chronic constrictive pericarditis are similar to those of chronic pericardial effusion. There tends to be predominantly right-

---

Differential diagnosis
Pericardial effusion

Infection
- Viral pericarditis
- Bacterial pericarditis (streptococcus)
- Tuberculous pericarditis

Myocardial infarction
- Peri-infarct pericarditis
- Cardiac rupture
- Dressler's syndrome

Malignant pericarditis
- Secondary (common) or primary (rare) tumours
- Leukaemia

Autoallergic
- Acute rheumatic fever
- Rheumatoid arthritis

Other
- Myxoedema
- Trauma (stab wounds)
- After cardiac surgery

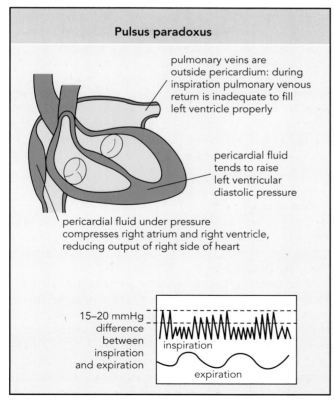

Pulsus paradoxus

pulmonary veins are outside pericardium: during inspiration pulmonary venous return is inadequate to fill left ventricle properly

pericardial fluid tends to raise left ventricular diastolic pressure

pericardial fluid under pressure compresses right atrium and right ventricle, reducing output of right side of heart

15–20 mmHg difference between inspiration and expiration

inspiration

expiration

Fig. 6.76 Pulses paradoxus or the apparent diminution of the pulse on inspiration is a feature of pericardial tamponade.

Symptoms and signs
Cardiac tamponade

Causes
- Any cause of pericardial effusion (see differential diagnosis box)
- Pneumonia
- Trauma

Clinical presentation
- Hypotension
- Oliguria
- Raised jugular venous pulse
- Paradoxical pulse

Diagnosis
- Chest radiograph: enlarged heart shadow
- ECG: small voltages, 'electrical alternans'
- Echo: effusion with collapse of right ventricle

Treatment
- Pericardiocentesis
- Surgical drainage

sided heart failure, often with massive oedema. The jugular venous pressure is elevated and often has a characteristic pulse waveform, with a very rapid dip in the pulse as the tricuspid valve opens, followed by an equally abrupt termination as filling of the ventricle is curtailed. In longstanding severe constrictive pericarditis, the pericardium may become adherent to the ribcage and the examiner can feel a tugging on the posterior ribs in time with the heart beat.

 Examination of elderly people
Cardiovascular examination

- General approach and techniques unaltered
- Some stress tests may be impractical but there are alternatives
- Likely to be multisystem disease
- Common problems are hypertension, ischaemic heart disease and peripheral vascular disease
- Ischaemic heart disease may be asymptomatic
- Acute myocardial infarction may be 'silent'
- Ankle swelling usually clue to venous insufficiency not heart failure
- Aortic stenosis is common and difficult to diagnose but worth treating if severe
- Cardiac arrhythmias are common and do not generally require investigation unless symptomatic
- Causes of dizziness or transient loss of consciousness include postural hypotension (often drug induced), vertebrobasilar insufficiency, arrhythmias (especially bradycardia)
- Multiple drug therapy may be the cause of the problem – nonsteroidals cause fluid retention and hypertension

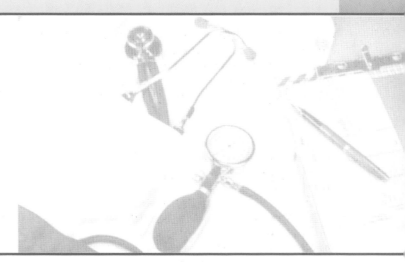

7.
The Abdomen

The abdominal examination follows that of the heart and lungs. Diseases of the abdominal organs may already be apparent from the general examination: for example, you may have noticed jaundice when examining the skin and eyes and in patients with obstructive jaundice, scratch marks may be apparent. You may have been aware of abnormal weight loss, signs of malnutrition or anaemia. Underlying iron deficiency may be revealed by a smooth, atrophic tongue and by cracks at the angles of the mouth (cheilosis), which may also suggest a vitamin B group deficiency.

STRUCTURE AND FUNCTION

The symptoms and signs of abdominal disease reflect disorder in the anatomy and physiology of the major abdominal organs. These organs are packed neatly into the abdominal cavity (Fig. 7.1) The liver, gallbladder and spleen lie protected under cover of the lower thoracic ribs, whereas the stomach, 6 m of small intestine and 1.5 m of large bowel cover and cushion the pancreas, kidneys and ureters. The urinary bladder, and in women the ovaries and adnexae, lie hidden deep in the protective wall of the pelvis.

GASTROINTESTINAL TRACT

Mouth and oesophagus

Digestion begins in the mouth where food is chewed and moistened with saliva. The salivary fluid is a cocktail of enzymes, including amylase and lingual lipase and bicarbonate and lysozyme. Saliva is secreted by the parotid, submandibular and sublingual glands, with a small contribution from the labial glands on the inner aspects of the lips.

Swallowing is controlled by a medullary centre in the brainstem which relays to and from the pharynx and

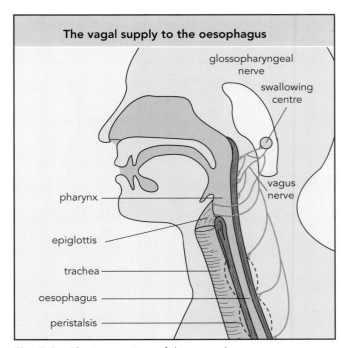

Fig. 7.1 The anatomical relationships of the major digestive organs.

Fig. 7.2 The innervation of the oesophagus.

oesophagus via the glossopharyngeal and vagus nerves (Fig. 7.2). There is also an intrinsic innervation within the smooth muscle of the oesophagus. There are three phases to the swallowing reflex: oral, pharyngeal and oesophageal. During the oral phase, the tongue presses the bolus up against the hard palate and drives the food into the pharynx. In the pharyngeal phase, the respiratory tract closes off, the upper pharyngeal sphincter (cricopharyngeus) relaxes and the upper, middle and lower pharyngeal constrictors propel the food into the oesophagus. In the oesophageal phase, a powerful peristaltic wave propels the bolus towards the stomach. The lower oesophageal sphincter has intrinsic tone that prevents regurgitation of the gastric contents: it relaxes in advance of the peristaltic wave and remains relaxed for a few seconds after the wave has passed.

Difficulty swallowing (dysphagia) may be caused by damage to the neural control, abnormalities of the oesophageal muscle or obstruction of the lumen.

Stomach

The churning action of the stomach continues the mixing process started in the mouth and prepares food for its journey into the duodenum. The parietal cells in the body of this muscular organ (Fig. 7.3) secrete hydrochloric acid, which sterilises the meal, and an intrinsic factor, which is necessary for the absorption of vitamin B_{12} in the terminal ileum. The chief cells secrete pepsinogen which is converted to the proteolytic enzyme pepsin by the low pH of the stomach lumen. The secretion of acid is stimulated by the vagus nerve, distension of the stomach with food and the secretion of the hormone gastrin from the G-cells of the gastric antrum (Fig. 7.4). A mucous layer coats the stomach mucosa, protecting it from self-inflicted injury by acid and pepsin.

Regurgitation of gastric contents into the oesophagus is prevented by an antireflux mechanism at the gastro-oesophageal junction. This includes the intrinsic tone of the lower oesophageal sphincter, the flap-valve effect of the angle of His and the squeezing effect of intra-abdominal pressure on the small segment of oesophagus that protrudes through the diaphragm into the abdomen (Fig. 7.5). If one or more of these antireflux mechanisms breaks down, gastric contents may regurgitate into the lower oesophagus, damaging the mucosa and causing heartburn.

Small intestine

The small intestine comprises the duodenum, the jejunum and the ileum. It fills most of the anterior

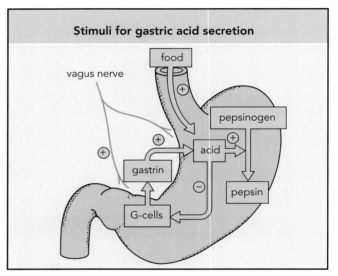

Fig. 7.4 The control of gastric acid secretion by food, vagal stimulation and gastrin. Pepsinogen is activated to pepsin at low pH.

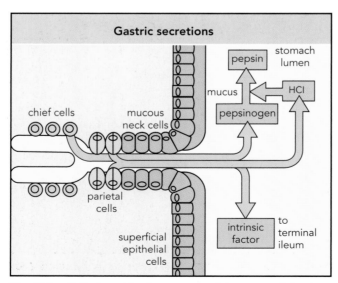

Fig. 7.3 Cells found in the mucosa of the stomach body are responsible for the principal gastric secretions.

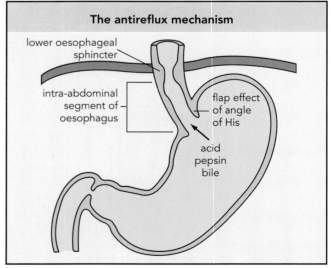

Fig. 7.5 The antireflux mechanism comprises the intrinsic tone of the lower oesophageal sphincter, the acute angle formed at the oesophagogastric junction (angle of His) and the pressure on the intra-abdominal oesophagus.

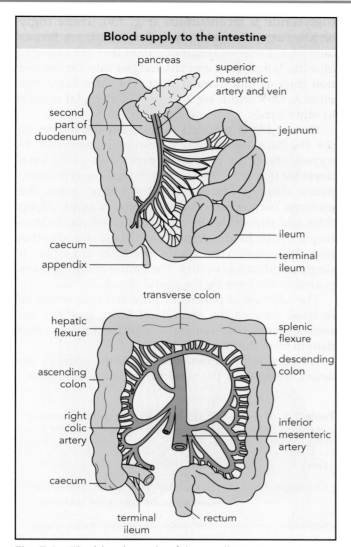

Blood supply to the intestine

pancreas

superior mesenteric artery and vein

second part of duodenum

jejunum

caecum

ileum

appendix

terminal ileum

transverse colon

hepatic flexure

splenic flexure

descending colon

ascending colon

right colic artery

inferior mesenteric artery

caecum

terminal ileum

rectum

Fig. 7.6 The blood supply of the small intestine, colon, sigmoid and rectum.

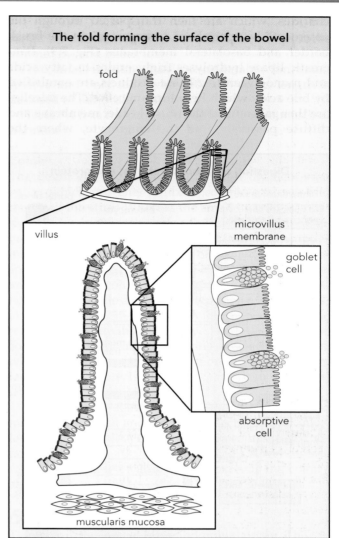

The fold forming the surface of the bowel

fold

villus

microvillus membrane

goblet cell

absorptive cell

muscularis mucosa

Fig. 7.7 The large surface area of the small intestine is formed by the duodenal folds, the villi and the microvillous membrane of the enterocyte.

abdomen and is framed by the ascending, transverse and descending colon. Blood is supplied by the superior mesenteric vessels (Fig. 7.6). The principal role of the small intestine is digestion and absorption, which is achieved by a combination of macroscopic and microscopic folds creating a vast absorptive area (Fig. 7.7).

Most of the enzymes necessary for the digestion of fat, protein and carbohydrate are present in the duodenum. Enterocytes develop in the base of the crypts of Lieberkuhn and migrate to the tip of the finger-shaped villi (Fig. 7.8). Both the enterocyte's capacity to produce specialised digestive enzymes on the brush border membrane and its absorptive properties develop progressively as the cell migrates towards the villous tip, at which point these functions are maximally developed.

Carbohydrate digestion is initiated by salivary and pancreatic amylase. Enzymes, such as lactase and sucrase, on the brush border membranes of the enterocytes, complete the digestion of complex polysaccharides and disaccharides to monosac-

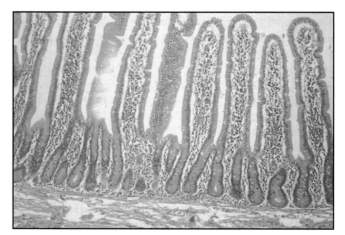

Fig. 7.8 Duodenal enterocytes develop in the crypts and migrate towards the villous tip.

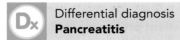 Differential diagnosis
Pancreatitis

- Idiopathic
- Toxic (alcohol, drugs)
- Common bile duct stone
- Abdominal trauma
- Mumps

of the organ. The pain can usually be localised to the epigastric, periumbilical or suprapubic areas, depending on whether the affected organ is derived from the embryological foregut, midgut or hindgut (Fig. 7.21). Pain arising from foregut is felt in the epigastrium; midgut pain is perceived around the umbilicus; and pain arising from the hindgut is felt in the suprapubic area. Visceral pain may also radiate to specific sites and this helps to establish its origin (Fig. 7.22). It is

Diagnostic features of abdominal pain

Disorder	Localisation	Character	Aggravating factors	Relieving factors	Visceral symptoms	Major physical signs	Diagnostic test
Acute pancreatitis	Epigastric and left hypochondrium radiating to back	Severe, constant pain		May improve when sitting forward	Nausea, vomiting	Tachycardia, shock, tender upper abdomen with guarding. Bruising in flanks	Raised serum and urinary amylase
Acute cholecystitis/ biliary colic	Right hypochondrium/ epigastrium radiating to right scapula and shoulder	Initially colicky, becomes continuous. Patient writhes	Palpation over the gallbladder bed (below 10th rib in right upper quadrant)		Nausea, vomiting, may have fever and rigors	Tender right hypochondrium, positive Murphy's sign, may be jaundiced	Biliary tract ultrasound, ERCP
Renal colic (ureteric stones)	Loin pain radiating to groin, and in males the scrotum	Very intense colicky pain. Patient writhes			Nausea, vomiting, frequency	Microscopic or obvious haematuria	Abdominal radiograph (90% stones visible), ultrasound intra-venous urogram
Intestinal obstruction	Large bowel: lower abdomen Small intestine: periumbilical	Colic	Food, drink		Large bowel: constipation, vomiting occurs later Small intestine: vomiting, constipation occurs later	Abdominal distension, empty rectum	Radiograph of abdomen shows air–fluid levels in bowel
Acute appendicitis	Initially, periumbilical pain, later localises to right iliac fossa	Initially dull, later intense	Movement, hip extension	Lying still	Nausea, anorexia, vomiting	Fever, tenderness and guarding in the right iliac fossa	Laparoscopy
Perforated peptic ulcer	Sudden onset of epigastric pain. May radiate to the shoulder and extend to whole abdomen	Severe, persistent	Movement	Lying still	Nausea, vomiting	Fever, tachycardia, hypotension, shock, rigid abdomen with rebound tenderness	Chest radiograph reveals air under the diaphragm
Ruptured ectopic pregnancy	Lower abdomen	Sudden onset, severe pain	Movement	Lying still		Tachycardia, hypotension, shock. Lower abdominal tenderness may become generalised. Guarding and rebound tenderness, tender cervix	Positive pregnancy test, anaemia, ultrasound
Ruptured aortic aneurysm	Pain radiating to the back	Moderately severe			Nausea, sweating	Pulsatile tender mass, hypotension, shock, oliguria/aneuria	Abdominal radiograph (calcification), ultrasound angiography

Fig. 7.20   The characteristics of abdominal pain which may help in making a differential diagnosis.

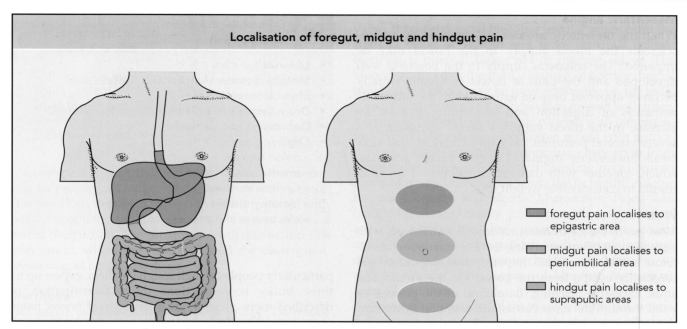

Fig. 7.21   Perception of visceral pain is localised to the epigastric, umbilical or suprapubic region according to the embryological origin of the diseased organ.

commonly accompanied by nonspecific, 'visceral' symptoms (e.g. anorexia, nausea, pallor, sweating).

Colic is a characteristic manifestation of visceral pain and is caused by concerted and excessive smooth muscle contraction. It signifies obstruction of a hollow, muscular organ, such as the intestine, gallbladder, bile duct or ureter, and consists of recurring bouts of intense, cramping, visceral pain which build to a crescendo and then fade away. When the smaller organs such as the gallbladder, bile duct or ureters are acutely obstructed by a stone, the cyclical nature of colic soon gives way to a continuous visceral pain caused by the inflammatory effect of the impacted stone or secondary infection. Movement does not aggravate visceral pain, so the patient may writhe or double-up in response to it.

Unlike the visceral peritoneum, the parietal peritoneum is innervated by pain-sensitive fibres. Therefore, pain arising from the parietal peritoneum is well localised to the area immediately overlying the area of inflammation or irritation. Parietal pain is aggravated by stretching or moving the peritoneal membrane; the patient lies as still as possible. Palpation over the area is extremely painful, with the overlying muscles contracting to protect the peritoneum (guarding). When the pressure of the examining hand is suddenly released, the pain is further aggravated and the patient winces. This sign is known as 'rebound tenderness'.

Abdominal pain may progress from a visceral sensation to a parietal pain. Acute appendicitis provides an excellent example of this transition. When this midgut structure becomes inflamed and obstructed, a dull pain localises to the periumbilical area and the patient may feel nauseous and sweaty. As the inflammation advances through the visceral covering to the parietal peritoneum, the pain appears to shift to the right iliac fossa where it localises over McBurney's point. The character of the pain also changes from dull to sharp. The area overlying the appendix is very tender and palpation causes reflex guarding and rebound tenderness.

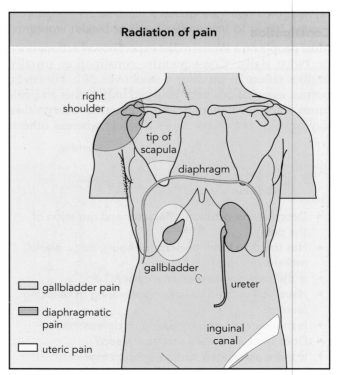

Fig. 7.22   Characteristic radiation of pain from the gallbladder, diaphragm and ureters. The pain is not always felt in the organ concerned.

Symptoms and signs
Some renal symptoms and their causes

Frequency
- Irritable bladder
  - infection, inflammation, chemical irritation
- Reduced compliance
  - fibrosis, tumour infiltration
- Bladder outlet obstruction
  - in prostatism, detrusor failure may limit the volume voided

Polyuria
- Ingestion of large volumes of water, beverages or alcohol
- Chronic renal failure (loss of concentrating power)
- Diabetes mellitus (osmotic effect of glucose in urine)
- Diabetes insipidus (caused by a lack of ADH or tubules insensitive to circulating ADH)
- Diuretic treatment

Dysuria
- Bacterial infection of the bladder (cystitis)
- Inflammation of the urethra (urethritis)
- Infection or inflammation of the prostate (prostatitis)

Incontinence
- Sphincter damage or weakness after childbirth
- Sphincter weakness in old age
- Prostate cancer
- Benign prostatic hypertrophy
- Spinal cord disease, paraplegia

Oliguria or anuria
- Hypovolaemia (dehydration or shock)
- Acute renal failure caused by acute glomerulonephritis
- Bilateral ureteric obstruction (retroperitoneal fibrosis)
- Detrusor muscle failure (bladder outlet obstruction or neurological disease)

Hesitancy
Hesitancy is a delay between attempting to initiate urination and the actual flow of urine. It is a characteristic sign of bladder outlet obstruction (e.g. as a result of prostatic hypertrophy).

Oliguria and anuria
Patients may complain of passing only small volumes of urine. The term oliguria is used if less than 500 ml of urine is passed over 24 h. The subjective assessment of urine volume is often inaccurate and requires confirmation by 24 h urine collection and measurement. Apparent oliguria may occur in patients with bladder muscle (detrusor) failure. Consequently, it may be necessary to pass a catheter to confirm true oliguria.

Pain
Pain may originate in the kidneys, ureter, bladder or urethra. Infection of the kidneys (pyelonephritis) causes pain and tenderness in the renal angles, usually associated with fever, anorexia and nausea. Obstruction of the ureters by stones, sloughed papillae or blood may cause intense pain in the renal angle. This pain may radiate towards the groins and, in men, into the testes. Renal 'colic' caused by stones in the ureters is extremely painful, often causing the patient to double-up or roll around in a futile attempt to find relief. Bladder pain may occur in severe cystitis. The pain is of moderate severity, localised to the suprapubic region and associated with urgency and frequency.

Dysuria
Dysuria describes a stinging or burning sensation that occurs when passing urine. It is often accompanied by frequency and urgency. The most common cause of dysuria is cystitis.

Haematuria
Blood in urine may be obvious, associated with a cloudy colour or only apparent on chemical testing (microscopic haematuria). Whether the passage of blood is painful or painless may be of diagnostic assistance.

Differential diagnosis
Haematuria

Painful
- Kidney stones
- Urinary tract infection
- Papillary necrosis

Painless
- Infection
- Cancer of the urinary tract
- Acute glomerulonephritis
- Contamination during menstruation

EXAMINATION OF THE ABDOMEN

Before beginning your examination ask the patient to lie flat, with the head resting comfortably on a pillow, arms lying loosely on either side. According to the demands of the particular procedure you are performing, try to expose the patient as little as possible. The 'classical' arrangement is shown in Figure 7.25 but until you gain experience it will help to have the visual clues provided by the landmarks of the entire abdomen and lower chest; subsequent illustrations reflect this.

The abdominal examination depends largely on the palpation and percussion of organs that normally lie out of reach of the examining hands. As with all other examinations, it is important to become completely familiar with the clinical anatomy of the abdomen.

The costal margin demarcates the superficial boundary between the chest and abdomen, although the domes of the diaphragm rise behind the ribs to accommodate the liver and spleen, so a full abdominal examination also includes examination of the lower half of the chest (Fig. 7.26). Familiarise yourself with the bony landmarks of the abdomen (Fig. 7.27). Feel the xiphisternum at the lower end of the sternum, then trace the outline of the costal margin formed by the seventh costal cartilage at the xiphisternum to the tip of the 12th rib. Note a distinct step in the costal margin which provides a useful landmark because it coincides with the tip of the 10th rib. Turn your attention to the bony margins of the lower abdomen. The iliac crest has a distinct anterior prominence, the anterior superior iliac spine, from which the inguinal ligament runs downward and medially to attach to a lateral prominence on the pubic bone (the pubic tubercle).

For descriptive purposes the anterior abdominal wall may be divided into four quadrants (Fig. 7.28). Trace the imaginary lines demarcating the left and right upper and lower quadrants. A vertical line extends from the xiphisternum to the pubic symphysis in the midline and a horizontal line is drawn through the umbilicus. The abdomen may also be divided into nine segments resembling a 'noughts and crosses' matrix (Fig. 7.29). These segments are useful landmarks for ensuring a complete and systematic examination of the abdomen. A vertical line is dropped from the mid-clavicular points on either side and these are crossed by a horizontal line drawn in the subcostal plane and by a line joining the anterior superior iliac spines.

When locating or describing the position of the abdominal organs it is useful to recognise the anterior anatomical planes and their correlation with vertebral levels (Fig. 7.30). The xiphisternum corresponds to the level of T9. The transpyloric plane lies midway between the suprasternal notch and the pubis, approximately a hand's breadth below the xiphoid cartilage. This plane corresponds to the vertebral level of L1 and passes through the pylorus, the long axis of the pancreas, the duodenojejunal flexure and the hila of the kidneys. The subcostal plane coincides with the level of L3 and is defined by a line joining the lowest point of the thoracic cage on either side. A line joining the highest points of the iliac crest corresponds to the level of L4.

INSPECTION OF THE ABDOMEN

Contours

Expose the patient to the groins and observe the symmetry of the abdomen from the foot of the bed. The normal abdomen is concave and symmetrical and moves gently with respiration. Next, move to the patient's right and view the abdomen tangentially. From this position it is easier to pick out the subtle changes of contour and shadow. In thin individuals you may notice the pulsation of the abdominal aorta in the midline above the umbilicus. Ask the patient to raise the head a few inches off the pillow. This tenses the rectus abdominis, which becomes firm and prominent on either side of the midline.

Abnormal contours and distention of the abdomen may be caused by a number of mechanisms (Fig. 7.31). Establish whether the swelling is generalised or localised. Fluid and gaseous distention is generalised and symmetrical (Fig. 7.32). Fluid gravitates towards the flanks causing the loins to bulge, and the

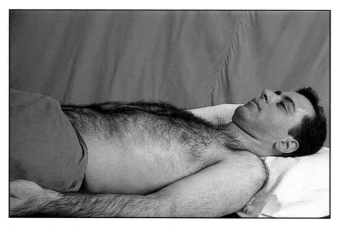

Fig. 7.25 The patient should be exposed as little as possible during your examination.

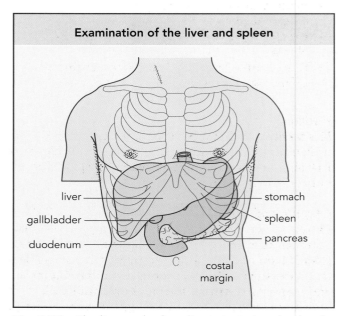

Fig. 7.26 The liver and spleen lie protected under the ribs and so the lower one-half of the chest must be exposed in order to examine them.

umbilicus, which is normally inverted, may become everted when massive ascites distends the abdomen beyond its normal compliance. In thin individuals, the contour of an enlarged liver may be visible below the right costal margin. A midline fullness in the upper abdomen may indicate disease of the stomach (e.g. carcinoma), pancreas (e.g. pancreatic cysts) or an abdominal aortic aneurysm. Suprapubic fullness

may reflect an enlarged uterus (pregnancy or fibroids), ovaries (cysts or carcinoma) or a full bladder. The periodic rippling movement of bowel peristalsis may be observed in intestinal obstruction, especially in thin individuals. This is referred to as a visible peristalsis.

Abnormal bulges may appear when intra-abdominal pressure is raised and may be revealed by

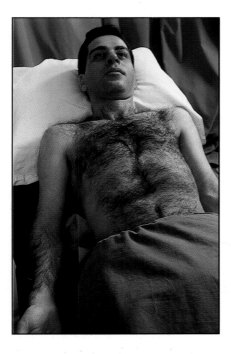

Fig. 7.27 The bony landmarks of the anterior abdominal wall.

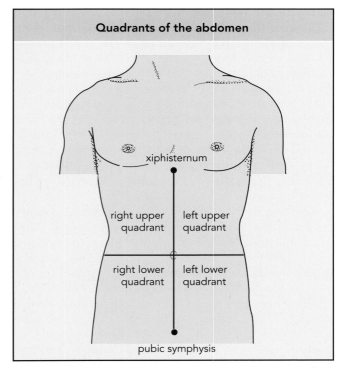

Fig. 7.28   The quadrants of the anterior abdominal wall.

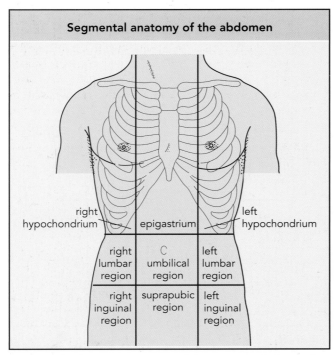

Fig. 7.29   The nine segments of the anterior abdominal wall.

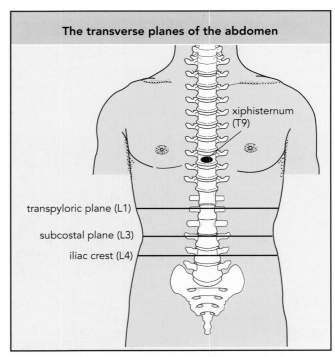

Fig. 7.30   The transverse planes and their equivalent vertebral levels.

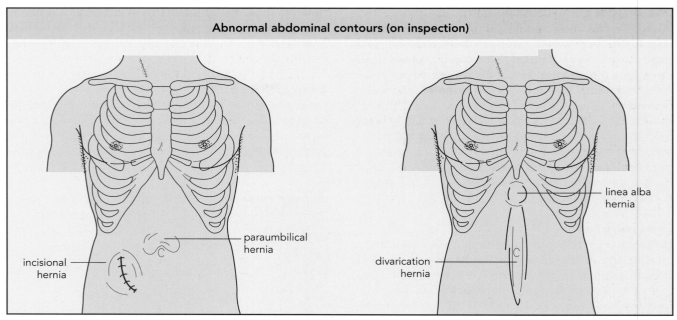

Abnormal abdominal contours (on inspection)

incisional hernia

paraumbilical hernia

divarication hernia

linea alba hernia

Fig. 7.31 Some abnormal abdominal contours.

tensing the abdominal muscles. If the muscles of the recti are abnormally separated on either side of the midline (divarication of the recti), tensing the abdominal muscles causes a longitudinal bulge to appear in the midline (Fig. 7.31). The appearance of a more localised bulge just above or below the umbilicus occurs with a paraumbilical hernia (Fig. 7.31). Direct and indirect inguinal herniae may also become prominent when intra-abdominal pressure is raised by coughing. Surgical scars are potential points of weakness in the abdominal wall and incisional herniae may develop under the scar.

Skin
During pregnancy the abdominal wall skin is stretched and after childbirth many women are left with tell-tale stretch lines (striae gravidarum) that arc across the mid- and lower abdominal wall on either side of the midline (Fig. 7.33). Stretch marks similar to those occurring after pregnancy may occur in patients successfully treated for ascites. In Cushing's syndrome, excessive adrenal corticoid secretion thins the skin and purplish striae appear on the abdominal wall even in the absence of a pregnancy. In acute haemorrhagic pancreatitis, there may be a bluish discoloration of either the flanks (Grey Turner's sign) or the periumbilical area (Cullen's sign), which results from seepage of bloodstained ascitic fluid along the fascial planes and into the subcutaneous tissue. A similar appearance may occur after rupture of an ectopic pregnancy.

Look for veins coursing over the abdominal wall: they are rarely prominent in health. If veins are visible, map the direction of flow by emptying the vein with the index finger of one hand while attempting to prevent refilling by applying occlusive pressure more proximally over the vein. The direction of flow helps distinguish normal from abnormal flow patterns (Fig. 7.34). In portal hypertension and inferior vena caval obstruction, the venous return to the liver or vena cava is redirected through abdominal wall collaterals that provide an alternative route to the right atrium. These veins dilate and may be seen coursing across the abdominal wall. It is possible to distinguish collaterals caused by portal hypertension from those caused by inferior vena caval obstruction by mapping the direction of flow in these vessels.

Look for surgical scars, which should have a fleshy red or pink colouring in the first year after an operation, becoming white as the scar tissue matures. Common locations of surgical scars are shown in Figure 7.35.

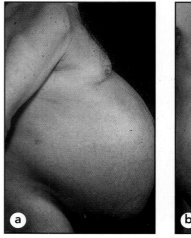
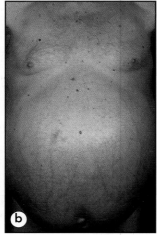

Fig. 7.32 The characteristic appearance of gross ascites.

PALPATION OF THE ABDOMEN

Although the intra-abdominal organs are normally impalpable, in diseased states palpation and percussion provide substantial clinical information. These procedures are difficult to perform if the patient is not relaxed. If the abdominal wall muscles are tense, ask the patient to bend the knees and flex the hips (Fig. 7.36). This helps to relax the abdomen. Always warm your hands before palpating the abdomen and use the fingertip and palmar aspects of the fingers; a single-handed technique may be used but you may prefer to use both hands, the upper hand applying pressure, while the lower hand concentrates on feeling (Fig. 7.37).

Light palpation

Before laying a hand on the abdomen ask the patient to localise any areas of pain or tenderness. If these are present, begin the examination in the segment furthest from the discomfort. Start light palpation by gently pressing your fingers into each of the nine segments, sustaining the light pressure for a few seconds while gently exploring each area with the fingertips. Tenderness may be reflected by grimacing, so with every move of your hand briefly look to see the patient's facial response.

Gentle palpation will detect tenderness caused by inflammation of the parietal peritoneum. In peritonitis, the patient flinches on even the lightest palpation and there is reflex rigidity, guarding and rebound tenderness. Light palpation may localise an area of peritoneal inflammation, thereby helping to establish a differential diagnosis. It is unusual to feel the abdominal organs or large masses on light palpation unless they are grossly enlarged.

Deep palpation

Once you have used light palpation to explore for areas of tenderness and muscle tension, the sequence is repeated using firm but gentle deep pressure with the palmar surface of the fingers. Deep palpation is helpful

Fig. 7.33 Striae gravidarum appear after childbirth.

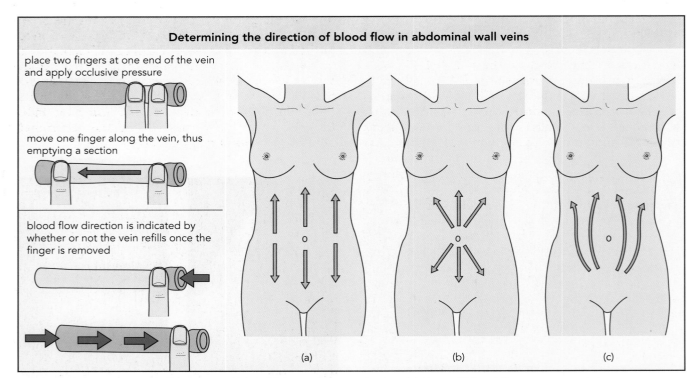

Determining the direction of blood flow in abdominal wall veins

place two fingers at one end of the vein and apply occlusive pressure

move one finger along the vein, thus emptying a section

blood flow direction is indicated by whether or not the vein refills once the finger is removed

(a)   (b)   (c)

Fig. 7.34 Determining the direction of blood flow in abdominal veins. (a) Normal blood flow pattern and those characteristic of (b) portal hypertension and (c) obstruction of the inferior vena cava.

Surgical incisions

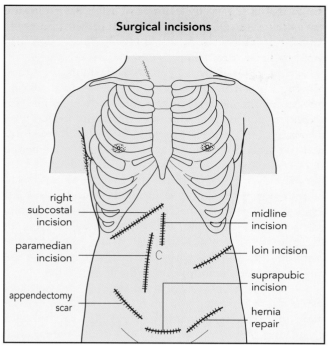

right subcostal incision

paramedian incision

appendectomy scar

midline incision

loin incision

suprapubic incision

hernia repair

Fig. 7.35 Surgical scars seen commonly on the abdomen.

Palpation of the abdomen

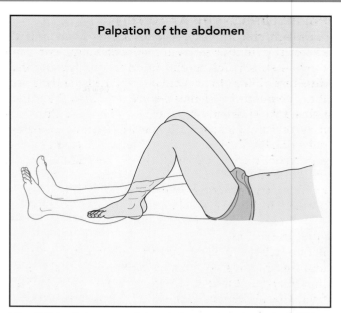

Fig. 7.36 Palpation of the abdomen may be aided if the patient is asked to flex the hips. This helps to relax the anterior abdominal wall.

for palpating abdominal masses, and healthy individuals often report pain on deep pressure of the abdomen. If the patient is relaxed it is usually possible to press deeply into the abdomen. While doing so try to imagine the anatomy underlying your hand (Fig. 7.38). In thin individuals, the descending and sigmoid colon may be felt as an elongated tubular structure in the left loin and lower quadrant. The sigmoid is mobile and can readily be rolled under the fingers. The colon can usually be distinguished from other structures because of its firm stool content. It has a putty-like consistency and can be indented with the fingertips. The 'mass' also becomes less obvious after the passage of stool. In thin individuals, the abdominal aorta may be felt as a discrete pulsatile structure in the midline, above the umbilicus. The rectus muscles may be mistaken for an abnormal fullness or the edge of a mass. Tensing the abdominal

muscles causes the rectus to become more prominent, whereas intra-abdominal masses are less easy to feel.

Abdominal masses and enlargement of the liver, spleen and kidneys may also be felt by deep palpation. Any abnormal fullness, firmness or discrete mass should be localised by careful palpation of shape, mobility, consistency and movement with respiration. Localisation helps determine which organ may be involved. Determine whether there is any deep tenderness, suggesting stretching of the capsule of either the liver or kidney, or early peritoneal inflammation or infiltration. A large pulsatile structure in the midline above the umbilicus indicates an aortic aneurysm or a transmitted impulse to a mass overlying the aorta. These can usually be distinguished using the index finger of either hand to sense whether the movement is pulsatile or transmitted (Fig. 7.39).

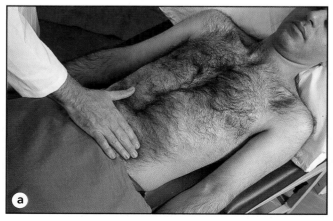

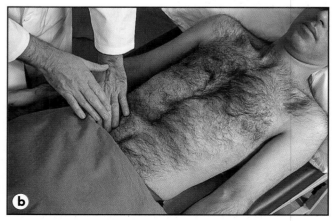

Fig. 7.37 Light abdominal palpation is performed using one (a) or both hands (b).

Palpation of the organs

The solid organs (liver, pancreas, kidneys and spleen) are normally out of reach of the examining hand. The stomach, small intestine and colon are soft, pliable and impalpable. In chronic fibrosing diseases of the liver (e.g. micronodular cirrhosis) or kidneys (e.g. chronic glomerulonephritis), these organs shrink even further from reach. However, they may become palpable when enlarged.

Palpating the liver

Examine the liver with the surface anatomy in mind. Visualise its upper margin as a line passing just below each nipple on either side and imagine the lower margin spanning a line from the tip of the 10th rib on the right to a point just below the left nipple (Fig. 7.40). The upper surface of the organ is tightly apposed to the undersurface of the diaphragm and examination takes advantage of the movement of the liver with respiration. The initial aim of the examination is to define the outline of the lower edge of the right lobe, which is normally tucked along the inner surface of the right costal margin. The edge of the smaller left lobe nestles under the lower left rib cage and is often impalpable even when the organ is generally enlarged.

Examine from the patient's right and use either the fingertips or the radial side of the index finger to explore for the liver edge under the costal margin. Point the ends of the index, middle and ring fingers in an upward position, facing the liver edge, at a point midway between the costal margin and iliac crests, lateral to the rectus muscle (Fig. 7.41). Press the fingertips inwards and upwards and hold this position while the patient takes a

deep inspiration. Near the height of inspiration relax the inward pressure slightly but maintain upward pressure. As the fingers drift upwards feel for the liver edge slipping under them as the organ descends. If no edge is felt, repeat the manoeuvre in a stepwise fashion, each time moving the starting position a little closer to the costal margin. If the liver is impalpable at this point, you should repeat the procedure more laterally in line with the anterior axillary line. In patients of thin or medium build a normal liver edge may be palpable just below the right costal margin at the height of inspiration. Repeat the palpation in the midline and below the left costal margin where the lower edge of the middle and left lobes should not be palpable. A single-handed technique may also be used (Fig. 7.41). The radial surface of the index finger is positioned below and parallel to the costal margin and this surface is used to explore for the lower liver edge as it descends during inspiration.

At this point in the examination it is useful to percuss for the lower liver edge. With the long axis of your middle finger positioned parallel to the right costal margin, percuss from the point where you started palpating for the liver (Fig. 7.42). This point normally overlies bowel and should sound resonant. Repeat the percussion in a stepwise manner, each time

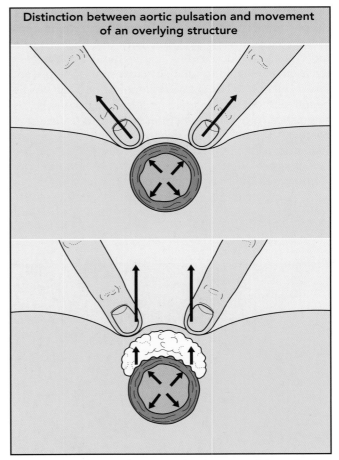

Distinction between aortic pulsation and movement of an overlying structure

Fig. 7.39 Palpating the aorta. The direction of the pulsation indicates whether it arises directly from the aorta (above) or is transmitted by a mass overlying the tissues (below).

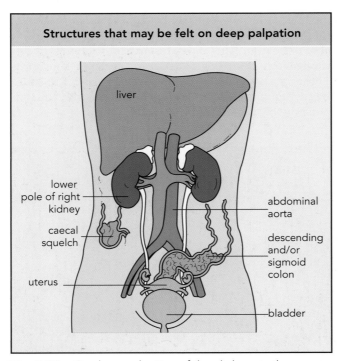

Structures that may be felt on deep palpation

liver

lower pole of right kidney

caecal squelch

uterus

abdominal aorta

descending and/or sigmoid colon

bladder

Fig. 7.38 On deep palpation of the abdomen, these structures may be felt.

moving the finger closer to the costal margin until the note becomes duller. This should coincide with the costal margin. Ask the patient to inspire deeply; the dullness should move down as the liver descends.

Next, find the position of the upper margin of the liver so that you can assess the liver span. The upper margin cannot be palpated because it lies high in the dome of the diaphragm, but it can be located by noting the change in percussion note from the resonance of the lungs to the dullness of the liver. The upper margin of the liver usually lies deep to the sixth intercostal space. Percuss the third space and then percuss each succeeding interspace until you detect the transition from resonance to dullness (Fig. 7.43). On deep inspiration the percussion interface should descend by either one or two interspaces as the lungs expand and the liver descends. Liver size is proportional to body size. Measure the liver span in the midclavicular line; in women this should measure 8–10 cm and in men, 10–12 cm.

Downward displacement of the liver In patients who have hyperinflated lungs (e.g. emphysema), the diaphragm is flattened and the liver is pushed down

so that the edge may be easily palpable below the costal margin (Fig. 7.44). Percussion reveals that the upper border of the liver is depressed and that the liver span is within normal limits.

Abnormal liver shape The right lobe of the liver may be abnormally shaped, with an elongated tongue-like projection pointing towards the right iliac crest

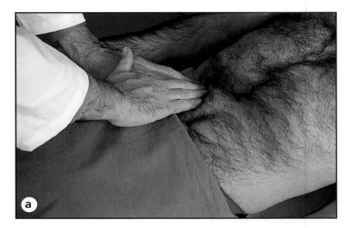

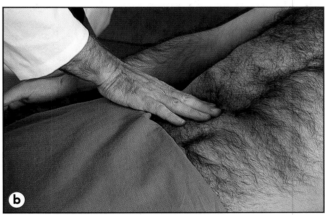

Fig. 7.41 Liver palpation. A two-handed (a) and single-handed (b) technique using the radial surface of the index finger(s) to feel for the lower liver edge as it descends during inspiration.

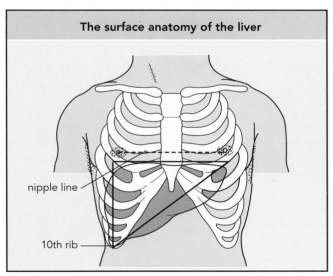

Fig. 7.40 The surface anatomy of the liver.

The surface anatomy of the liver

nipple line

10th rib

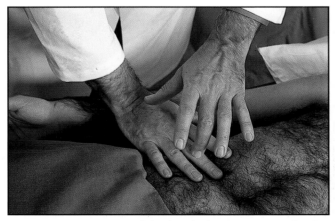

Fig. 7.42 Positioning of the hand when percussing for the lower border of the liver.

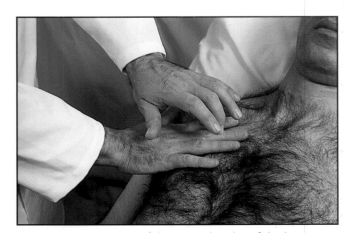

Fig. 7.43 Percussion of the upper border of the liver.

(Fig. 7.45). This anatomical variant, known as a Riedel's lobe, is more common in women and feels like a mobile mass on the right side of the abdomen arising from under the costal margin and moving with respiration. A Riedel's lobe is commonly mistaken for an enlarged right kidney and if in doubt this can be resolved by ultrasound scanning.

Enlargement of the liver Liver enlargement is usually described as mild, moderate or massive (Fig. 7.46). If the liver is enlarged, trace the shape of the liver edge and decide whether it is smooth or irregular, whether the consistency is soft, firm or hard and whether or not the organ is tender. The presence of a palpable spleen suggests cirrhosis with portal hypertension or infiltrating diseases of the reticuloendothelial and haemopoietic systems.

Small livers The lower margin of the liver may not be palpable because of fibrosis or atrophy of the organ. This may be difficult to detect clinically but should be suspected if the liver edge is not palpable and if, on percussion, the dullness of the lower liver margin is detected well above the costal margin (Fig. 7.47). Atrophy of the liver may be the result either of severe acute liver damage, perhaps caused by fulminant

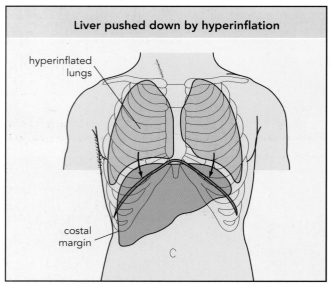

Fig. 7.44 When the lung fields are markedly hyperinflated, the liver is pushed down and the lower border may be readily palpable, although the span is normal.

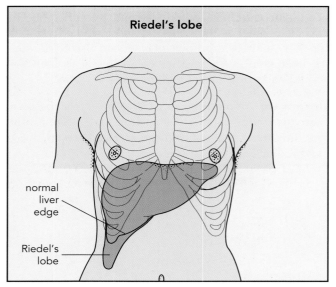

Fig. 7.45 A Riedel's lobe is a normal variant of shape. The elongated 'tongue' is palpable and must be distinguished from a pathological cancer.

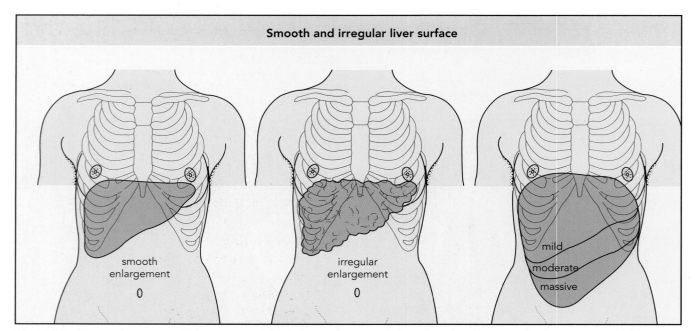

Fig. 7.46 Liver enlargement. Enlargement of the liver can be smooth (e.g. fatty liver) or irregular (e.g. macronodular cirrhosis, tumour infiltration).

viral hepatitis or hepatotoxic poisons, or of chronic disease causing fibrosis and micronodular cirrhosis (e.g. alcoholic cirrhosis).

General signs of liver disease

The liver has considerable functional reserve but as this is exhausted the patient develops characteristic signs of liver failure. Look for jaundice in the sclerae, which are normally a brilliant white colour. Mild jaundice may be difficult to discern in artificial light and in dark-skinned patients the sclerae may be slightly pigmented. With deepening jaundice the skin becomes yellow, and in chronic, severe obstructive jaundice the skin may appear almost green in colour.

In patients with chronic liver disease, localised vascular dilatation results in the appearance of vascular spiders (spider naevi) (see Fig. 3.11). These consist of a central arteriole from which branch a series of smaller vessels, in a pattern resembling spider legs. Spider naevi are found in the territory drained by the superior vena cava; common sites include the neck, face and dorsa of the hands. The central arteriole can be occluded with a pencil tip and on release of the pressure the vessels rapidly refill from the centre.

Severe hepatocellular disease associated with portosystemic shunting can result in hepatic encephalopathy.

Differential diagnosis
Hepatomegaly

- Macronodular cirrhosis
- Neoplastic disease (primary and secondary cancer, myeloproliferative disorders)
- Infections (viral hepatitis, tuberculosis, hydatid disease)
- Infiltrations (iron, fat, amyloid, Gaucher's disease)

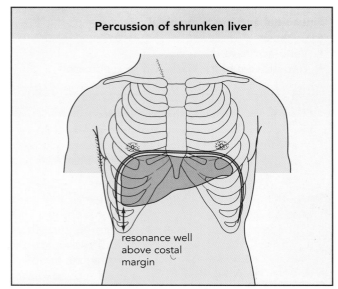

Percussion of shrunken liver

resonance well above costal margin

Fig. 7.47 Atrophy of the liver may be detected by percussing the lower border. The area of resonance will extend above the costal margin.

Often there are accompanying signs of portal hypertension, such as splenomegaly and ascites, but the physical sign characteristic of hepatic encephalopathy is a 'flapping tremor'. Ask the patient to stretch out both arms and hyperextend the wrists with the fingers held separated (Fig. 7.48). A coarse, involuntary flap occurs at

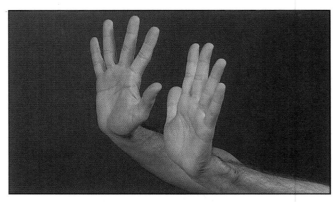

Fig. 7.48 To elicit a flapping tremor in hepatic encephalopathy, ask the patient to outstretch the arms with the hands extended at the wrist and metacarpophalangeal joints. This position is held for 20 s.

Symptoms and signs
Signs of liver disease

General examination
- Nutrition status
- Pallor (blood loss)
- Jaundice
- Breath fetor of liver failure
- Xanthelasmata (chronic cholestasis)
- Parotid swelling (alcohol abuse)
- Bruising (clotting diathesis)
- Spider naevi
- Female distribution of body hair

Mental state
- Wernicke's or Korsakoff's psychosis
- Flapping tremor of hepatic encephalopathy
- Inability to copy a five-pointed star

Hands
- Leuconychia (hypoproteinaemia)
- Liver flap
- Palmar erythema
- Dupuytren's contractures
- Mild finger clubbing

Chest
- Gynaecomastia
- Right-sided pleural effusion

Abdomen
- Dilated veins
- Liver or spleen enlargement
- Ascites
- Testicular atrophy

days (see differential diagnosis box – acute renal failure). When renal failure develops over weeks, months or years, systemic signs appear (see differential diagnosis and symptoms and signs boxes – chronic renal failure).

Palpating the kidneys

Pole to pole the kidneys extend from the vertebral level of T12 to L3 and the larger right lobe of the liver displaces the right kidney 2 cm lower than the left. Viewed from the rear, the kidneys lie in the renal angle formed by the 12th rib and the lateral margin of the vertebral column (Fig. 7.54). The adrenal glands perch on the upper pole of each kidney.

The kidneys are not usually palpable through the thickness of the abdominal wall and abdominal contents, although in thin individuals a normal-sized kidney may be felt. The right kidney is easier to palpate because it lies lower than the left. A normal kidney has a firm consistency and a smooth surface.

When examining the kidneys, position the patient close to the edge of the bed and examine each kidney from the patient's right, bearing in mind the surface anatomy. The kidneys are retroperitoneal organs and deep bimanual palpation is required to explore for them. When examining the left kidney, tuck the palmar surfaces of the left hand posteriorly into the left flank and nestle the fingertips in the renal angle (Fig. 7.55a). Position the middle three fingers of the right hand below the left costal margin, lateral to the rectus muscle and at a point opposite the posterior hand (Fig. 7.55b). To examine the right kidney, tuck your left hand behind the right loin and position the fingers of your right hand below the right costal margin, lateral to rectus abdominis. Palpate for the lower pole of each kidney in turn. The aim of the manoeuvre is briefly to trap the lower pole of the kidney between the fingers of both hands as the organ moves up and down with deep respiration. The spleen is closely associated with the diaphragm and thus moves early in respiration but the kidneys lie lower down and they only descend towards the end of inspiration. Ask the patient to inspire deeply; press the fingers of both hands firmly together, attempting to capture the

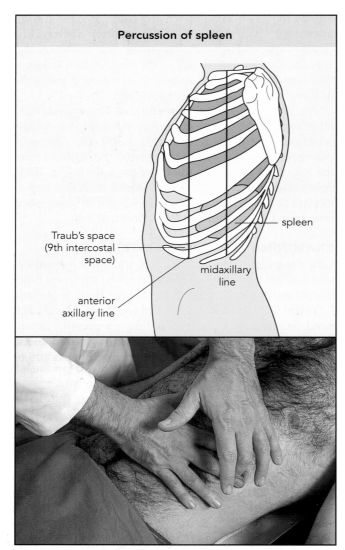

Fig. 7.52 After palpating for the spleen, percuss for the enlarged organ in the 9th intercostal space anterior to the anterior axillary line.

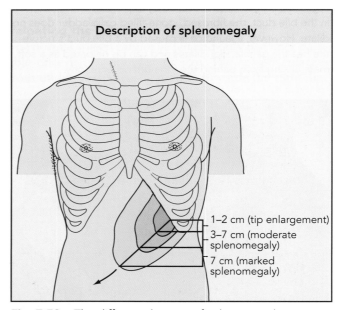

Fig. 7.53 The different degrees of splenomegaly.

> **Dx** Differential diagnosis
> **Splenomegaly**
>
> - Portal hypertension
> - Infections (malaria, subacute bacterial endocarditis, tuberculosis, typhoid)
> - Chronic lymphatic leukaemia
> - Chronic myeloid leukaemia
> - Myelofibrosis
> - Gaucher's disease
> - Haemolytic anaemia

lower pole as it slips through the fingertips. This technique is known as balloting the kidney (Fig. 7.55b). If the kidney is palpable the rounded lower pole can be felt slipping between the opposing fingers as the patient breathes in and out.

The kidney may be tender, especially when acutely infected (pyelonephritis) or obstructed (hydronephrosis). This may be apparent on bimanual palpation, although a more specific sign is 'punch' tenderness over the renal angles. To test this response sit the patient forward and place the palm of the left hand over the renal angle. Then, using moderate force, punch the dorsal surface of the hand with the ulnar surface of the clenched right fist (Fig. 7.56). Perform this test for each kidney in turn and assess the patient's reaction.

It is important to distinguish kidney enlargement from splenomegaly on the left and hepatomegaly on the right. The principal cause of bilateral enlargement is polycystic disease of the kidney, whereas

Differential diagnosis
Acute renal failure

- Shock (hypovolaemic, septic or cardiogenic)
- Acute glomerulonephritis
- Toxins or drugs (ethylene glycol, carbon tetrachloride)
- Acute haemoglobinuria or myoglobinuria
- Acute renal vein thrombosis

Differential diagnosis
Chronic renal failure

- Chronic glomerulonephritis
- Systemic hypertension
- Diabetes mellitus with nephropathy
- Chronic obstructive uropathy
- Polycystic disease of the kidneys
- Analgesic nephropathy

Symptoms and signs
Signs of chronic renal failure

- Sallow complexion
- Anaemia (normocytic, normochromic)
- Uraemic fetor
- Deep acidotic breathing (Kussmaul respiration)
- Hypertension
- Mental clouding
- Uraemic encephalopathy (flapping tremor)
- Pleural and pericardial effusion
- Pericardial rub (pericarditis)
- Evidence of fluid overload or depletion
- Renal masses (polycystic kidneys)
- Large bladder (chronic bladder outlet obstruction)

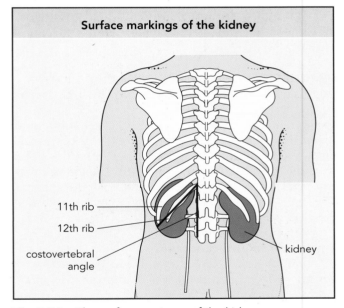

Surface markings of the kidney

11th rib
12th rib
costovertebral angle
kidney

Fig. 7.54 The surface anatomy of the kidneys.

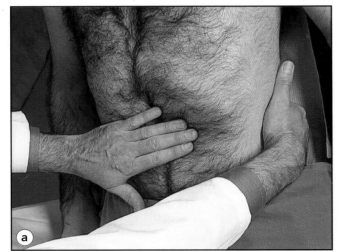

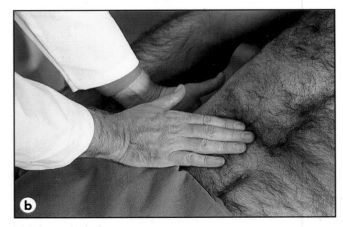

Fig. 7.55 Positioning the hands when palpating (a) the left and (b) the right kidney.

unilateral enlargement suggests a malignant tumour (e.g. hypernephroma).

Palpating the aorta

The descending aorta emerges through the aortic hiatus in the diaphragm and hugs the vertebral bodies until it bifurcates into the common iliac arteries at the level of L4, which approximates to a point just below the umbilicus. It lies adjacent to the inferior vena cava and gives off a number of major tributaries that feed the major abdominal organs (Fig. 7.57). The aorta can be palpated between the thumb and finger of one hand or by positioning the fingers of both hands on either side of the midline at a point midway between the xiphisternum and the umbilicus (Fig. 7.58). Press the fingers posteriorly and slightly medially and feel for the pulsation of the abdominal aorta against your fingertips. This pulsation can be felt in thin individuals but it is usually impalpable in muscular or obese patients.

An abdominal aortic aneurysm may be felt as a large pulsatile mass above the level of the umbilicus. The abdominal aorta may also become abnormally prominent in elderly people when marked curvature of the spine displaces it anteriorly and laterally.

PERCUSSION OF THE ABDOMEN

At this stage of the examination you will have percussed the liver and spleen. General percussion of the abdomen is used to establish whether abdominal distension is caused by gas or fluid. Percussion is also used to detect an overfilled bladder. The stomach, small bowel and colon fill the entire anterior abdomen and the percussion note of the anterior abdomen wall between the costal margins and iliac crests is normally tympanic.

Percussion to detect ascites

Abdominal distension is usually caused either by gaseous dilatation of the bowel or abnormal accumulation of fluid. In the supine position, gas accumulates more centrally, whereas fluid gravitates into the flanks. The gas-filled normal bowel tends to float

above ascites, so the gas–fluid interface characteristic of ascites is detected by a change in the percussion note from the resonance overlying bowel to the dullness of fluid. The presence of ascites can be confirmed by altering the patient's posture and demonstrating a change in the position of the gas–fluid interface.

A change in percussion note (shifting dullness) is easiest to assess by percussing from an area of reso-

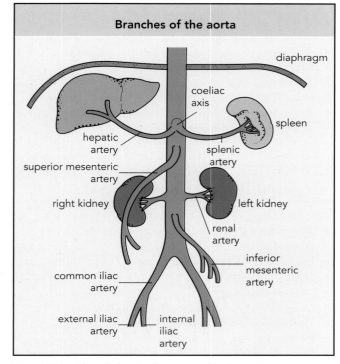

Fig. 7.57   The abdominal aorta and its branches.

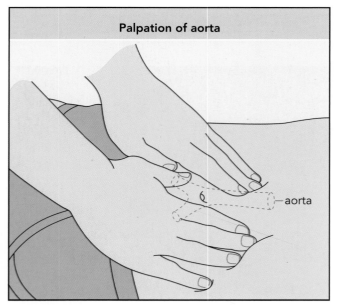

Fig. 7.58   Palpation of the aorta at a point midway between the umbilicus and the xiphisternum.

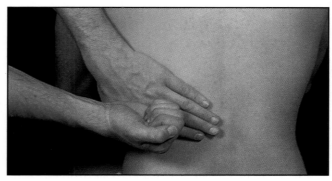

Fig. 7.56   Assessing the punch tenderness over the renal angles.

nance to an area of dullness. With the patient supine, percuss in the midline at the level of the umbilicus with the fingers parallel to the lateral wall of the abdomen (Fig. 7.59a). This point overlies gas-filled bowel and the percussion note should be tympanic. Progressively reposition your hand approximately 2 cm to the left and repeat the percussion towards the left flank (Fig. 7.59b). The note should remain tympanic until you reach the lateral abdominal wall. A distinct transition zone between tympany and dullness, a gas–fluid interface, should be marked lightly with a water-soluble marking pen. Now ask the patient to roll into the right lateral position. This allows the fluid to gravitate to the right flank and the gas-filled bowel to rise into the left flank (Fig. 7.60). Repeat the percussion from the midline towards the left flank. The tympany should extend well lateral to the interface marked in supine examination.

Percussion to detect a distended bladder
If the bladder outlet is obstructed and the detrusor muscle fails, the organ distends and emerges above the pubic bone from its usual position deep within the

pelvis. The suprapubic area is usually tympanic and a dull sound on percussion here is a useful clinical sign of bladder distension.

Use the general principle of percussing from resonance to dullness to check for bladder enlargement. Percuss from the level of the umbilicus, parallel to the pubis (Fig. 7.61) and progress down the midline towards the pubic bone. The note should remain tympanic to the pubic bone. A level of dullness above this landmark indicates the upper margin of a distended bladder or possibly enlargement of the uterus. An enlarged bladder is felt as a rounded fullness, whereas an enlarged uterus is felt as a more distinct solid structure.

AUSCULTATION OF THE ABDOMEN
The sounds generated by the abdomen are gurgling noises caused by the intestinal peristalsis moving gas and fluid through the bowel lumen. These are best assessed by auscultation.

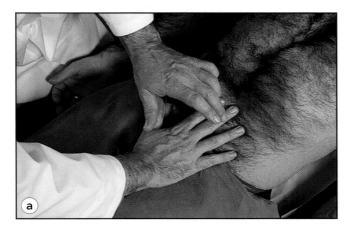

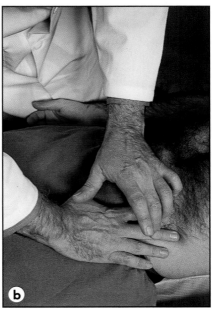

Fig. 7.59 When percussing for ascites, (a) begin in the midline with your finger parallel to the lateral wall of the abdomen and (b) continue towards the left flank. A change in the percussion note indicates a gas–fluid interface.

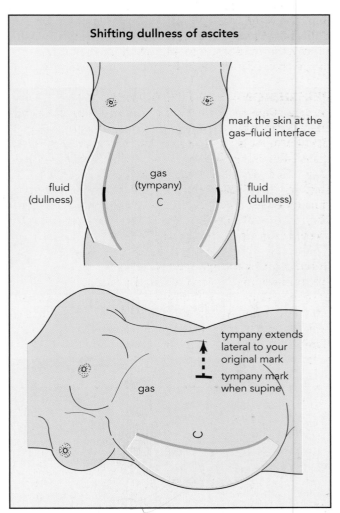

Fig. 7.60 To confirm the presence of ascites, roll the patient into the right lateral position because this causes fluid to settle in the dependent right flank, whereas gas-filled bowel floats above to fill the left flank. A shift in the positions of dullness and tympany indicates free fluid.

Listening for bowel sounds

Place the diaphragm of the stethoscope on the mid-abdomen and listen for intermittent gurgling sounds (borborygma). These peristaltic sounds occur episodically at 5–10 s intervals, although longer silent periods may occur. Keep listening for approximately 30 s before concluding that bowel sounds are reduced or absent.

The absence of any bowel sounds can indicate intestinal paralysis (paralytic ileus); this is always associated with abdominal distension. Rapidly repetitive bowel sounds (often termed 'active' bowel sounds) may be normal but they may also be an early sign of mechanical obstruction if they are associated with a colicky abdominal pain. In progressive bowel obstruction, large amounts of gas and fluid accumulate and the bowel sounds change in quality to a higher pitched 'tinkling'. This is an ominous sign of impending bowel paralysis.

Auscultation may also be helpful when diagnosing obstruction of gastric outflow. In pyloric obstruction, the stomach distends with gas and fluid; this can be detected by listening for a 'succussion splash'. Steady the diaphragm of the stethoscope on the epigastrium and shake the upper abdomen for the splashing sound characteristic of gastric outflow obstruction (Fig. 7.62).

Listening for arterial bruits

Position the diaphragm of the stethoscope over the abdominal aorta and apply moderate pressure (Fig. 7.63a). The heart sounds may be transmitted to this area but aortic flow should be silent. A distinct systolic murmur (a bruit) indicates turbulent flow and suggests arteriosclerosis or an aneurysm.

Listen for renal arterial bruits at a point 2.5 cm above and lateral to the umbilicus (Fig. 7.63b). The presence of a renal bruit suggests congenital or arteriosclerotic renal artery stenosis or narrowing caused by fibromuscular hyperplasia.

AUSCULTATION OVER THE LIVER AND SPLEEN

Conclude the auscultation by listening over the liver (Fig. 7.64) and spleen. A soft and distant bruit heard over an enlarged liver is always abnormal, suggesting either primary liver cell carcinoma or acute alcoholic hepatitis. Secondary liver tumours do not transmit bruits. Occasionally, a creaking 'rub' may be

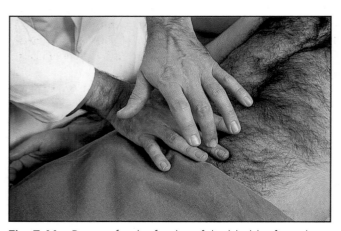

Fig. 7.61 Percuss for the fundus of the bladder from the level of the umbilicus.

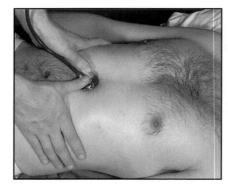

Fig. 7.62 If you suspect obstruction of the pyloric outlet, check for a 'succussion splash' by simultaneously listening in the epigastrium and shaking the upper abdomen from side to side.

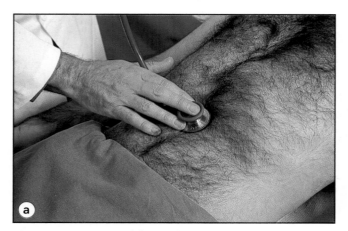
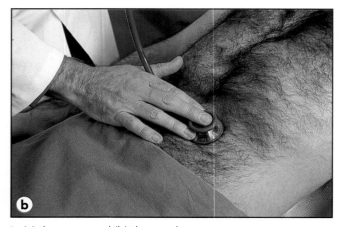

Fig. 7.63 Position of the stethoscope when listening for bruits in (a) the aorta and (b) the renal artery.

heard over the liver or spleen. This indicates inflammation of the outer capsule of the organ and adjacent peritoneum, perhaps caused by perihepatitis or perisplenitis. More rarely, carcinomatous infiltration of the capsule and surrounding structures may be the cause.

EXAMINING THE GROINS

The spermatic cord, inguinal lymph nodes and femoral artery occupy the groin. A swelling in the groin is usually the result of either an inguinal or femoral hernia or due to enlarged lymph nodes.

INGUINAL CANAL AND FEMORAL SHEATH
During male fetal development the testis and spermatic cord migrate from the abdomen into the scrotum

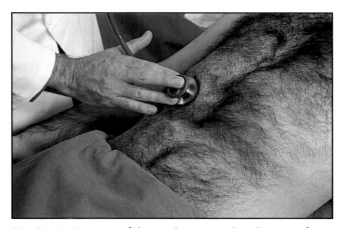

Fig. 7.64   Position of the stethoscope when listening for a liver bruit.

through the inguinal canal. This passage occludes after the descent of the testes but it remains a potential route through which the bowel can herniate in later life, causing an inguinal hernia.

The inguinal canal passes downward and medially from the internal to the external ring, running above and parallel to the inguinal ligament, which forms its lower border (Fig. 7.65). The internal ring lies immediately above the point at which the inguinal ligament and femoral artery intersect. The femoral artery lies at the midfemoral point, which is located midway between the anterior superior iliac spine and the symphysis pubis. The external ring lies immediately above and medial to the pubic tubercle. The femoral artery enters the femoral triangle from behind the inguinal ligament and is enclosed in a fascial sheath. This sheath also accommodates the femoral vein, which lies medial to the artery, and the femoral canal, which is a small gap immediately adjacent and medial to the vein. The femoral canal is plugged with fat and a lymph node (Cloquet's gland) and it is a potential pathway for the formation of a direct femoral hernia.

Examining herniae
An indirect inguinal hernia forms when bowel or omentum protrudes through a lax internal ring and finds its way into the inguinal canal. Bowel may force its way through the external ring and may even slip into the scrotum (Fig. 7.66).

An inguinal hernia usually presents as a lump in the groin or the scrotum that is most prominent when the intra-abdominal pressure is raised (e.g. when standing or coughing). The hernia may reduce spontaneously when the patient lies down, so it is best to

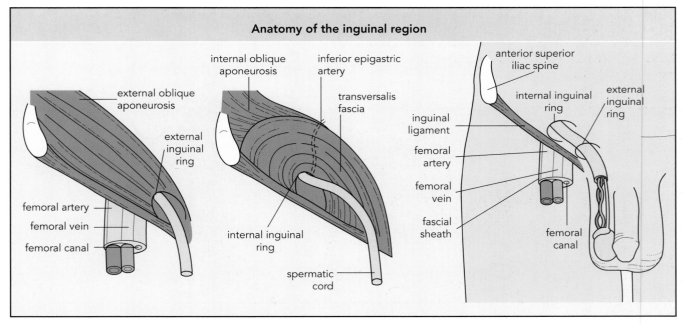

Anatomy of the inguinal region

external oblique aponeurosis

internal oblique aponeurosis

inferior epigastric artery

transversalis fascia

anterior superior iliac spine

internal inguinal ring

external inguinal ring

inguinal ligament

femoral artery

femoral vein

fascial sheath

femoral canal

external inguinal ring

femoral artery

femoral vein

femoral canal

internal inguinal ring

spermatic cord

Fig. 7.65   The anatomy of the inguinal canal and femoral sheath.

examine the hernia with the patient standing. Place two fingers on the mass and ascertain whether or not an impulse is transmitted to your fingertips when the patient coughs. Most herniae can be reduced manually, so attempt this by gently massaging the mass towards the internal ring. Once the hernia is fully reduced, occlude the internal ring with a finger pressing over the femoral point. Ask the patient to cough. An indirect inguinal hernia should not reappear until you release the occlusion of the internal ring.

A direct inguinal hernia develops through a weakness in the posterior wall of the inguinal canal. These herniae seldom force their way into the scrotum and, once reduced, their reappearance is not controlled by pressure over the internal ring.

When an inguinal hernia extends as far as the external ring it may be confused with a femoral hernia. The distinction is made by establishing the relationship of the hernia to the pubic tubercle: an inguinal hernia lies above and medial to the tubercle, whereas a femoral hernia lies below and lateral.

EXAMINING THE ANUS, RECTUM AND PROSTATE

RECTUM AND ANUS

The rectum is a curved segment of the bowel, approximately 12 cm long, lying in the concavity of the mid- and lower sacrum (Fig. 7.67). The upper two-thirds of the anterior rectum but not the posterior surface is covered by peritoneum. The anterior rectal peritoneum reflects onto the bladder base in men, it forms the rectouterine pouch (known as the pouch of Douglas) in women and is filled with loops of bowel. Anterior to the lower one-third of the rectum lie the prostate, bladder base and seminal vesicles in men and the vagina in women. The anus is 3–4 cm long and joins the rectum to the perineum. The anal wall is supported by powerful sphincter muscles, the voluntary external and involuntary internal sphincters, which constrict to provide tone and continence (Fig. 7.68). The rectal mucosa can be directly visualised through a proctoscope or sigmoidoscope but a great deal may be learned by palpation of the anus, rectum and prostate.

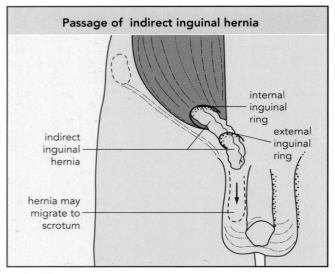

Fig. 7.66   An indirect hernia enters through the internal ring and exits through the external ring.

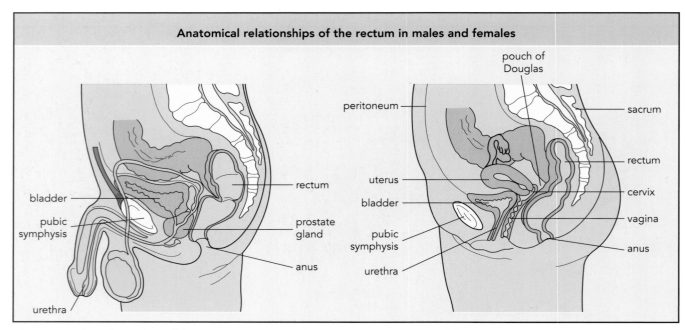

Fig. 7.67   The relationship of the anterior rectum to the prostate gland and bladder base in men (left) and the posterior vaginal wall and uterine cervix in women (right).

Rectal examination should not be unduly painful and it is important to explain this to the patient, along with your reasons for performing it. The examination will promote a feeling of rectal fullness and it may stimulate a desire to evacuate. Tell the patient to expect this. Always work with an assistant and always glove both hands.

Position the patient in the left lateral position with the hips and knees well flexed and the buttock positioned at the edge of the bed (Fig. 7.69). The positions around the anal opening are described by the positions around the clock face (Fig. 7.70). Gently separate the buttocks to expose the natal cleft and anal verge (Fig. 7.71). Inspection of the natal cleft and anal verge may reveal skin tags, pilonidal sinuses, warts, fissures, fistulas, external haemorrhoids or prolapsed rectal mucosa (Fig. 7.72). A bluish discoloration of the perineal skin suggests Crohn's disease. The anal skin is innervated with pain fibres and anal pain and tenderness are suggestive of infection (e.g. perianal abscess), fissure and fistula in ano or thrombosis of an external haemorrhoid.

Lubricate your index finger with a clear, water-soluble gel (e.g. K-Y jelly) and press the fingertip against the anal verge with the pulp facing the 6 o'clock position (Fig. 7.71). Slip your finger into the anal canal and then insert it into the rectum, directing the tip posteriorly to follow the sacral curve (Fig. 7.73). With your finger fully introduced, check on anal tone by asking the patient to squeeze your

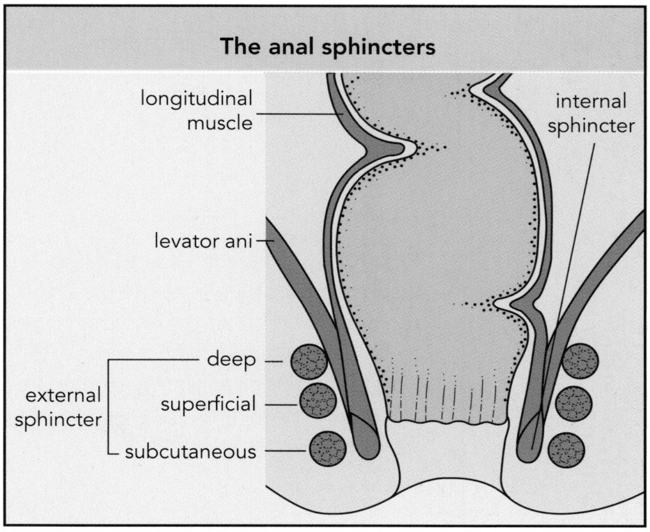

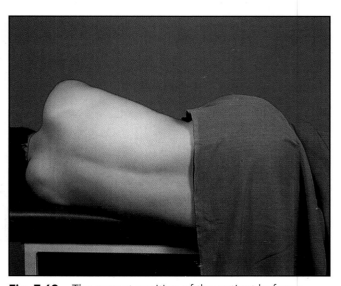

Fig. 7.68   The internal and external anal sphincters.

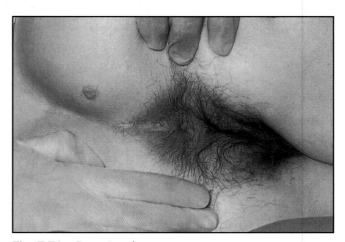

Fig. 7.69   The correct position of the patient before a rectal examination.

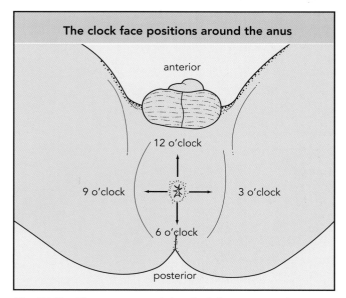

Fig. 7.70   The positions of the clock face are used to describe positions around the anus.

Fig. 7.71   Exposing the anus.

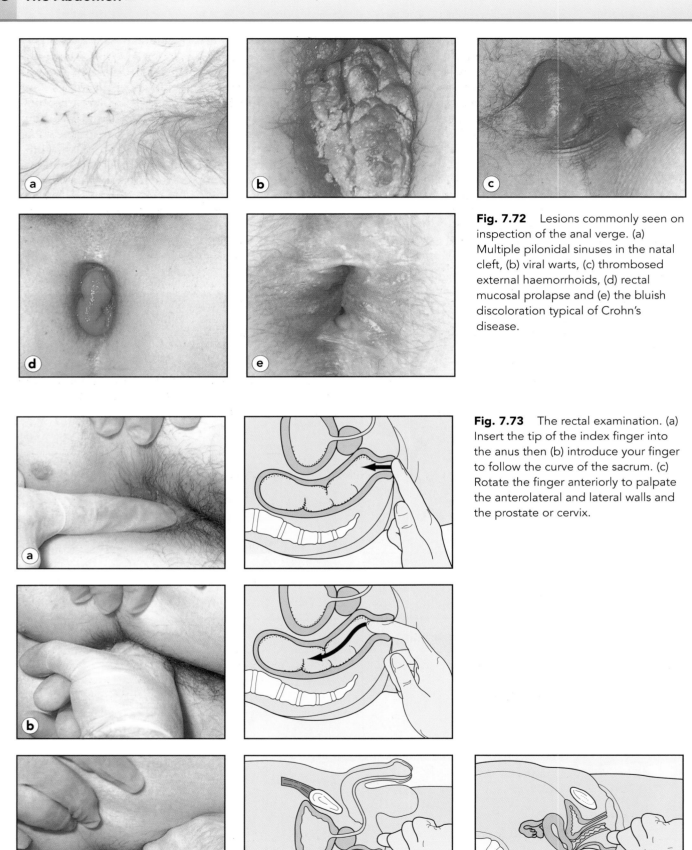

Fig. 7.72 Lesions commonly seen on inspection of the anal verge. (a) Multiple pilonidal sinuses in the natal cleft, (b) viral warts, (c) thrombosed external haemorrhoids, (d) rectal mucosal prolapse and (e) the bluish discoloration typical of Crohn's disease.

Fig. 7.73 The rectal examination. (a) Insert the tip of the index finger into the anus then (b) introduce your finger to follow the curve of the sacrum. (c) Rotate the finger anteriorly to palpate the anterolateral and lateral walls and the prostate or cervix.

finger with the anal muscles. Then gently sweep the finger through 180° using the palmar surface of the finger to explore the posterior and posterolateral walls of the rectum. Rotate the finger round to the 12 o'clock position. This is accomplished more easily by adopting a half-crouched position and simultaneously pronating your wrist. This position allows you to sweep the finger across the anterior and anterolateral walls of the rectum. The normal rectum feels uniformly smooth and pliable. In men, the prostate can be felt anteriorly and in women it may be possible to feel the cervix as well as a retroverted uterus.

On rectal palpation you may feel an intrinsic tumour caused by a carcinoma or polyp. Perirectal sepsis causes marked rectal wall tenderness and an abscess may be felt pointing into the lumen. The anterior rectal peritoneal reflection straddles both the anterior rectum itself and the structures lying in front of it. Consequently, malignant or inflammatory lesions of the peritoneum may be felt through the anterior wall of the rectum.

Withdraw your finger from the rectum and anus and check the glove tip for stool. There may be melaena, blood or pus and you may notice the pale, greasy stools characteristic of malabsorption.

PROSTATE

The prostate gland is examined during the rectal examination. The normal prostate measures approximately 3.5 cm from side to side and protrudes 1 cm into the rectum (Fig. 7.74a). The gland has a rubbery, smooth consistency and a shallow longitudinal groove separates the right and left lobes. It should not be tender to palpation but the patient may experience the urge to urinate.

Palpation of the prostate aims to assess size, consistency, nodularity and tenderness. The assessment of prostatic size is learnt through experience. Benign hypertrophy of the prostate is common in men over 60 years old. The enlargement is smooth and symmetrical and the gland feels rubbery or slightly boggy (Fig. 7.74b). A cancerous prostate may feel asymmetric, with a stony hard consistency, and discrete nodules may be palpable (Fig. 7.74c). Marked prostatic tenderness suggests acute prostatitis, a prostatic abscess or inflammation of the seminal vesicles. If prostatic infection is suspected, attempt to massage the organ from within the rectum in order to squeeze prostatic fluid towards the urethral meatus, where it can be collected for microscopy and culture.

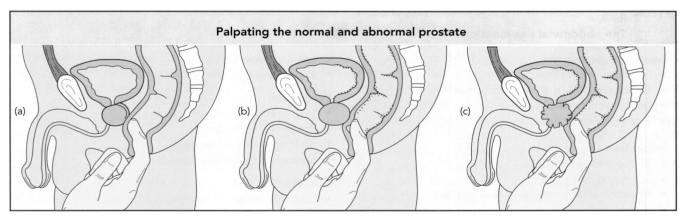

Palpating the normal and abnormal prostate

(a) (b) (c)

Fig. 7.74 (a) The normal prostate felt through the anterior rectal wall has a median sulcus separating the two lateral lobes. (b) The median sulcus may become indistinct in a benign hypertrophied prostate and the gland feels firm and smooth and bulges more than 1 cm into the lumen. (c) A carcinomatous prostate feels hard and irregular and the median sulcus is obliterated.

 Differential diagnosis
Causes of faecal incontinence

Severe constipation with overflow

Diseases of the colon and rectum
- Acute diarrhoeal illness
- Inflammatory bowel disease
- Colorectal cancer
- Hypotonic sphincter following difficult vaginal delivery

Neurological disorders
- Dementias and depressive illness
- Cerebrovascular disease and stroke
- Spinal cord disease
- Autonomic neuropathy

characterised by fever as well as redness and tenderness over the infected segment. Ask about local trauma, as fat necrosis may cause pain, and also consider thrombophlebitis of the veins (Mondor's disease).

DISCHARGE

Patients may present with an abnormal nipple discharge. Determine whether the fluid is clear, opalescent or bloodstained. In men, and women who have never conceived, a discharge is always abnormal. However, after childbearing, some women continue to discharge a small secretion well after lactation has stopped. The inappropriate secretion of milk (galactorrhoea) is caused by a deranged prolactin physiology. A blood discharge should always alert you to the likelihood of an underlying breast cancer.

BREAST LUMPS

A patient may present after discovering a breast lump by self-examination. This discovery causes great alarm because the patient will usually associate the lump with breast cancer.

EXAMINATION OF THE BREAST

You will usually examine the breast in the course of the chest examination. In asymptomatic women, you will need to decide whether to include a full breast examination as part of your routine examination. Male doctors must always examine in the presence of a female nurse or chaperone. The aim of examination is to check for breast lumps and it is reasonable to recommend a formal breast examination in asymptomatic women over the age of 40 years. Before examining the patient, suggest to her that the general examination of the chest offers a good opportunity to check the breasts for lumps. Remember to inform her of your findings (reassurance is the best of all medicines). Many techniques have been described, yet the principles remain similar.

INSPECTION

The patient should undress to the waist. Position yourself in front of the patient, who should be sitting comfortably with her arms at her side (Fig. 8.13). Note the size, symmetry and contour of the breasts, the colour and venous pattern of the skin. Observe the nipples and note whether they are symmetrically everted, flat or inverted. If there is unilateral flattening or nipple inversion, ask whether this is a recent or long-standing appearance. In fair-skinned women, the areola has a pink colour but darkens and becomes permanently pigmented during the first pregnancy. Ask the patient to raise her arms above her head and then press her hands against her hips (Figs 8.14, 8.15). These movements tighten the suspensory ligaments, exaggerating the contours and highlighting any abnormality. In men, the nipple should lie flat on the pectoralis muscle.

Dx Differential diagnosis
Breast lumps

Benign
- Fibroadenoma (mobile)
- Simple cyst
- Fat necrosis
- Fibroadenosis (tender 'lumpy' breasts)
- Abscess (painful and tender)

Malignant
- Glandular
- Areolar

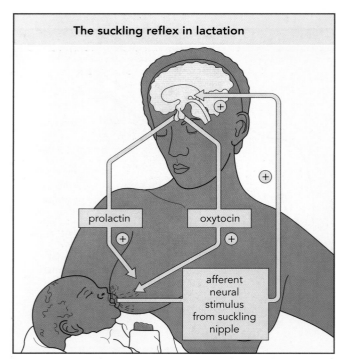

The suckling reflex in lactation

prolactin

oxytocin

afferent neural stimulus from suckling nipple

Fig. 8.12 Sucking sends an afferent stimulus to the anterior and posterior pituitary, resulting in the release of prolactin and oxytocin.

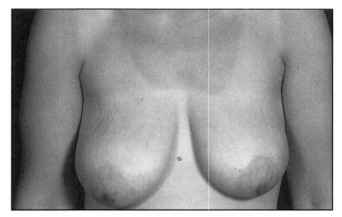

Fig. 8.13 Initially, inspect the breast from the front with the patient sitting with her arms comfortably resting at her sides.

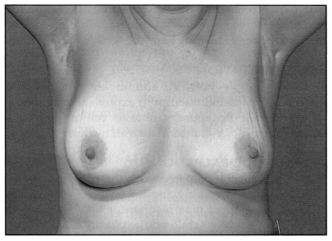

Fig. 8.14   To accentuate any asymmetry of the breast ask the patient to raise her arms above her head.

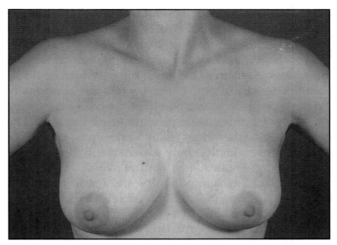

Fig. 8.15   Another technique for accentuating the breast contours is by pressing the hands against the hips.

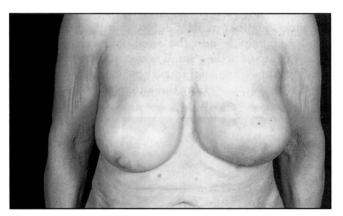

Fig. 8.16   Asymmetry of the breast.

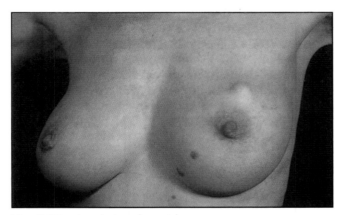

Fig. 8.17   An obvious breast lump.

ABNORMALITIES ON INSPECTION

In normal women there may be some asymmetry of the breast and nipples, ranging from unilateral hypoplasia to a mild but obvious asymmetry (Fig. 8.16). You may be struck by an obvious lump (Fig. 8.17), retraction or gross deviation of a nipple (Fig. 8.18), prominent veins or oedema of the skin with dimpling like an orange skin (peau d'orange). Abnormal reddening, thickening or ulceration of the areola should alert you to the possibility of Paget's disease of the breast, a specialised form of breast cancer (Fig. 8.19). Male gynaecomastia is an important physical sign and may be spotted on inspection as a swelling of the areola or, in more florid cases, the development of obvious breasts (see Ch. 9).

BREAST PALPATION

During the chest examination the patient will be lying on the examination couch with her arms resting comfortably at her side or held above her head. Palpate the breast tissue with the palmar surface of the middle three fingers, using an even rotary movement to compress the breast tissue gently towards the chest wall

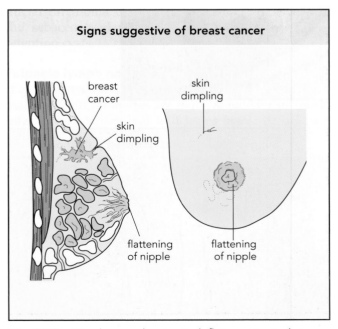

Fig. 8.18   Nipples may be everted, flat or retracted.

Questions to ask
The menstrual cycle

- Age of menarche?
- Age of telarche?
- Do you use the contraceptive pill or hormone replacement therapy?
- Length of cycle?
- Days of blood loss?
- Number of tampons or pads used per day?
- Are there clots?
- Has there been a change in the periodicity of the cycle?

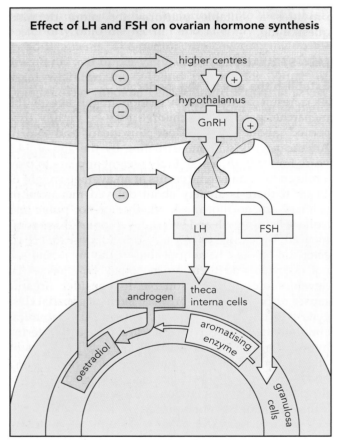

Effect of LH and FSH on ovarian hormone synthesis

Fig. 8.35 Effect of gonadotrophins on the theca interna and granulosa cells which produce the ovarian hormones.

cators: women with heavy periods saturate rather than stain tampons or pads, whereas the passage of large and frequent clots suggests excessive bleeding. The only accurate method for assessing menstrual loss is to weigh absorbent pads before and after each change.

Attempt to classify any change or abnormality in the menstrual cycle. First establish whether the cycles are regular and, if so, calculate the cycle length and attempt to assess whether the periods are scanty or heavy. Bear in mind contraceptive practices because the patient's intrinsic rhythms will be masked if she is taking a cyclical contraceptive pill or undergoing hor-

mone replacement therapy (HRT) (Fig. 8.35). The most common irregularities include failure to menstruate at the expected time (secondary amenorrhoea). Cycles may be infrequent and scanty (oligomenorrhoea), unusually frequent (polymenorrhoea), excessively heavy (menorrhagia) or frequent and heavy (polymenorrhagia). Bleeding after intercourse is termed postcoital bleeding. If regular cycles are interrupted by days of spotting or blood-tinged discharge, this is known as intermenstrual bleeding.

Secondary amenorrhoea

Develop the case history by considering possible causes of secondary amenorrhoea. Pregnancy and lactation are the most common causes. The patient may suspect a pregnancy: there may be clues such as early morning nausea and vomiting, urinary frequency and tender enlarged breasts. Stress, anxiety, depression, bereavement and a change of environment may interrupt the cyclical release of sex hormones by the hypothalamic–pituitary axis. Consider fear of pregnancy, which is a common cause of delayed menstruation. Not only do patients with excessive weight loss due to anorexia nervosa present with amenorrhoea but highly trained long-distance athletes may also stop menstruating. Enquire about contraceptive practices as 'post pill' amenorrhoea is well recognised. Consider the menopause in women entering the climacteric years. This is often heralded by a change in the cyclical pattern, reduced menstrual flow and the onset of menopausal symptoms such as hot flushes and dryness of the introitus and vagina. In the absence of

Differential diagnosis
Secondary amenorrhoea

Physiological
- Pregnancy
- Lactation

Psychological
- Anorexia nervosa
- Depression
- Fear of pregnancy

Hormonal
- Postcontraceptive pill
- Pituitary tumours
- Hyperthyroidism
- Adrenal tumours

Ovarian
- Polycystic ovaries
- Ovarian tumour
- Ovarian tuberculosis
- Constitutional disease
- Severe acute illness
- Chronic infections or illnesses
- Autoimmune diseases

an obvious cause for amenorrhoea, consider diseases of the hypothalamus, pituitary and ovary.

Abnormal patterns of uterine bleeding

Oligomenorrhoea Oligomenorrhoea is the term used to describe infrequent or scanty menstrual periods. This pattern may be normal between the menarche and the establishment of a regular menstrual pattern and is also a feature of the climacteric as the menopause approaches. In some women, the oligomenorrhoea of puberty persists into adult life. Ascertain whether the infrequent, scanty periods are a change from the normal pattern or a pattern present from puberty. If oligomenorrhoea presents as a distinct change in the menstrual pattern, consider the same factors implicated in the differential diagnosis of secondary amenorrhoea.

Dysfunctional uterine bleeding This term is used to describe frequent bleeding or excessive menstrual loss that cannot be ascribed to local pelvic pathology (e.g. fibroids, pelvic inflammatory disease, carcinoma, polyps). Establish whether the abnormal cyclical pattern is regular or irregular. Regular dysfunctional bleeding may present as menorrhagia, epimenorrhoea or polymenorrhoea. The predictability of these abnormal cycles usually implies that ovulation is occurring, although this needs to be confirmed. Irregular dysfunctional bleeding usually implies that ovulation has ceased; the menstrual rhythm is lost and the cyclical pattern is replaced by unpredictable bleeding of varying severity.

Intermenstrual and postmenopausal bleeding Patients may complain of vaginal bleeding unexpectedly between normal periods or after the menopause. Enquire about sex hormone therapy, as 'breakthrough bleeding' may occur with hormone treatment. Diseases of the uterus and cervix may present with abnormal bleeding, so consider disorders of the mucosa (e.g. endometritis, carcinoma, endometrial polyps) or submucosa (e.g. submucosal leiomyomas, fibroids). Postcoital bleeding usually indicates local cervical or uterine disease (carcinoma or a cervical polyp).

Vaginal discharge

Vaginal discharge is a common complaint during the child-bearing years. Many women notice slight soiling of the underwear at the end of the day; this is a normal physiological response to the cyclical changes occurring in the glandular epithelium of the genital tract and it is likely to become more profuse in pregnancy. A physiological discharge is scanty, mucoid and odourless. Pathological discharge is usually trichomonal or candidal vaginitis. The discharge may irritate the vulval skin causing itching (pruritus vulvae) or burning. Attempt to assess the severity of the dis-

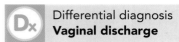

Dx Differential diagnosis
Vaginal discharge

Physiological
- Pregnancy
- Sexual arousal
- Menstrual cycle variation

Pathological
- Vaginal
  - candidosis (thrush)
  - trichomoniasis
  - *Gardnerella* associated
  - other bacteria (e.g. caused by a retained tampon)
  - postmenopausal vaginitis
- Cervical
  - gonorrhoea
  - nonspecific genital infection
  - herpes
  - cervical ectopy
  - cervical neoplasm (e.g. polyp)
  - intrauterine contraceptive device

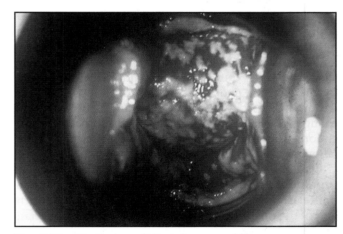

Fig. 8.36 Vaginal candidiasis has a curd-like appearance.

charge by ascertaining whether the discharge merely stains the underwear or is heavier and requires protective pads.

The nature of the discharge may be helpful. With vaginitis caused by *Candida albicans* the discharge is white, has a curd-like appearance and consistency (Fig. 8.36) and causes intense itching. Vaginitis caused by *Trichomonas vaginalis* usually presents with a profuse opaque or cream-coloured, frothy discharge that has a characteristic 'fishy' smell (Fig. 8.37). The trichomonal discharge may cause vulval irritation and is occasionally accompanied by burning on micturition: this is caused by inflammation of the urethral meatus. If the patient complains of a profuse, foul-smelling discharge, consider a retained foreign body (e.g. a tampon). Cervical infection due to gonorrhoea, *Chlamydia trachomatis* or nonspecific cervicitis may masses (Figs 8.45, 8.46). Most genital warts are caused by a human papillomavirus. The lesions usually occur on the fourchette and may extend onto the labia, into the vagina, and posteriorly onto the perineum. Flat, round or oval papules covered by a grey exudate suggests lesions of secondary syphilis (condylomata lata) (Fig. 8.47).

Vulval ulceration has a wide differential diagnosis. The most common ulcerating lesions include carcinoma of the vulva or macerated, ulcerating herpetic warts. Acute vulval ulceration occurring with mouth and tongue ulcers and inflamed red eyes suggests Behçet's syndrome. A firm painless labial ulcer suggests the chancre of primary syphilis, whereas broad, moist ulcerating papules covered by grey slough suggest secondary syphilis. Suspect granuloma inguinale (caused by *C. trachomatis*) in women from tropical and subtropical regions presenting with vulval nodules and inguinal lymphadenopathy. The nodules coalesce and ulcerate, forming a large ulcer with rolled edges which must be distinguished from carcinoma. Chancroid, caused by *Haemophilus ducreyi*, is another sexually-transmitted ulcerating disease affecting the vulva.

Leucoplakia is a potentially malignant, hypertrophic skin lesion affecting the labia, clitoris and perineum. The skin thickens, feels hard and indurated and is distinguished from surrounding tissue by its white colour.

Bartholin's glands are palpable if the ducts obstruct. This results in a painless cystic mass or an acute (Bartholin's) abscess: a hot, red, tender swelling in the posterolateral labia majora deep to the posterior end of the labia minora (Fig. 8.48).

Differential diagnosis
Vulval ulceration

Squamous cell carcinoma

Infections
- Syphilitic chancre
- Secondary syphilis
- Granuloma inguinale (chlamydia)
- Chancroid (*Haemophilus ducreyi*)
- Ulcerating herpetic warts

Behçet's syndrome

EXAMINATION OF THE VAGINA

If the patient has an intact hymen, you may choose to examine the genitalia indirectly through the rectum. If the woman has an intact hymen but uses vaginal tampons, it is usually possible to perform a single digit vaginal examination.

Before proceeding with the internal examination, separate the labia to expose the vestibule and ask the

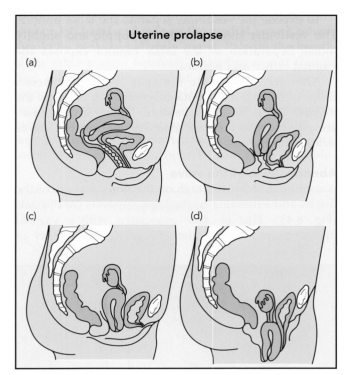
Fig. 8.49 Uterine prolapse. (a) Normal uterus. (b) First- and (c) second-degree prolapse of the uterus. (d) Complete prolapse of the uterus.

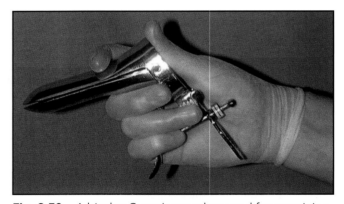
Fig. 8.50 A bivalve Cusco's speculum used for examining the vaginal walls and cervix.

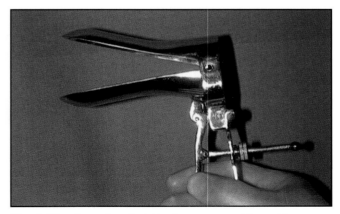
Fig. 8.51 Speculum held in the open position with a lock-nut.

patient to 'bear down' and exert a downward force on the vulva. If the pelvic floor is stable and the muscles intact, bulges and swellings should not appear through the vaginal walls below the introitus. If there is muscle weakness, the posterior bladder wall may prolapse, causing a bulge (a cystocele) along the anterior vaginal wall (Fig. 8.34). If the rectum prolapses, this may cause a bulge (a rectocele) in the posterior vaginal wall. Uterine prolapse may also occur (Fig. 8.49).

A full vaginal examination includes inspection with a speculum, followed by a bimanual examination of the uterus and adnexae. Before continuing the examination, explain that you are about to inspect the vagina and cervix with a speculum.

SPECULUM EXAMINATION

The speculum is designed for inspection of the cervix and vaginal walls. In addition, the speculum provides access to the cervix and fornices for bacteriological swabs and cervical smears. If you anticipate taking samples, use water as a lubricant for your gloved fingers and the speculum because lubricant gels may interfere with the processing and analysis of samples.

A bivalve speculum (e.g. Cusco's) is the instrument most commonly used to insepct the vagina (Fig. 8.50). Thoroughly familiarise yourself with its operation before examining a patient. The instrument is made of either stainless steel or plastic, and is available in different sizes. There are two blunt, rounded, elongated blades hinged at the base. In the closed position, the tips of the blades appose, allowing the closed blades to slide safely into the slit-shaped introitus and into the tubular vagina. The blades open when the thumbpiece is squeezed (Fig. 8.51) and, once positioned in the vagina, a hinged screw and nut arrangement fixes the blades in the open position.

Warm the blades under a stream of tepid water. The most convenient hand position for holding the speculum is illustrated in Figure 8.50. Explain to the patient that you are about to insert the instrument and reassure her that the procedure should be painless. Use the index and middle fingers of the free hand to separate the labia and expose the introitus (Fig. 8.52a). Position these two fingers just inside the introitus, pressing gently towards the perineal body. Slide the closed blades obliquely over the fingers into the introitus and introduce the instrument into the vagina, directing it to follow the line of the long axis of the vagina, maintaining a posterior angulation of approximately 45° (Fig. 8.52b). While inserting the instrument, rotate it in a clockwise direction until the anterior and posterior blades run along the length of the anterior and posterior vaginal walls with the handles pointing towards the anus (Figs 8.52c,d). Maintain a downward pressure on the speculum and press on the thumbpiece to hinge the blades open (Fig. 8.52e) to expose the vaginal vault and cervix (Fig. 8.52f).

Adjust the light source to illuminate the vagina. If the cervix is not immediately visible, arc the blades anteriorly to bring the cervix into view. If you have difficulty finding the cervix, withdraw the blades a little and reposition the speculum in a more horizontal plane. Make any minor adjustments necessary to establish the optimal position for visualising the cervix, then tighten the thumbscrew to secure the position.

EXAMINATION OF THE CERVIX

The position of the cervix relates to the position of the uterus (Fig. 8.32). The cervix usually points posteriorly and the uterus lies in an anterior plane (anteversion). Conversely, the cervix may point anteriorly with the uterus in a posterior retroverted position. There are also intermediate positions between these two. The

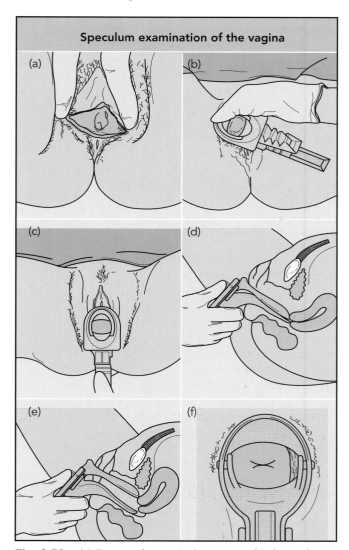

Fig. 8.52 (a) Expose the vaginal opening, (b) direct the closed speculum into the vagina, (c) rotate the speculum as it penetrates the long axis. (d) Final position of the fully inserted speculum. (e). Open the blades. (f) Search for the cervix and os.

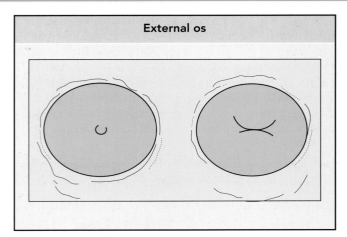

Fig. 8.53   In nulliparous women, the external os is round (left); it becomes slit-shaped (right) after birth of a child.

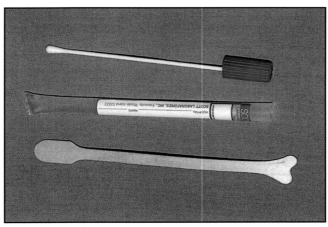

Fig. 8.54   Spatula with bifid end used for cervical cytology. Transport medium for microbiology, and swab.

cervix should lie centrally along the long axis of the vagina projecting 1–3 cm into the vagina. The shape of the external os changes after childbirth. In nulliparous women, the os is round, whereas after childbirth, the os may be slit-like or stellate (Fig. 8.53).

Inspect the colour of the cervix. The colour varies according to the position of the meeting point, usually in the region of the external os, of the squamous epithelium covering the vaginal surface of the cervix and the mucosal lining of the cervical canal. The surface of the cervix is pink, smooth and regular, and resembles the epithelium of the vagina. In early pregnancy the cervix has a bluish colour caused by increased vascularity (Chadwick's sign). During pregnancy, the squamocolumnar junction may migrate beyond the external os and onto the cervix, retreating back, a few months after childbirth, into the cervical canal. Periodically, after pregnancy, the squamocolumnar junctions fail to regress into the os, giving the appearance of an erosion (ectopy). Failure to regress during fetal development may give rise to a congenital erosion. Cervical 'erosions' are not ulcerated surfaces but a term used to describe the appearance of the cervix when the endocervical epithelium extends onto the outer surface of the cervix. The columnar epithelium appears as a strawberry-red area spreading circumferentially around the os or onto the anterior or posterior lips. Cervical ectopy cannot be confidently distinguished from early cervical cancer, so cytology should always be performed.

ABNORMALITIES OF THE CERVIX

An eccentric cervix suggests disease of the uterus or the adnexae. Nabothian cysts may develop if there is obstruction of the endocervical glands. These are seen as small, round, raised white or yellow lesions which only assume importance if they become infected. There may be a cervical discharge. If there is a pungent odour, suspect an infective cause and swab the area.

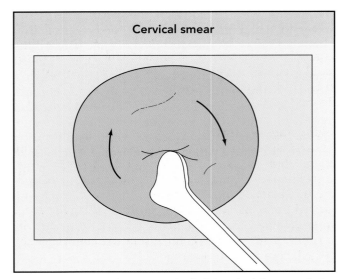

Fig. 8.55   Cervical meatus. The bifid end of the spatula is advanced to the external os and cervical cells are harvested by rotating the spatula around the circumference of the os.

An inflamed cervix covered by a mucopurulent discharge or slough is characteristic of acute and chronic cervicitis; the mucosa looks red rather than pink and, if the cervicitis follows pregnancy, you may notice laceration and pouting of the endocervical mucosa (ectropion). Cherry-red friable polyps may grow from the cervix (a source of vaginal bleeding after intercourse). Ulceration and fungating growths suggest cervical carcinoma.

Cervical smear

Cytologists can detect premalignant cells or established cervical cancer by examining a preparation of cells scraped from the surface of the cervix. The technique is routine in the course of the speculum examination. The demonstration of premalignant cells provides the opportunity for cancer prevention: the early detection of cancer allows for a higher, successful cure rate.

Before proceeding with the smear, prepare three clean glass microscope slides. Accurate labelling of the specimens is critical: slides with frosted glass at one end are preferable, for this allows you to write the patient's name and number clearly on the slide. Prepare the slide, mark with the patient's details, and label 'cervical smear'. Explain to the patient that you are about to take a smear. The cervical smear is performed after inspecting the cervix. A specially-designed disposable wooden spatula with a bifid end at one side and a rounded end at the other is used (Fig. 8.54). The bifid end is used to harvest the cervical cells. Introduce the spatula through the speculum and position the bifid end at the os (Fig. 8.55). The desquamating cells are collected by rotating the spatula around the circumference of the os and the lips of the cervix. Withdraw the spatula and spread the cervical material onto the labelled glass slide by stroking each side of the bifid end of the spatula along the glass. The cervical cells and some mucus should cling to the glass. Immediately spray the slides with fixative or fix them by immersion in 95% alcohol.

Taking vaginal swabs

If the patient has a vaginal discharge, use the speculum examination to take a swab for culture. You can use a conventional throat swab; insert the cotton wool end into the secretion (e.g. the region of the cervical os and vaginal pool) and allow the tip sufficient time to soak up secretion. Remove the swab, place it in a suitable transport medium and send the specimen immediately to the laboratory for processing.

Removing the speculum

After inspecting the cervix, undo the thumbscrew and simultaneously withdraw the speculum and rotate the open blades in an anticlockwise direction to ensure that the anterior and posterior walls of the vagina can be inspected. Near the introitus, allow the blades to close, taking care not to pinch the labia or any hairs while withdrawing the speculum.

INTERNAL EXAMINATION OF THE UTERUS

The speculum examination is followed by the vaginal examination. Explain that you are about to perform an internal examination of the uterus, tubes and ovaries. Again, expose the introitus by separating the labia with the thumb and forefinger of the gloved left hand and gently introduce the gloved and lubricated right index and middle fingers into the vagina, remembering that the organ is directed backwards in the direc-

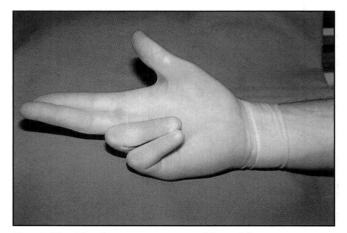

Fig. 8.56 The finger position used for performing a vaginal examination.

tion of the sacrum. The thumb is abducted to allow maximum use of the length of the index and middle fingers; the ring and little finger are flexed into the palm (Fig. 8.56). Palpate the vaginal wall as you introduce your fingers. The walls are slightly rugose, supple and moist.

CERVIX

Locate the cervix with the pulps of your fingertips. The cervix should feel firm, rounded and smooth. Assess the mobility of the cervix by moving it gently and palpate the fornices. This procedure should be painless.

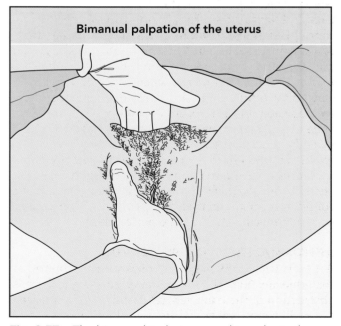

Fig. 8.57 The bimanual technique used to palpate the uterus. The vaginal fingers lift the cervix, while the other hand dips downwards and inwards to meet the fundus.

Abnormalities of the cervix

In pregnancy, the cervix softens (Hegar's sign). If there is tenderness on movement (known as 'excitation tenderness'), suspect infection or inflammation of the uterus or adnexae; or if the patient is shocked, suspect an ectopic pregnancy. You may palpate an ulcer or tumour already noted on the speculum examination.

UTERUS

Next, palpate the uterus. A bimanual technique is used to assess the size and position of the organ (Fig. 8.57). Position the palmar surface of your free hand on the anterior abdominal wall about 4 cm above the symphysis pubis. Attempt to 'capture' the uterus gently between your apposing fingers. Use your internal fingers to elevate the cervix and uterus in the direction of the external hand while simultaneously pressing the fingertips of the external hand in the direction of the internal fingers. Using this displacement technique an anteverted fundus should be palpable just above the symphysis. Assess its size, consistency and mobility, and note any masses and tenderness.

Further exploration may be helped by re-examining the uterus with your fingers positioned in the anterior fornix (Fig. 8.58); this permits the vaginal fingers to examine the anterior surface of the uterus while the abdominal fingers explore the posterior wall. If the uterus is retroverted, the fundus is more difficult to feel through the abdominal wall; nevertheless, it might become more readily palpable if the vaginal fingers are positioned in the posterior fornix.

Abnormalities of the uterus

If the uterus appears to be uniformly enlarged, consider a pregnancy, fibroid or endometrial tumour. Fibromyomas (fibroids) are common benign uterine tumours which may be single or multiple and may vary in size. Single, large uterine fibroids are felt on abdominal examination as a firm, nontender, well-defined rounded mass arising from the pelvis. On bimanual palpation, the mass appears contiguous with the cervix: the two structures move together. Multiple fibroids give the uterus a lobulated feel. Occasionally, the fibroid is pedunculated and is felt as a mobile pelvic mass which is readily confused with a mass arising from the adnexae.

ADNEXAE

Palpate the left and right adnexae in turn. Note, the adnexae are difficult to palpate in obese women. Place the fingers of your abdominal hand over the iliac fossa while readjusting the vaginal fingers into the lateral fornix and positioning the finger pulps to face the abdominal fingers (Fig. 8.59). Remembering the anatomy of the ovaries and fallopian tubes, gently but firmly appose the fingers of either hand by pressing the abdominal hand inward and downward, and the vaginal fingers upwards and laterally. Feel for the adnexal structures as the interposed tissues slip between your fingers. The manoeuvre should be relatively painless, although palpation of the ovaries might elicit some tenderness. Yet again, reassure you patient that any discomfort she feels is normal. If you feel an adnexal structure, assess its

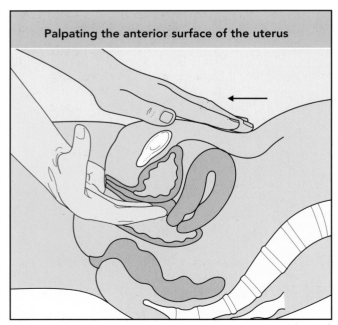

Fig. 8.58 By placing the vaginal fingers in the anterior fornix it is possible to examine the anterior surface of the uterus.

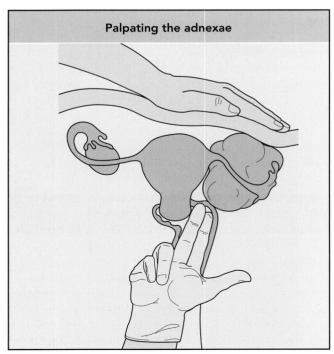

Fig. 8.59 Positioning the vaginal and abdominal fingers to palpate the adnexal structures.

Review
The gynecological examination

General examination
- Endocrine syndrome
- Hirsutism, acne
- Breast examination
- Routine abdominal examination
- Inguinal lymph nodes

Vulva
- Inspection and palpation of the vulva
- Bartholin's gland palpation

Vagina
- Digital examination
  - cervix
  - cervical tenderness
  - fornices
  - pouch of Douglas

Uterus
- Bimanual palpation
  - body and fundus
  - adnexal region
  - ovaries

Speculum
- Inspect cervix and os
- Take cervical smear
- Bacterial swab for culture
- Inspect vaginal mucosa as speculum withdrawn

size, shape, mobility and tenderness. Ovaries are firm, ovoid, and often palpable. Normal fallopian tubes are impalpable.

Abnormalities of the adnexal structures

The most common causes of enlarged ovaries include benign cysts (e.g. follicular or corpus luteal cysts) and malignant ovarian tumours. Ovarian tumours are either unilateral or bilateral. Cysts feel smooth and the wall may be compressible. Occasionally, ovarian tumours are large enough to be palpable on abdominal examination and may fill the lower and mid-abdomen, creating the impression of ascites.

In acute infections of the fallopian tubes (salpingitis), there is lower abdominal tenderness and guarding, and, on vaginal examination, marked tenderness of the lateral fornices and cervix. The acute pain makes palpation of the adnexae difficult. In chronic salpingitis, the lower abdomen and lateral fornices are tender, yet the uterus and adnexae may be amenable to examination. If the uterus is retroverted and fixed by adhesions, it may be possible to feel thickening and swelling of the tubes extending to the ovaries. If the tubes are blocked, there may be cystic swelling of the tubes (hydrosalpinx) or they may become infected and purulent (pyosalpinx).

After completing the bimanual examination, withdraw your fingers from the vagina and inspect the glove tips for blood or discharge. Redrape the genital area and reassure the patient that the examination is complete and that you will discuss the findings in the consulting room once she is dressed.

Examination of elderly people
Breasts and genital tract

- There is rapid fall in sex hormone synthesis after the menopause, resulting in changes in the structure and function of the genitalia
- There is progressive involution of the breast tissue and, as the acinar tissue atrophies, the breasts become more pendulous
- The risk of breast cancer remains at any age, including the very old
- After the menopause there is loss of vulval adipose tissue, and reduction in vaginal secretion results in drying of the mucosal surface
- The atrophy of tissue of the introitus results in vestibular narrowing, increased susceptibility to urinary tract infection and dyspareunia
- Loss of sex hormones results in altered hair distribution and androgen dominance may be apparent with male pattern facial hair growth, mild to moderate male pattern baldness and loss of the female pattern labial hairline
- Despite involutional changes, many older women maintain libido and remain sexually active into the later years of life
- Atrophy of the vagina and introitus can be prevented by hormone replacement therapy and topical oestrogen application
- Vaginal lubrication can be enhanced by using water-soluble lubricant jellies

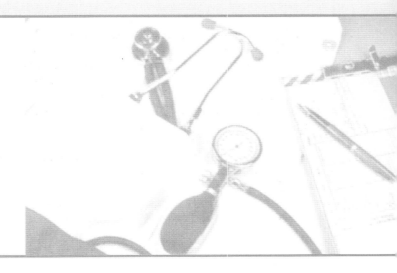

9.
The Male Genitalia

Unlike the female genitalia, the male organs are readily accessible for examination. As for women, taking a sexual case history and examining a male is embarrassing and intrusive, so care must be taken to ensure confidentiality, privacy and comfort. An overview of structure and function will help you gain confidence when taking a history and examining the genitalia and will aid the interpretation of symptoms and signs.

STRUCTURE AND FUNCTION

The male genitalia include the penis, scrotum, testes, epididymides, seminal vesicles and prostate gland (Fig. 9.1). The penis provides a common pathway to the exterior for both urine and semen. In fetal devel-

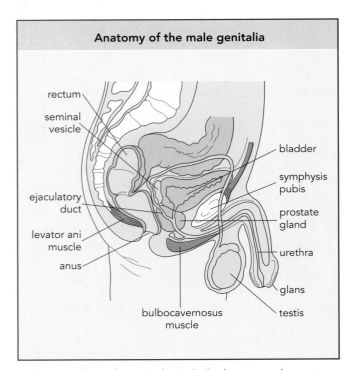

Anatomy of the male genitalia

rectum
seminal vesicle
ejaculatory duct
levator ani muscle
anus
bulbocavernosus muscle
bladder
symphysis pubis
prostate gland
urethra
glans
testis

Fig. 9.1 The male genitalia include the external organs, seminal vesicles and the prostate gland.

opment, the testes develop close to the kidneys and slowly migrate caudally, emerging at the external inguinal ring in the eighth month of development and descending into the scrotum in the ninth month. The neural, vascular and lymphatic supply to the testes also arise from near the kidney and the migrating testes drag these structures through the inguinal canal into the scrotum. This has important clinical implications, as renal pain is often referred to the scrotum and the natural route for lymphatic spread of testicular cancer is to para-aortic (rather than inguinal) nodes.

PUBERTY
In boys, puberty starts 1–2 years later than in girls. The onset of male puberty is signalled by an increase in testicular volume and this is followed approximately 1 year later by a spurt in linear growth and an increase in muscle bulk.

Hormonal changes in puberty
Testosterone feedback to the hypothalamus can inhibit the hypothalamic–pituitary axis release of luteinising hormone (LH) and follicle-stimulating hormone (FSH). In the child, this feedback is especially sensitive and even low levels of circulating gonadal steroids are sufficient to inhibit the secretion of FSH and LH. Male puberty is initiated by a fall in the sensitivity of the hypothalamus to inhibition at low levels of circulating sex hormones. By resetting the sensitivity of the feedback to the hypothalamus, FSH and LH are released, thereby exerting their trophic effects on their target cells in the testes.

Throughout male puberty, LH levels increase slowly and steadily (Fig. 9.2), whereas FSH levels increase more sharply in early puberty, with a more gentle increase afterwards. FSH stimulates the Sertoli cells and regulates the growth of seminiferous tubules and spermatogenesis. As most of the testis is formed of tubules, the increased testicular volume in puberty is largely under the control of FSH. LH stimulates the Leydig (interstitial) cells which synthesise testosterone from cholesterol (Fig. 9.3). Testosterone circulates bound to sex hormone-binding globulin (SHBG). The linear growth spurt follows closely behind the surge of testosterone. Some testosterone is converted to oestrodiol in the Leydig cells and other extragonadal tissue sites. The effects of testosterone are in Table 9.1 shown. The importance of oestrogen in males remains unclear, although it does regulate the synthesis of SHBG.

Development of secondary sexual characteristics

Tanner described the pubertal development of the male genitalia and pubic hair growth (Fig. 9.4). Initially, the testes enlarge and the scrotal skin becomes thin and red (stage 2). The enlargement of the phallus occurs later in the growth spurt and is associated with thickening, crinkling and pigmentation of the scrotal skin (stage 3). Increasing levels of gonadal and adrenal androgens stimulate the growth of pubic, axillary and facial hair. Pubic hair begins to develop as sparse, long, slightly curly hair at the base of the phallus (stage 4). Later, coarser, curlier hair extends to cover the symphysis pubis and finally extends to the inner thigh and along the linea alba (this constitutes the male escutcheon) (stage 5).

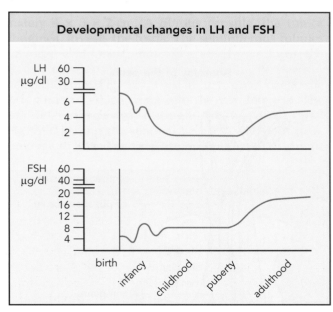

Fig. 9.2 Changes in LH and FSH secretion before, during and after puberty.

Table 9.1 Effects of testosterone

- Stimulates the development of secondary sexual characteristics
- Controls libido
- Anabolic effect causes muscle growth and fat deposition
- With growth hormone, stimulates linear growth in adolescence
- With erythropoietin, stimulates red cell production

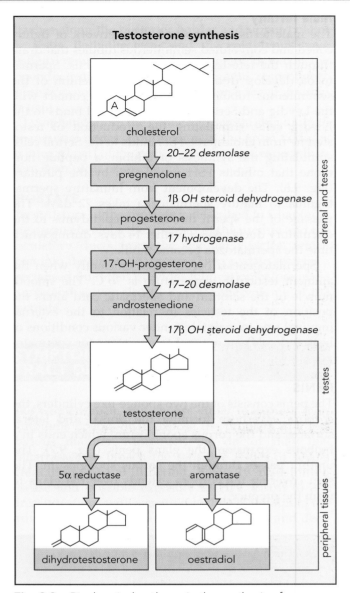

Fig. 9.3 Biochemical pathway in the synthesis of testosterone from cholesterol.

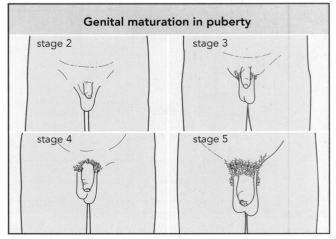

Fig. 9.4 Tanner's five stages of male genital maturation. (Stage 1 preadolescence is not shown.)

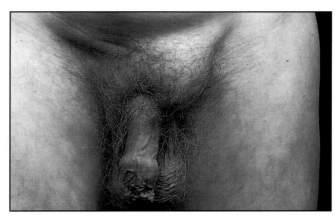

Fig. 9.11 Hernias may only become apparent when the patient stands.

confidence, or lack of it, soon becomes apparent to the patient. If you have a good knowledge of the anatomy and physiology already outlined, you will soon master a quick but thorough examination. It is advisable for women doctors to examine the genitalia with a chaperone close at hand.

It is usual practice to wear disposable plastic gloves for hygienic reasons and to emphasise the strictly clinical nature of the examination. The genitalia are usually examined with the patient lying but remember that varicoceles and scrotal hernias may only be apparent when the patient stands; it is advisable to check for scrotal swellings in the standing position if the diagnosis is unclear with the patient lying down (Fig. 9.11). Avoid creating a feeling of total nakedness by covering part of the thighs.

GENERAL EXAMINATION

You will already have performed a general examination and noted the distribution of facial, axillary and abdominal hair. In testicular malfunction (hypogonadism), there may be loss of axillary hair, the pubic hair distribution may start to resemble the distinctive

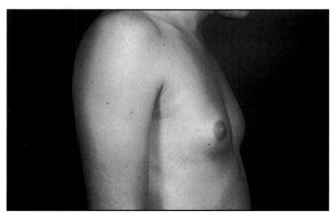

Fig. 9.12 Typical appearance of male gynaecomastasia.

female pattern and there is a typical facial appearance with wrinkling around the mouth. You will have also checked the breast and noted whether or not gynaecomastia was evident (Fig. 9.12).

NORMAL PENIS

The length and thickness of the flaccid penis vary widely and bear no relationship either to potency or to fertility. The dorsal vein of the penis is usually prominent along the dorsal midline. Gently retract the foreskin (prepuce) to expose the glans penis. The foreskin should be supple, allowing smooth and painless retraction. There is often a trace of odourless, curd-like smegma underlying the foreskin. Examine the external urethral meatus, which is a slit-like orifice extending from the ventral pole of the tip of the glans. Use your index finger and thumb to squeeze the meatus gently open. This should expose healthy, glistening pink mucosa. If the patient has complained of a urethral discharge, try to elicit this sign. The patient may be able to 'milk' the shaft of the penis to express the secretion; if not, you may try to express a discharge by 'milking' the shaft of the penis from the base towards the glans. If a discharge appears, swab the area with a sterile bud and immerse the specimen in a transport medium for quick dispatch to the microbiology laboratory.

 Differential diagnosis
Male gynaecomastia

Physiological
- Puberty
- Old age

Pathological
- Hypogonadism
- Liver cirrhosis
- Drugs (spironolactone, digoxin, oestrogens)
- Tumours (bronchogenic carcinoma, adrenal carcinoma, testicular tumours)
- Thyrotoxicosis

ABNORMALITIES OF THE PENIS

Prepuce The prepuce may be too tight to retract over the glans (phimosis). If the prepuce is tight but retracts and catches behind the glans, oedema and swelling may occur, preventing the return of the foreskin (paraphimosis). If left untreated, the swelling and congestion may result in gangrene.

Glans Hypospadias (Fig. 9.13) is a developmental abnormality causing the urethral meatus to appear on the inferior (ventral) surface of the glans (primary hypospadias), penis (secondary hypospadias) or even the perineum (tertiary hypospadias). Inflammation of the glans is termed balanitis (Fig. 9.10); if there is

Hypospadias

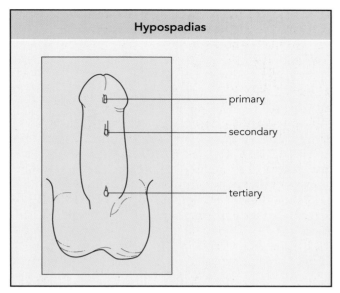

- primary
- secondary
- tertiary

Fig. 9.13 Hypospadias: a developmental abnormality. The urethral meatus opens on the ventral surface of the penis.

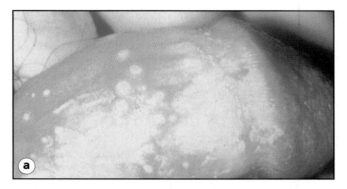

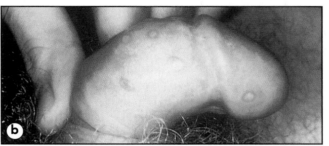

Fig. 9.14 After 4–5 days incubation, a crop of relatively painless herpetic vesicles appear on the penis (a). Vesicles rupture, with the development of painful superficial erosions with a characteristic erythematous halo (b).

inflammation of the glans and prepuce, the term balanoposthitis is used. Genital (herpetic) warts may be seen on the glans.

Urethral discharge This is one of the most common genital disorders in men and is caused by urethral inflammation (urethritis). The cause of a urethral discharge cannot be confidently predicted from appearance, although gonorrhoea is likely to cause a profuse purulent discharge. Nongonococcal urethritis may also be caused by urethral infection or be associated with Reiter's syndrome.

Penile ulcers Ulceration of the glans or, more rarely, the shaft of the penis may occur in a number of disorders. Examine the ulcer and always palpate the groins

for inguinal lymph node involvement because the skin of the penis drains to this group of nodes. The most common cause is herpetic ulceration. Characteristic painless vesicles occur 4–5 days after sexual contact (Fig. 9.14). The vesicles often rupture, causing painful superficial erosions with a characteristic erythematous halo. The confluence of these erosions may cause discrete ulcers that can become secondarily infected. The urethral meatus may be affected causing dysuria. If there is a possible history of sexually transmitted disease, consider syphilis (primary chancre) (Fig. 9.15) and in the tropics consider chancroid, lymphogranuloma venereum and granuloma inguinale. Infrequently, fixed drug reactions may cause penile ulceration. Squamous cell carcinoma may present as an ulcer of the penis or the scrotum.

 **Differential diagnosis
Genital ulcers**

Infections
- Genital herpes
- Syphilis (chancre, mucous patches, gumma)
- Tropical ulcers

Balanitis
- Severe candidiasis
- Circinate balanitis (Reiter's syndrome)

Drug eruption
- Localised fixed drug eruption
- Generalised (Stevens–Johnson syndrome)

Carcinoma
Behçet's syndrome

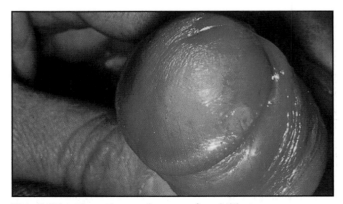

Fig. 9.15 The primary chancre of syphilis may occur on the glans, prepuce or shaft.

Priapism Occasionally, a patient may present with a painful and prolonged erection. This pathological erection is termed priapism. Most often there is no obvious cause but predisposing factors such as leukaemia, haemoglobinopathies (e.g. sickle cell anaemia) and drugs (aphrodisiacs) should be considered.

EXAMINATION OF THE SCROTUM

Inspect the scrotal skin, which is pigmented when compared with body skin. The left testis lies lower than the right but the impression of both testes is readily identified (Fig. 9.16). The tone of the dartos muscle is influenced by ambient temperature. Consequently, the normal scrotal appearance varies with temperature.

Ensure that your hands are warm before palpating the testis. Use gentle pressure, sufficient to explore the bulk of the tissue without causing pain. Throughout the examination, watch the patient's facial expression, for this should reassure you that the examination is not causing undue discomfort. Compare the left and right

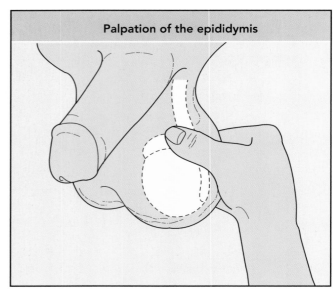

Palpation of the epididymis

Fig. 9.18 The epididymis is felt along the posterior pole of the testis.

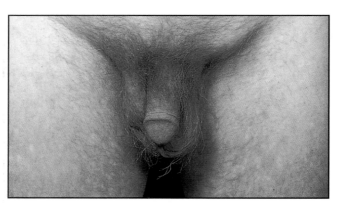

Fig. 9.16 The left testis lies lower than the right.

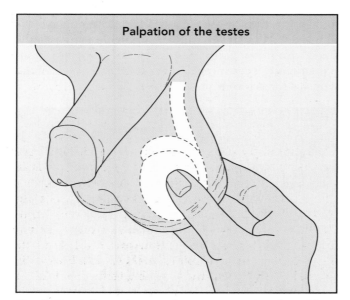

Palpation of the testes

Fig. 9.17 Palpate the testis between your thumb and first two fingers.

testes because many testicular disorders are unilateral. Feel the testicle between your thumb and first two fingers (Fig. 9.17). Note the size and consistency of the testis. The organ has a pliant, soft rubbery consistency and there should not be much tenderness. Next, palpate the epididymis, which is felt as an elongated structure along the posterolateral surface of the testicle (Fig. 9.18). The epididymis normally feels smooth and is broadest superiorly at its head.

Finally, roll with the finger and thumb the vas deferens, which passes from the tail of the epididymis to the inguinal canal through the external inguinal canal. This structure is smooth and nontender and is felt leading from the epididymis to the external inguinal ring.

Abnormalities of the scrotum

If one-half of the scrotum appears smooth and poorly developed, consider an undescended testis (cryptorchidism). This appearance of the scrotum helps to distinguish a maldescent from a retractile testis, in which the testis has descended but retracts vigorously towards the external inguinal ring. The retracted testis will be difficult to palpate.

The scrotal skin may be red and inflamed; a common cause is candidiasis (Fig. 9.19). Small yellowish scrotal lumps or nodules are common and usually represent sebaceous cysts.

Swellings in the scrotum

Decide whether the swelling arises from an indirect inguinal hernia or from the scrotal contents. It is possible to 'get above' a testicular swelling but not a scrotal hernia (Fig. 9.20). An intrinsic swelling may arise from enlargement of the testis, testicular appendages and

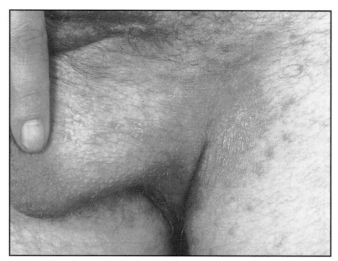

Fig. 9.19 Candida infection of the scrotum often extends to the groin and thigh.

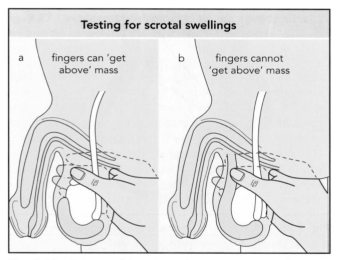

Testing for scrotal swellings

a | fingers can 'get above' mass

b | fingers cannot 'get above' mass

Fig. 9.20 It is possible to 'get above' a true scrotal swelling (a), whereas this is not possible if the swelling is caused by an inguinal hernia that has descended into the scrotum (b).

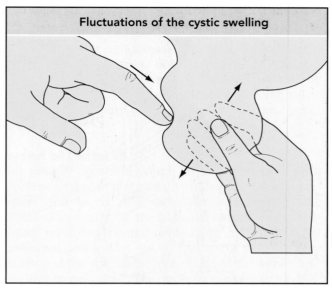

Fluctuations of the cystic swelling

Fig. 9.21 To distinguish a solid from a cystic mass, fix the swelling between finger and thumb of one hand and use the index finger of the other hand to invaginate at right angles.

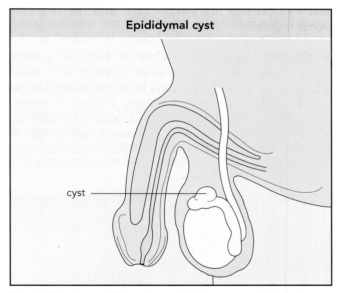

Epididymal cyst

cyst

Fig. 9.22 An epididymal cyst is felt separately from the testis and lies posteriorly.

epididymis or by an accumulation of fluid in the tunica vaginalis, the double membrane that invests the testes.

Palpate the swelling between the thumb and first two fingers and decide whether the swelling is solid or cystic.

Cystic swelling Cystic accumulations are caused by entrapment of fluid in the tunica vaginalis (a hydrocele) or accumulation of fluid in an epididymal cyst and are typically fluctuant. Steady the mass between the thumb and first two fingers of one hand and use the index finger of the other hand to invaginate the mass in a second plane (Fig. 9.21). The tense fluid-filled cyst will fluctuate between finger and thumb in response to the pressure change. Cystic lesions usually transilluminate. Darken the room and place a pen-

torch light up against the swelling. A fluid-filled cyst spreads a bright red glow into the scrotum, whereas this does not occur with solid tumours. Remember that if the cyst wall is abnormally thickened or the effusion is bloodstained, transillumination may not occur. Next, try to distinguish between a hydrocoele and an epididymal cyst. As the epididymis lies behind the body of the testis, an epididymal cyst is felt as a distinct swelling behind the adjoining testis (Fig. 9.22). In contrast, a hydrocele surrounds and envelops the testis, which becomes impalpable as a discrete organ (Fig. 9.23). The distinction between an epididymal cyst

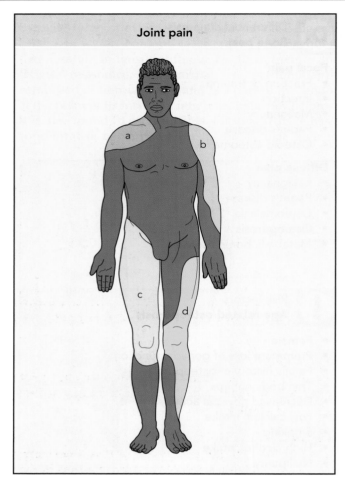

Joint pain

Questions to ask
Joint pain

- Where is the maximal site of pain?
- Does the pain change during the course of the day?
- Has the pain been there for a short or long time?
- Does the pain get better or worse with movement?

For certain joint disorders (e.g. at the shoulder), pain is apparent only during a specific range of movement. If confirmed by examination, this selectivity can be valuable in differential diagnosis.

Swelling and crepitus

If the patient has noticed joint swelling, elicit for how long it has been present, whether there is associated pain and whether the swelling fluctuates. A noisy joint is not necessarily pathological. Introspective individuals are likely to interpret periodic clicking in a joint, in the absence of pain, as having pathological signifi-

Differential diagnosis
Joint pain

- Inflammatory
  - rheumatoid arthritis
  - ankylosing spondylitis
- Mechanical
  - osteoarthritis
- Infective
  - pyogenic
  - tuberculosis
  - brucellosis
- Traumatic

Questions to ask
Muscle weakness

- Is the weakness global or focal?
- Is the weakness secondary to a painful limb?
- Does the weakness fluctuate?
- Is the weakness increasing in severity?

cance. It does not. Crepitus is a grating noise or sensation; it can have both auditory and palpable qualities. Fine crepitus is more readily felt than heard, but crepitus stemming from advanced degeneration of a large joint (e.g. the hip) is readily audible.

Locking

A joint locks if ectopic material becomes interposed between the articular surfaces. It is particularly associated with damage to the knee cartilages. Ascertain if the locking occurs at a particular point during movement of the joint.

MUSCLE

Muscle symptoms include pain and stiffness, weakness, wasting, abnormal spontaneous movements and cramps.

Pain and stiffness

Muscle pain tends to be deep, constant and poorly localised. If caused by local muscle disease, it is likely to be exacerbated by contraction of the muscle and relieved by rest. If the patient complains more of muscle stiffness (particularly of the lower limbs) than pain, suspect the possibility of spasticity caused by an upper motor neuron lesion.

Weakness

A complaint of global weakness is more likely in neurotic individuals than in patients with neurological disorders.

Important questions to ask include the distribution of the weakness, whether it appears related to any pain in the limb, whether it fluctuates and whether it is static or progressive. A complaint of predominant

Differential diagnosis
Muscle pain

- Inflammatory
  – polymyositis
  – dermatomyositis
- Infective
  – pyogenic
  – cysticercosis
- Traumatic
- Polymyalgia rheumatica
- Neuropathic
  – e.g. Guillain–Barré syndrome

proximal weakness suggests the possibility of primary muscle disease (e.g. polymyositis or myopathy). A predominantly distal weakness is more likely to be neuropathic. If the weakness is fluctuant, and particularly if it worsens during the course of activity, you will need to consider myasthenia gravis when you come to examine the patient (see also Ch. 11). Weakness caused by sudden entrapment of a peripheral nerve (e.g. a traumatic radial nerve palsy) will be stable or even improving by the time the patient seeks medical attention. In other conditions the weakness is progressive (e.g. motor neuron disease).

Wasting and fasciculation

Both these features form an important part of the examination, but both may have been noticed by the patient and volunteered during history-taking. If the patient describes muscle twitching, ascertain whether the movement has occurred in several different muscles or whether it has been confined to one area, most likely the calf.

Cramps

Cramps are seldom of pathological significance. They are usually confined to the calves and can be triggered by forced contraction of the muscle.

GENERAL PRINCIPLES OF EXAMINATION

BONE

Whichever structure is being examined, ensure that it is completely exposed and that the patient is comfortably positioned. Determine whether there is any abnormal angularity. Is there limb shortening? Look for tenderness by gently palpating those parts of the bone close to the skin surface.

JOINTS

You need to follow a strict routine with joint examination, incorporating inspection, palpation and assessment of the movement of the joint.

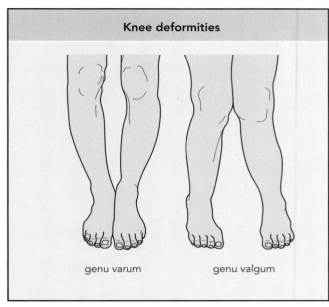

Fig. 10.6 Genu varum (left) and genu valgum (right).

Inspection

Things you are looking for include swelling, joint deformity, overlying skin changes and the appearance of the surrounding structures.

Swelling

Causes of joint swelling include effusions, thickening of the synovial tissues and of the bony margins of the joint. Differentiation of these causes is achieved by palpation. If you suspect joint swelling, compare it with the joint of the opposite limb. Particularly note if the swelling appears to be of the joint itself or of the adjacent structures.

Deformity

Deformity results either from misalignment of the bones forming the joint or from alteration of the relationship between the articular surfaces. If misalignment exists, a deviation of the part distal to the joint away from the midline is called a valgus deformity and a deviation towards the midline a varus deformity (Fig. 10.6). If a deformity exists you will need later to determine whether it is fixed or mobile. Partial loss of contact of the articulating surfaces is called subluxation, and complete loss dislocation. Although these are usually traumatic, they can also be seen in inflammatory joint disease, particularly rheumatoid arthritis. Swan neck, Boutonnière and mallet are descriptive terms used for deformities of the metacarpophalangeal and interphalangeal joints of the hand (Fig. 10.7).

Skin changes

You should palpate the skin over a joint to assess its temperature rather than relying simply on its colour. Redness of the skin over a joint implies an underlying acute inflammatory reaction (e.g. gout) (Fig. 10.8).

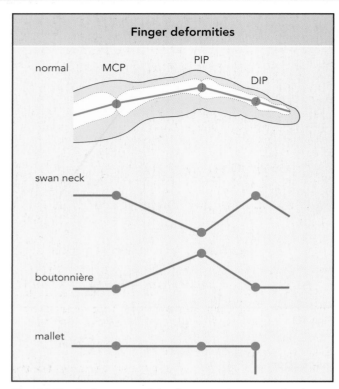

Finger deformities

normal   MCP   PIP   DIP

swan neck

boutonnière

mallet

Fig. 10.7   Deformities of the finger in rheumatoid arthritis.

Changes of adjacent structures

The most striking change adjacent to a diseased joint is wasting of muscle. Assess muscle bulk above and below the affected joint, making a comparison with the opposite limb if that is spared. Wasting of quadriceps is particularly conspicuous in severe disease of the knee joint.

Palpation

During palpation of a joint, assess the nature of any swelling, whether there is tenderness and whether the joint is hot.

Swelling

The method of examining for an effusion will be described for the individual joints. Your first step is to

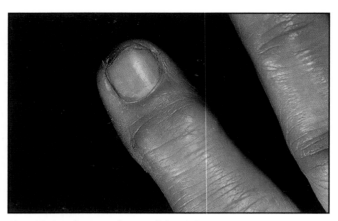

Fig. 10.9   Osteoarthritis of the DIP joint.

determine the consistency of any swelling. Is the swelling hard, suggesting bone deformities secondary to osteoarthritis? Certain sites are particularly susceptible to osteoarthritic change (e.g. the distal interphalangeal joints of the hand) (Fig. 10.9). A slightly spongy or boggy swelling suggests synovial thickening and is particularly associated with rheumatoid arthritis. An effusion is fluctuant, that is, the fluid can be displaced from one part of the joint to another. Swellings may also arise adjacent to a joint. Again determine their consistency. Soft fluctuant swellings suggest enlarged bursae. Harder swellings occur in rheumatoid arthritis and gout.

Tenderness

Carefully palpate the joint margin and adjacent bony surfaces together with the surrounding ligaments and tendons. Your task is to discover whether any tenderness is within the joint or outside it, and whether the tenderness is focal or generalised. In an acutely inflamed joint, the whole of its palpable contours will be tender. If there is derangement of a single knee cartilage, tenderness will be confined to the margin of that cartilage. In degenerative joint disease, you may find tenderness in structures adjacent to the joint. Tenderness close to the joint may reflect primary pathology in bone (e.g. osteomyelitis) or in the tendon

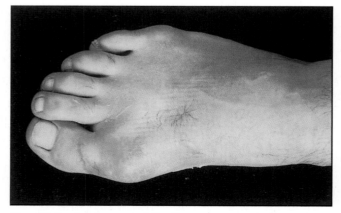

Fig. 10.8   Acute gout of the first metatarsophalangeal joint.

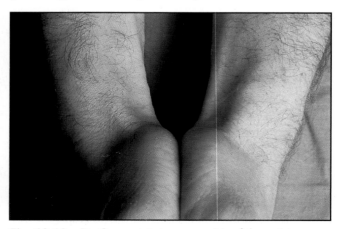

Fig. 10.10   De Quervain's tenosynovitis of the wrist.

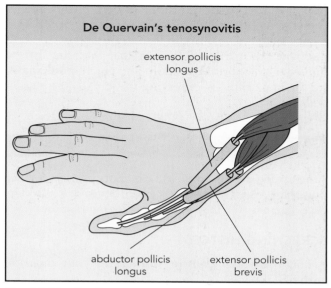

Fig. 10.11   De Quervain's tenosynovitis.

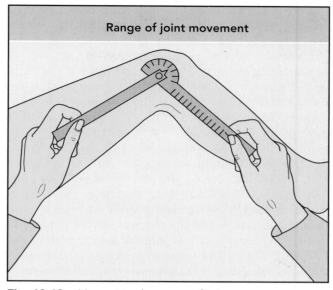

Fig. 10.13   Measuring the range of joint movement.

sheath (e.g. De Quervain's tenosynovitis) (Figs. 10.10, 10.11).

Temperature

For a small joint, for example, in the finger, assess temperature with the finger tips, using an unaffected joint in the same or the other hand for comparison. For a larger joint, for example, the knee, rub the back of your hand across the joint then compare with the other limb. If the contralateral joint is also affected, carry your hand above and below the joint margins to make the comparison.

Joint movement

Next proceed to examine the range of movement of the joint, whether movement is limited by pain and whether there is instability.

To define the range of joint movement, start with the joints in the neutral position, defined as the lower limbs extended with the feet dorsiflexed to 90°, and the upper limbs midway between pronation and supination with the arms flexed to 90° at the elbows (Fig. 10.12). For accurate measurement of joint movement you will need a goniometer (Fig. 10.13) but for routine purposes your eye should allow a reasonably true estimate. Movement of a joint is either active (i.e. induced by the patient) or passive (i.e. induced by the examiner). Sometimes you need to assess both but you will generally assess active movements in the spine but

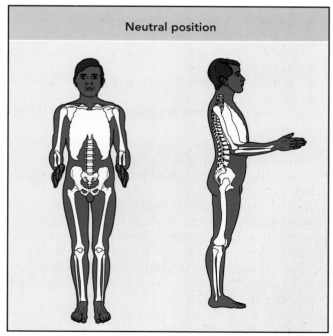

Fig. 10.12   The neutral position from which joint measurement is performed.

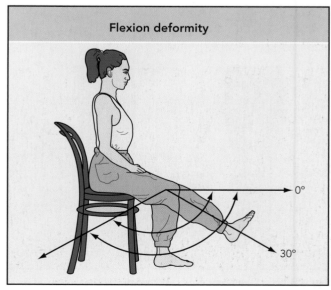

Fig. 10.14   30° flexion deformity of the knee.

passive movements in the limb joints. Restriction of active compared with passive movement is usually due to muscle weakness.

From the neutral position, record the degrees of flexion and extension. If extension does not normally occur at a joint (e.g. the knee) but is present, describe the movement as hyperextension and give its range in degrees. Sometimes there is restriction of the range of movement. For example, if the knee fails by 30° to reach the extended position, describe this as either a 30° flexion deformity or as a 30° lack of extension (Fig. 10.14). For the ankle and wrist, extension is described as dorsiflexion and flexion as plantar and palmar flexion, respectively. For a ball and socket joint, you will need to record the range of flexion, extension, abduction, adduction and internal and external rotation (Fig. 10.15). The range of joint movement varies between individuals: an excessive range of movement can be constitutional as well as pathological. Carefully note if pain occurs during joint movement. In joint disease, pain is likely to occur throughout the range of movement. In certain disease processes around the joint (e.g. in the ligaments or bursae), pain can be restricted to a particular range or type of movement. Damage of either the articular surfaces or of the ligaments related to a joint can lead to instability. You will discover this partly by finding that the joint can be moved into abnormal positions and partly, particularly for the knee joint, by observing the joint as the patient walks.

GALS

A screening history and examination process for the musculoskeletal system has been devised for undergraduate use (GALS – gait, arms, legs and spine).

SCREENING HISTORY

- Have you any pain or stiffness in your muscles, joints or back?
- Can you dress yourself completely without difficulty?
- Can you walk up and down stairs without difficulty?

If the answers to all three questions are negative, significant musculoskeletal abnormality is unlikely.

SCREENING EXAMINATION

- Gait – Inspect the patient walking, turning and walking back.
- Spine – Inspect the patient from three positions from behind, from the side, then asking the patient to bend forwards and touch the toes, and finally from in front asking the patient then to try to place the relevant ear on each shoulder in turn (lateral neck flexion).
- Arms – From in front ask the patient to place both hands behind the head, elbows back.
  Place both hands by the side, elbows straight.
  Place both hands out in front, palms down, fingers straight.
  Turn both hands over. Make a tight fist with each hand.
  Place the tip of each finger onto the tip of the thumb in turn.
  The examiner then squeezes across the second to the fifth metacarpals to elicit tenderness.
- Legs – Inspect from in front (with the patient standing).
  Inspect with the patient lying flat.
  Flex each hip and knee while holding the knee (confirming full knee flexion without knee crepitus).
  Passively internally rotate each hip in flexion (checking for pain and restricted movement).
  Press on each patella for tenderness and palpate for an effusion.
  Squeeze across the metatarsals for tenderness due to metatarsophalangeal disease.
  Inspect both soles for callosities reflecting abnormal weight-bearing.

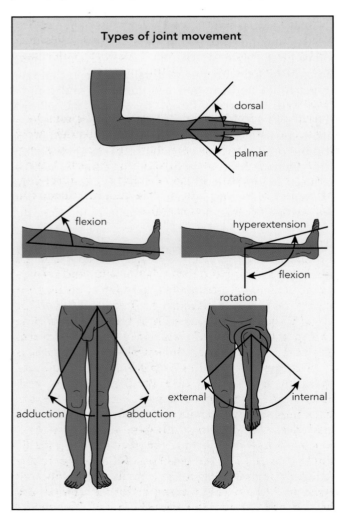

Types of joint movement

dorsal
palmar
flexion
hyperextension
flexion
rotation
external
internal
adduction
abduction

Fig. 10.15 Description of joint movement according to the type of joint.

RECORDING FINDINGS

Normal response to the screening questions can be recorded as:

Pain   0
Dress   ✓
Walk   ✓

Results of the physical examination can be recorded if gait (G) is normal, there are no abnormalities to the appearance (A) of the areas inspected (i.e. no swelling, deformity, wasting, abnormal position or skin change) and no abnormalities of movement (M) of the arms (A), legs (L) or spine (S) as follows:

	A	M
G	✓	
A	✓	✓
L	✓	✓
S	✓	✓

Any abnormality is recorded as an X and described in more detail.

MUSCLE

The methods for examining individual muscles will be given in the section on regional examination. Initially your assessment will include inspection, palpation, then testing of muscle power.

Inspection

Look for evidence of muscle wasting, for signs of abnormal muscle bulk and for spontaneous contractions.

Wasting

Remember that striking muscle wasting can accompany joint disease (e.g. wasting of the small hand muscles in rheumatoid arthritis and wasting of the quadriceps in virtually any arthropathy affecting the knee joint). If there is no significant joint disease, wasting (other than caused by a profound loss of body weight) reflects either primary muscle disease or disease of its innervating neuron. Make allowances for the age of the patient and his or her occupation. Some thinning of the hand muscles occurs in elderly people but is not accompanied by weakness. If you suspect wasting of one limb, measure the circumference of that limb and compare it with its fellow. For example, for the thigh, mark the line of the medial cartilage of the knee joint, measure up, for example, 20 cm, on each thigh and record the circumference of the legs at that point.

Increased muscle bulk

Usually abnormal muscle bulk reflects the patient's obsession with his own bodily strength (it is almost always a man). There are rare conditions that lead to muscle hypertrophy. If the enlargement is due to increase in muscle bulk, it is called true hypertrophy and is seen, for example, in congenital myotonia. If the increased bulk is due to fatty infiltration (and you will then discover the muscle is actually weak), it is called pseudohypertrophy. This finding is characteristic of certain of the muscular dystrophies (e.g. Duchenne's).

Spontaneous contractions

Completely expose the muscle when looking for evidence of spontaneous contraction. Make sure the patient is warm and relaxed. Shivering brought on by cold can be difficult to distinguish from fasciculation. Spontaneous movements can occur with both upper and lower motor neuron lesions. In the former, particularly at the spinal level, you may see either flexor or extensor spasms of the legs, either at the hips or knees. The movements can occur spontaneously or be triggered by attempting to move the patient and are often painful. Fasciculation produces episodic muscle twitching that can be subtle in small muscles. It is a feature of lower motor neuron lesions but can also be seen in normal individuals. Fasciculation is intermittent. Wait for a few minutes before deciding it is absent. It is particularly important to determine whether the fasciculation is confined to a single muscle or whether it is more widely distributed. The former may reflect the result of cervical radiculopathy or be physiological (particularly if confined to the calves); the latter suggests a diagnosis of motor neuron disease.

Palpation

Muscle palpation is of limited value. If the muscle is infected or inflamed it is likely to be tender. Most myopathies are painless but there are exceptions (e.g. the acute myopathy occurring in alcoholics). Muscle tenderness can also occur in neurogenic disorders (e.g. the peripheral neuropathy of thiamine deficiency can lead to marked calf tenderness).

Testing muscle power

You should follow the UK Medical Research Council classification (see page 348) when testing and recording muscle power. Remember to make allowance for sex, age and the patient's stature. If the muscle itself or the joint that it moves, is painful then power will be correspondingly limited. Patterns of muscle weakness are particularly important in neurological diagnosis. Is the weakness global, does it predominate distally or proximally in the limb, does its distribution fit with either a peripheral nerve or root distribution? Sometimes muscle power is decidedly fluctuant: there is a sudden give, alternating with more effective contraction. Although this pattern can occur in myasthenia gravis, it is usually the reflection of a nonorganic disability. If muscle fatigue is a prominent symptom assess it objectively. For example, for the deltoid, ask the patient to abduct the shoulder to 90°. Test power immediately, then after the patient has held that posture for 60 s.

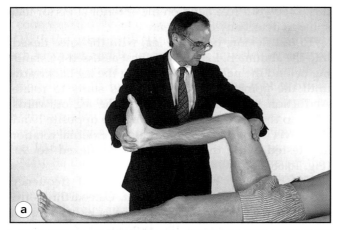

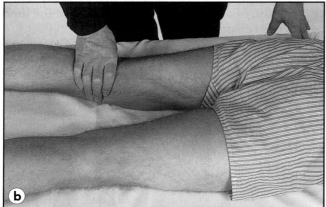

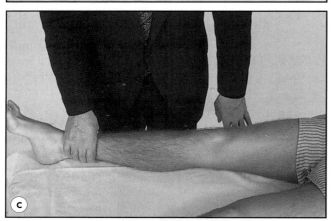

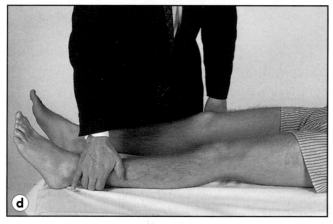

Fig. 10.70 Testing the muscles acting at the hip joint: (a) flexion, (b) extension, (c) adduction, (d) abduction.

is a potential complication. Fractures of the neck of the femur are commonplace in elderly people. The leg may be shortened and externally rotated. The condition carries a high morbidity for elderly people and has a capacity to progress to avascular necrosis of the femoral head. Fractures of the femoral shaft are either traumatic or pathological. Traction is the preferred treatment option in children but internal fixation is used for adults.

Slip of the upper femoral epiphysis occurs in adolescents, leading to pain and inability to weight bear.

Groin strains are common in people involved in sporting activities. The pain is dull, exacerbated by hip movement and is likely to be the result of tears in the fibres of the hip flexors.

Muscle function

Test the power of hip flexion, extension, abduction and adduction (Fig. 10.70). Sciatic palsies are associated with pelvic trauma, injuries to the buttock or thigh or infiltration by tumour. The muscles supplied by the lateral popliteal component of the nerve tend to be more affected than those supplied by the medial popliteal branch (Fig. 10.71).

THE KNEE

STRUCTURE AND FUNCTION

Although principally a hinge joint, a limited range of rotation is possible at the knee. Anteriorly, the capsule is formed by the tendon of the quadriceps femoris and the patella. At the sides, the capsule is strengthened by the medial and lateral collateral ligaments. Within the joint are the anterior and posterior cruciate ligaments passing from the tibia to the lateral and medial condyles of the femur, respectively (Fig. 10.72). Interposed between the femoral condyles and the tibia are the fibrocartilagenous semilunar cartilages. The joint capsule is lined by synovium that partly surrounds the cruciate ligaments. Communicating with the synovial cavity are bursae that are related to the insertions or

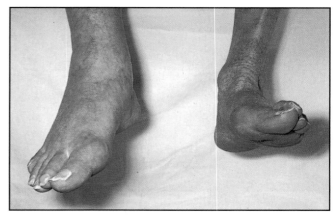

Fig. 10.71 Right sciatic palsy.

origins of some of the tendons around the joint (Fig. 10.73).

Flexion–extension occurs between approximately 0° and 150° (Fig. 10.74). A minor degree of hyperextension can occur in some normal individuals. As full

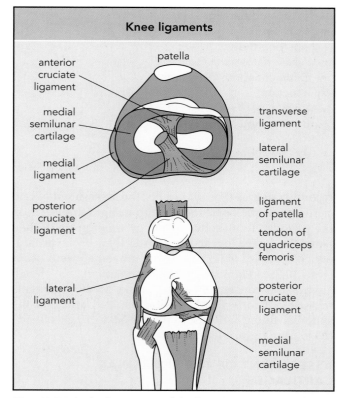

Knee ligaments

anterior cruciate ligament

patella

medial semilunar cartilage

transverse ligament

medial ligament

lateral semilunar cartilage

posterior cruciate ligament

ligament of patella

tendon of quadriceps femoris

lateral ligament

posterior cruciate ligament

medial semilunar cartilage

Fig. 10.72   The ligaments of the knee joint.

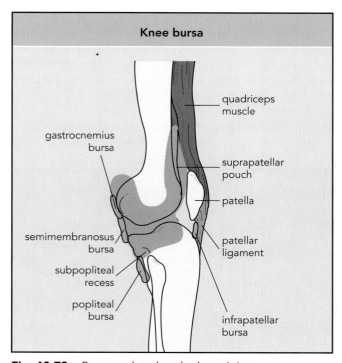

Knee bursa

quadriceps muscle

gastrocnemius bursa

suprapatellar pouch

patella

semimembranosus bursa

patellar ligament

subpopliteal recess

popliteal bursa

infrapatellar bursa

Fig. 10.73   Bursae related to the knee joint.

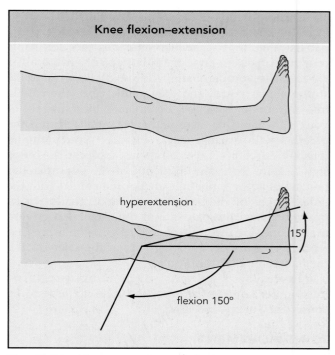

Knee flexion–extension

hyperextension

15°

flexion 150°

Fig. 10.74   Flexion–extension at the knee joint.

extension is reached, the femur rotates medially because of the longer articular surface of the medial condyle, tightening the capsular ligments in the process. Flexion is produced by the hamstrings and extension by the quadriceps femoris.

INSPECTION AND PALPATION

With the patient standing, look for a knee deformity, either genu valgum (knock-knee) or genu varum (bow leg). Now continue your inspection with the patient lying supine. The bulk of the quadriceps muscle is a sensitive guide to the presence of knee joint pathology. If necessary measure the thigh of each leg at a comparable distance from the joint margin. Next look for

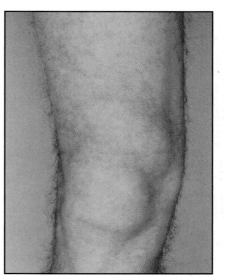

Fig. 10.75
Effusion in the suprapatellar pouch in a patient with rheumatoid arthritis.

an effusion. If this is large, the swelling will extend from the suprapatellar region down either side of the patella (Fig. 10.75). Smaller effusions are detectable only by palpation. First, try ballottement: the pattellar tap test. Use your left hand to force any fluid out of the suprapatellar pouch and then gently press the patella into the femur with the second and third fingers of your right hand. If there is a substantial effusion the patella will spring back against your fingers (Fig. 10.76a). For smaller effusions, look for the bulge sign. Again, force any fluid out of the suprapatellar pouch but at the same time anchor the patella with the index finger of the same hand. Next, gently stroke down between the patella and the femoral condyles, first on one side then the other. If an effusion is present, a bulge appears on the other side of the knee during the manoeuvre (Fig. 10.76b).

Palpate the joint and surrounding structures, looking for any tenderness and also to assess the consistency of any swelling.

JOINT MOVEMENT

Test the range of movement with the patient lying supine. Flexion occurs to approximately 150°. A small degree of extension can occur in some normal individuals. As you record the movement, palpate the joint for any crepitus. In addition, move the patella laterally and medially across the femoral condyles. Is the movement painful or does it elicit crepitus?

STABILITY

There are several important procedures that allow you to determine the integrity of the collateral and cruciate ligaments.

To test the collateral ligaments, attempt to abduct and adduct the lower leg. If there is lateral instability,

Differential diagnosis
Knee pain

- Trauma
  - fracture
  - dislocation
  - ligament damage
  - cartilage damage
- Arthritis
  - osteoarthritis
  - rheumatoid arthritis
- Osteochondritis dissecans
- Infection
  - e.g. osteomyelitis
- Bone tumours
- Referred
  e.g. from the hip

record its degree (Fig. 10.77). For the assessment of cruciate ligaments, bend the knee to a slight angle, sit on the patient's foot (better to ask permission first!) then tense the lower leg first forwards then backwards. If either ligament is lax, excessive movement will occur (Fig. 10.78). Damage to these ligaments is almost always the consequence of trauma. If the ligaments rupture, a bloodstained effusion results. Damage to the synovial lining will allow the blood to track outside the joint margin.

ASSESSMENT OF THE SEMILUNAR CARTILAGES

Damage to the cartilages is common. In order to test their integrity, bend the hip and knee to 90° and grip the heel with your right hand while pressing on the medial then lateral cartilage with your left (Fig. 10.79). Now internally and externally rotate the tibia while extending the knee. If there is a cartilage tear, its engagement between the tibia and femur during the manoeuvre leads to severe pain, a clunking noise and, sometimes, actual locking of the joint (McMurray's test).

In osteoarthritis, periarticular tenderness, particularly at the insertion of the capsule and collateral ligaments, is an important diagnostic clue. Later, bony

Questions to ask
Knee pain

- Is the pain unilateral or bilateral?
- Has the patient noticed swelling of the joint?
- Does the knee lock in certain positions?

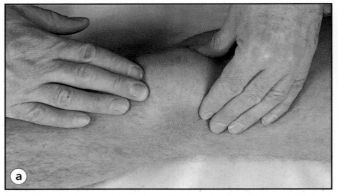

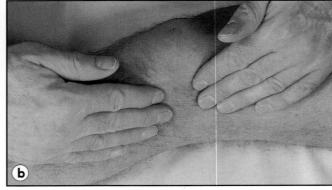

Fig. 10.76   Detection of an effusion. (a) Patellar tap. (b) Bulge sign.

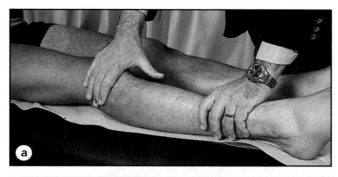

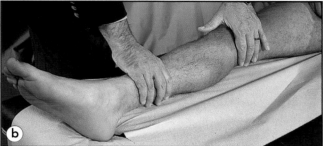

Fig. 10.77 Testing the collateral ligaments of the knee.

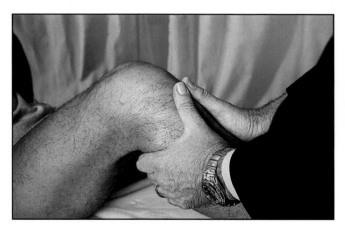

Fig. 10.78 Testing the cruciate ligaments.

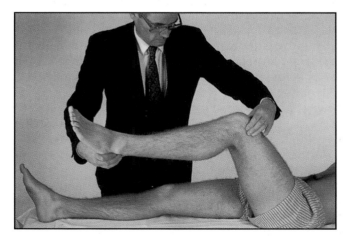

Fig. 10.79 McMurray's test.

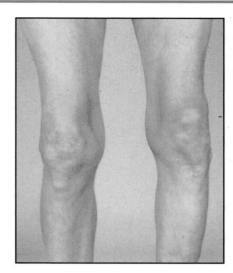

Fig. 10.80 Osteoarthritis of the knee. Bony swellings associated with quadriceps wasting.

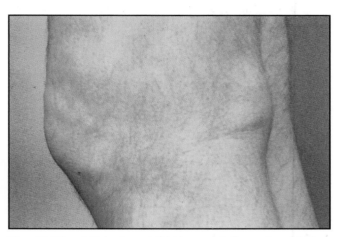

Fig. 10.81 A Baker's cyst that has partially ruptured into the calf.

swellings around the joint and secondary quadriceps wasting are common (Fig. 10.80). Remember to look at the back of the joint: the popliteal fossa. Posterior synovial protrusions (Baker's cysts) are visible here. They can complicate rheumatoid arthritis, in which additional features include effusions, synovial swelling and deformity (Fig. 10.81).

TRAUMATIC LESIONS

Ligament sprains are not associated with detectable laxity and are treated with a support bandage or plaster. With ligament rupture, the consequent joint instability necessitates surgical repair. Meniscal tears tend to occur in young people as the consequence of a twisting injury. The medial meniscus is usually affected. Effusion appears and the knee may lock, inhibiting complete extension. The torn elements are removed arthroscopically.

Patellar dislocation occurs laterally and tends to be recurrent. Total knee dislocation is unusual and generally the consequence of a road traffic accident. Fractures of the lower femur or upper tibia that involve the knee joint are complicated by joint stiffness and accelerated degenerative changes.

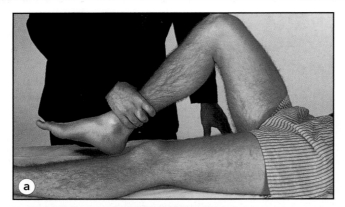

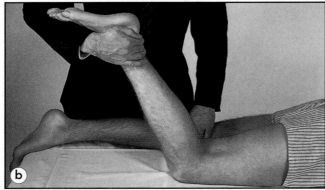

Fig. 10.82 Testing knee extension (above) and flexion (below).

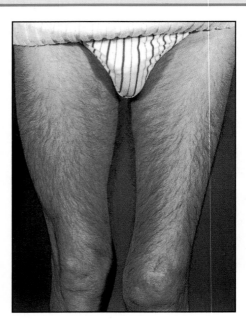

Fig. 10.84 Left femoral neuropathy after profundoplasty.

L3 syndrome		
Muscle weakness	Segmentary sensory change	Reflex depression
quadriceps hip adductors		Knee

Fig. 10.83 L3 root syndrome. Motor, sensory and reflex abnormalities.

MUSCLE FUNCTION

Test the muscles responsible for knee extension and flexion, the quadriceps and hamstrings, respectively (Fig. 10.82). Both quadriceps weakness and wasting can accompany joint disease. If the knee joint is normal, unilateral quadriceps weakness suggests either a femoral neuropathy or an L3 root syndrome. In the latter, there is weakness of both quadriceps and the hip adductors, associated with a depressed knee jerk and sensory change over the medial aspect of the thigh and knee (Fig. 10.83). A femoral neuropathy can result from thigh trauma or haemorrhage into the psoas sheath. In diabetes mellitus, wasting of the thigh is more often the result of ischaemia of the lumbar roots rather than being caused by a femoral neuropathy. Consequently, the thigh adductors are also affected. Femoral neuropathy leads to weakness and wasting of the quadriceps, loss of the knee jerk and sensory change over the anterior thigh and the medial aspect of the lower leg (Fig. 10.84). If the nerve is damaged at the level of the psoas sheath, hip flexion is also affected. An obturator nerve palsy can follow surgery or pelvic fracture or be secondary to an obturator hernia. Weakness is confined to the thigh adductors, with altered sensation over the thigh's inner aspect.

Meralgia paraesthetica

It is worth mentioning meralgia paraesthetica. The patient complains of pain, tingling and numbness over the anterolateral aspect of the thigh. There are no motor changes. The condition is caused by compression of the lateral cutaneous nerve of the thigh at the

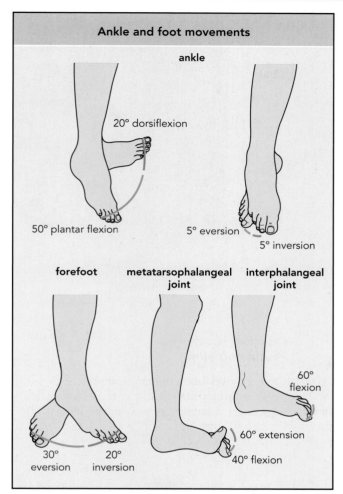

Fig. 10.85   Movements of the ankle, foot and big toe.

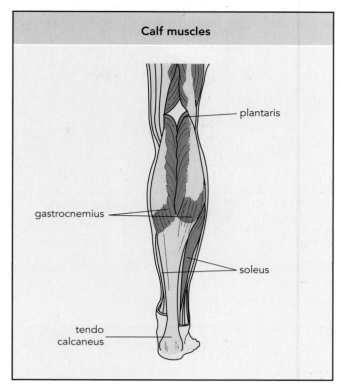

Fig. 10.86   Muscles of the calf.

level of the groin, and is the commonest entrapment neuropathy of the lower limb.

THE ANKLE AND FOOT

STRUCTURE AND FUNCTION

Movements of the ankle are essentially confined to extension (dorsiflexion) and flexion (plantar flexion). Inversion and eversion of the foot are partly achieved by movement at the subtalar joint (approximately 5°) and partly by movement at the midtarsal joints (20°). The predominant movements of the toes are dorsiflexion and plantar flexion (Fig. 10.85).

The main muscles of the calf are the soleus and gastrocnemius. The soleus acts purely as a flexor of the ankle, while the gastrocnemius flexes both the ankle and the knee. Of the other muscles in the posterior compartment, the tibialis posterior inverts the foot, whereas flexor digitorum longus and flexor hallucis longus flex the toes and big toe, respectively (Fig. 10.86).

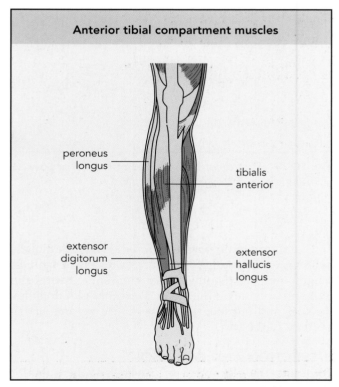

Fig. 10.87   Muscles in the anterior compartment of the leg.

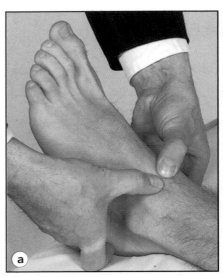
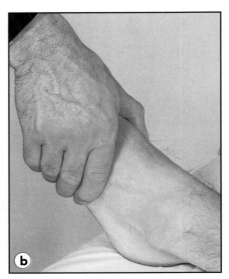
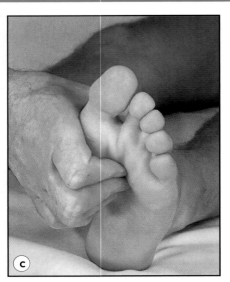

Fig. 10.88   Palpating (a) the anterior aspect of the ankle joint and (b) and (c) testing for tenderness of the metatarsophalangeal joints.

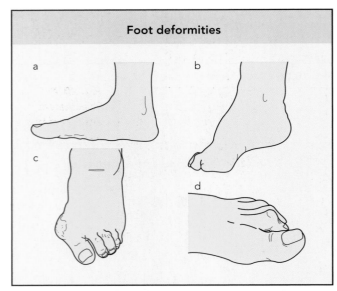

Fig. 10.89   Foot deformities. (a) Pes planus, (b) pes cavus, (c) hallux valgus and (d) hammer toe.

?   Questions to ask
Foot deformities

- Has the deformity been present from birth?
- Does it affect both feet?
- Is it associated with joint pain or tenderness?

ated or absent? Is there deformity or swelling of the toe joints? Remember to inspect the sole of the foot as well as its dorsal aspect. Now palpate the margins of the ankle joint. In an inflammatory arthropathy, the whole joint is likely to be tender, with corresponding pain on all movement. In ankle strain, the tenderness is likely to be confined to one site with pain predominantly occurring when the joint is moved in one direction. Next palpate the heel and Achilles tendon. The latter is a fairly common site for rheumatoid nodules. To detect tenderness in the metatarsophalangeal joints, compress each one between your thumb and finger (Fig. 10.88). To test the integrity of the Achilles tendon, squeeze the calf just below its maximal circumference. If the tendon is intact, the foot plantar flexes; if ruptured, no movement occurs.

Deformity of the foot is common. In flat foot, the longitudinal arch is lost with the consequence that most or the whole of the sole comes into contact with the ground (Fig. 10.89a). In pes cavus, the arch of the foot is exaggerated, with accompanying hyperextension of the toes (Fig. 10.89b). Hallux valgus predominates in women. It consists of abnormal adduction of the big toe at the metatarsophalangeal joint, with a bursa at the pressure point over the head of the first metatarsal (Fig. 10.89c). A hammer toe is characterised by hyperextension at the metatarsophalangeal joint with flexion

The anterior compartment muscles include tibialis anterior, extensor digitorum longus, extensor hallucis longus and the peronei. Tibialis anterior inverts the foot and dorsiflexes the ankle. The other two dorsiflex the toes and big toe, respectively. The peronei act as evertors of the foot.

INSPECTION AND PALPATION

To assess the alignment of the feet at the subtalar joints, look at the ankles from behind with the patient standing. In a varus deformity, the foot will be deviated towards the midline, in a valgus deformity away from it. With the patient still standing, look for any foot deformity. Is the arch of the foot exagger-

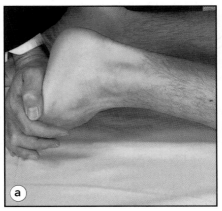

Fig. 10.90 Gouty tophi.

at the interphalangeal joint. Painful thickenings of the skin (corns) are liable to develop at the pressure points (e.g. over the proximal interphalangeal joints) (Fig. 10.89d).

JOINT MOVEMENT

The ankle joint proper is concerned with plantar and dorsiflexion. Inversion and eversion of the foot occur both at the subtalar and midtarsal joints. To test this movement, hold the heel firmly with one hand while inverting and everting the foot with the other hand. You have already looked for tenderness in the metatarsophalangeal joints. Now test the range of flexion and extension.

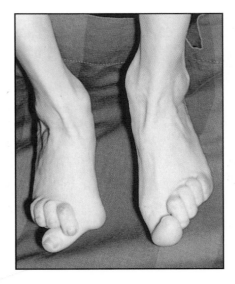

Fig. 10.91 Rheumatoid arthritis of the feet.

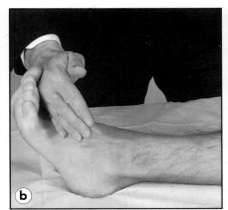
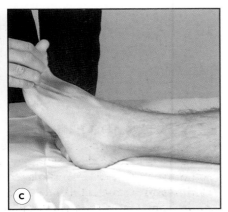

Fig. 10.92 Testing (a) and (b) plantar flexion and dorsiflexion of the ankle and (c) dorsiflexion of the toes.

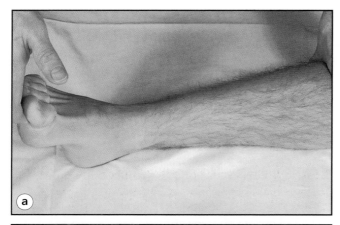

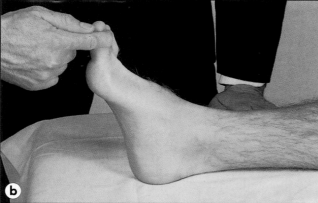

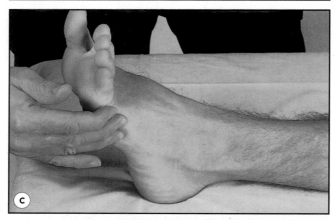

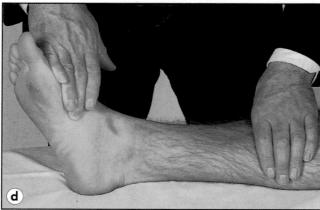

Fig. 10.93 Testing the (a) long toe flexors, (b) extensor hallucis longus, (c) peroneus longus and brevis and (d) tibialis posterior.

TRAUMATIC LESIONS

Ankle sprains result from an inversion force typically damaging the anterior talofibular ligament. Swelling develops with pain on weight-bearing. The condition is treated by a support bandage.

Pott's fracture is a fracture–dislocation of the ankle, sometimes requiring open reduction and fixation.

Rupture of the Achilles tendon results in pain in the heel. The calf is swollen with a palpable gap in the tendon. Open operation is called for if the condition is detected early.

Osteoarthritis can affect both the ankle and the foot. In the foot, involvement of the first metatarsophalangeal joint leads either to deformity (hallux valgus) or fixation (hallux rigidus). Gout typically affects the same joint. In an acute attack, there is intense pain associated with swelling and erythema of the overlying skin (Fig. 10.8). The reaction is secondary to deposition of urate salts within the connective tissues. If the hyperuricaemia is inadequately treated, urate deposits appear in periarticular and subcutaneous tissues. Typical sites include the first metatarsophalangeal joint, the elbow, the Achilles tendon and the ear (Fig. 10.90).

Rheumatoid arthritis involves both the ankle and the foot. When the disease is established, subluxation of the metatarsophalangeal joint is associated with flexion deformity at the proximal interphalangeal joints (Fig. 10.91). A variety of other inflammatory reactions can affect the ligamentous and tendon insertions around the heel. Causative agents include trauma and the seronegative arthritides.

L5 and S1 syndromes		
Muscle weakness	Sensory change	Reflex depression
L5 extensor hallucis longus eversion hip extension	anterior posterior	none
S1 plantar flexion knee flexion hip extension and abduction		ankle

Fig. 10.94 L5 and S1 root syndromes.

MUSCLE FUNCTION

Test the individual muscles concerned with movement at the ankle and foot. Start with the plantar and dorsi-flexors of the ankle, then of the toes. Specifically test the extensor of the big toe, extensor hallucis longus (Figs. 10.92, 10.93). Finally, test the evertors and invertors of the foot.

Lumbar spondylosis commonly affects the L5 and S1 roots. The motor deficit with the former is often confined to extensor hallucis longus. There is no reflex change but there may be sensory change over the medial aspect of the foot. In an S1 root syndrome, there is weakness of plantar flexion of the foot (and potentially also of the calf and buttock muscles) together with a depressed or absent ankle jerk and sensory loss over the lateral border of the dorsal and plantar aspects of the foot (Fig. 10.94).

In lateral popliteal palsy, there is weakness of dorsi-flexion of the foot and toes and of the foot everters. The sensory change is often relatively inconspicuous, sometimes being confined to a small area of loss over

Questions to ask
Patterns of weakness

- Is the weakness associated with sensory symptoms or signs?
- Is there a family history of muscle disease?
- Is the weakness symmetrical?
- Is the weakness predominantly proximal or distal?

the dorsum of the foot around the base of the first and second toes. There are no reflex changes.

PATTERNS OF WEAKNESS IN MUSCLE DISEASE

The pattern of weakness found in primary muscle disease differs from that seen in nerve root or peripheral nerve disorders. Conditions primarily affecting

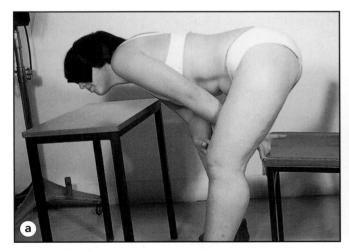

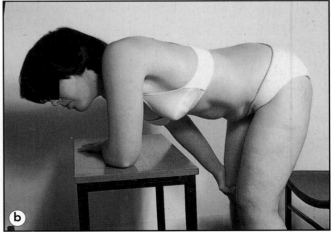

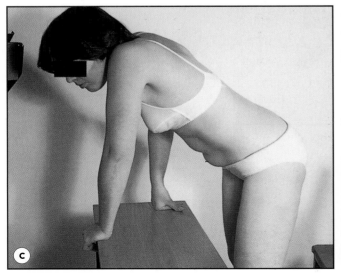

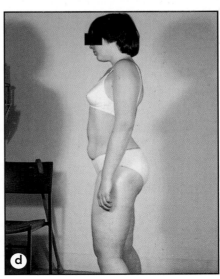

Fig. 10.95
Gowers' manoeuvre. The patient having reached a flexed position has to extend the trunk, partly by pressing on the table and partly by pressing on her thighs.

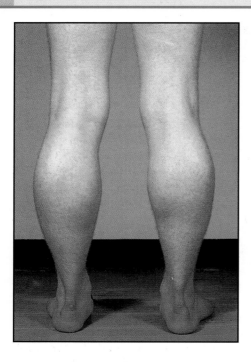

Fig. 10.96
Pseudohypertrophy of the calves.

muscle include a group of genetically determined disorders (the muscular dystrophies), a group of inflammatory disorders (e.g. polymyositis), various biochemical and endocrinological dysfunctions and, finally, a further genetically determined group associated with myotonia.

Certain characteristics support a clinical diagnosis of primary muscle disease. The weakness, which is usually symmetrical, tends to predominate proximally. In the upper limbs, the periscapular muscles and deltoid are weak but the hand muscles are spared. In the lower limbs, weakness of hip flexion and extension is often conspicuous. The patient adopts a lordotic posture and has a waddling gait.

Trendelenburg's sign is likely to be positive bilaterally (see Fig. 10.64). There is particular difficulty getting upright from a lying position. Typically, the patient turns into the prone position, kneels then climbs up the legs using the upper limbs in order to extend the trunk (Gowers' manoeuvre) (Fig. 10.95). Muscle wasting and loss of tendon reflexes are late features of the myo-

Gait disorders

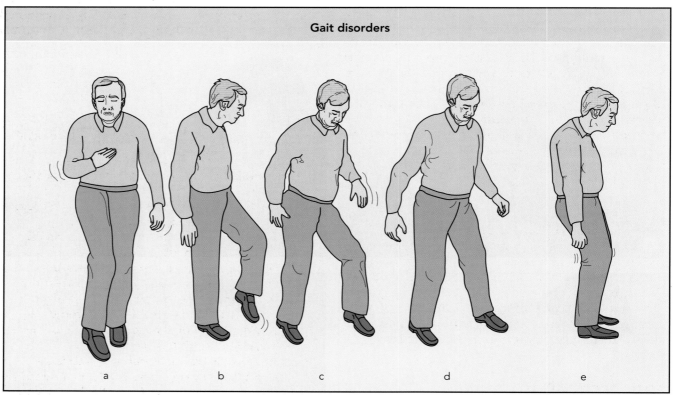

Fig. 10.97   Gait disorders. (a) Hemiplegic, (b) unilateral foot drop, (c) sensory ataxia, (d) cerebellar ataxia and (e) parkinsonism.

pathies. In some of the muscular dystrophies, pseudo-hypertrophy of muscle occurs because of infiltration by fat and connective tissue (Fig. 10.96). Distal weakness sometimes occurs in primary muscle disease, often then showing a characteristic distribution. Weakness of the hands is a prominent feature of dystrophia myotonica, in which muscle weakness is accompanied by myotonia, particularly of grip.

You will have noticed how the patient walks when entering the consulting room. Having completed your limb assessment of joint and muscle you can now examine the gait formally. Remember that disease of the joints of the lower limbs can affect walking. The possibility will have been raised by the history and suggested by the joint examination. If the patient has described a substantial problem with gait, be ready to provide support when the patient starts to walk. Ask the patient to walk for a few metres, then turn and walk back towards you. You should observe both the pattern of leg movement and the posture of the arms together with control of the trunk. If gait appears normal, ask the patient to walk heel–toe, that is, 'as if on a tightrope'. If the patient appears nervous, walk alongside them.

SPASTIC GAIT
In a hemiplegia (Fig. 10.97a), the arm is held flexed and adducted while the leg is extended. In order to move the leg, the patient tilts the pelvis, which produces an outward and forward loop of the leg (circumduction). Failure to dorsiflex the foot leads to it scraping along the ground. If both legs are spastic, for example, because of spinal cord disease, the whole movement is stiff, with thrusts of the trunk being used to assist locomotion.

FOOT DROP GAIT
Foot drop (Fig. 10.97b) can be either unilateral or bilateral. The former is usually the result of a lateral popliteal palsy, the latter is the consequence of a peripheral neuropathy. Increased flexion at the hip and knee allows the plantar flexed foot to clear the ground.

ATAXIC GAIT
An ataxic gait (Figs 10.97c, d) can reflect either loss of sensory information from the feet or a disorder of cerebellar function. In the former case, the patient stamps the feet down in order to overcome the instability. Consequently, patients with this problem are much more unstable in the dark or with the eyes closed (positive Romberg's test).

Cerebellar disease leads to a broad-based gait that is unaffected by the presence or absence of visual information. Loss of truncal control produces erratic body movement. With unilateral cerebellar disease the patient staggers to the affected side.

WADDLING GAIT
Patients with substantial proximal lower limb weakness waddle from side-to-side as they walk, from a failure to tilt the pelvis when one leg is raised from the ground. There is usually an exaggerated lumbar lordosis. The findings suggest a proximal myopathy.

PARKINSONIAN GAIT

Patients with Parkinson's disease develop an increasingly flexed posture (Fig. 10.97e). Stride length diminishes and one or both arms fail to swing. There may be a problem initiating or arresting gait. Turning is difficult and requires an exaggerated number of steps.

APRAXIC GAIT

In certain conditions (e.g. normal pressure hydrocephalus) there is a particular problem with the organisation of gait even though other skilled lower limb movements are spared. The patient is liable to freeze to the ground, unable to initiate movement.

HYSTERICAL GAIT

Here, walking is erratic and unpredictable. The patient staggers wildly, often with an exaggerated movement of the arms. Falls and injuries do not exclude the possibility of a hysterical conversion reaction. There is often a violently positive Romberg's test which the patient self-corrects.

 Examination of elderly people
Bones, muscles and joints

- Muscle strength declines with age; for example, grip strength falls by approximately 50% between the ages of 25 and 80 years
- Muscle bulk declines with age, for example, in the small hand muscles
- Some degree of ulnar deviation at the wrists can occur with ageing

- The range of joint movement lessens with age
- Gait becomes less certain in elderly people, with a tendency for the steps to shorten
- Elderly people tend to stand with slightly flexed hips and knees

11.
The Nervous System

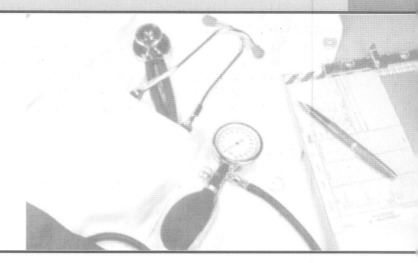

Medical students often approach the neurological examination with trepidation and, indeed, there is no denying the complexities of the nervous system or the difficulties sometimes experienced in attempting anatomical localisation on the basis of abnormal physical signs. The problem for the student, however, often begins with a failure to acquire the skills necessary to elicit those signs. If they are not identified correctly, mistakes in interpretation and diagnosis inevitably follow.

This chapter summarises the examination of the central and peripheral nervous systems, although it will seldom be necessary to examine all the areas covered. Selection is influenced partly by the patient's history but also by cooperation, conscious state and level of fatigue. Certain examination techniques demand a good deal of both patient and examiner and if responses become erratic it is better to return to the examination later. Students, and sometimes doctors, are prone to examine only those areas immediately accessible with the patient supine. Remember to turn the patient over in order to assess the spine and the muscles of the shoulder and pelvic girdles. Always record your findings in full, avoiding irritating acronyms (e.g. PERLA for pupils equal, reacting to light and accommodation) and, if your examination has been limited, state exactly what you have done (rather than just 'CNS' followed by a tick). Remember that physical signs can alter, sometimes rapidly, and repeating your examination can give you useful insight into the mechanisms of certain disorders.

THE CORTEX

STRUCTURE AND FUNCTION
On the basis of differences in histological structure, distinct areas can be identified within the cerebral cortex (Fig. 11.1). Tracts within the cortex comprise efferent pathways such as the pyramidal system, afferent pathways such as the thalamocortical projec-

tions, association fibres passing from regions within the hemisphere and commissural fibres connecting regions contralateral to one another. Surrounding the primary cortical areas for movement, sensation and vision are the cortical association areas. For example, the lateral geniculate body projects not just to the visual cortex (area 17) but also to areas 18 and 19, parts of the visual association cortex (Fig. 11.1).

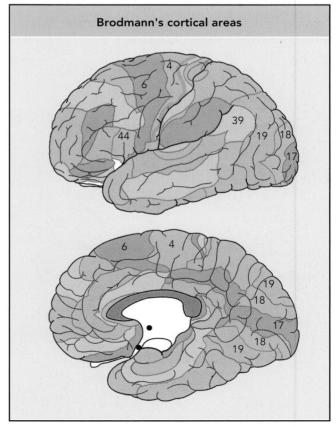

Fig. 11.1 Lateral and medial aspects of the cerebral hemisphere showing some of Brodmann's cortical areas.

The frontal lobe is separated from the parietal lobe posteriorly by the central (rolandic) sulcus, whereas the temporal lobe lies below the lateral (sylvian) sulcus. The boundaries of the parietal, temporal and occipital lobes are not defined by a specific sulcus (Fig. 11.2).

The brain is supplied by paired internal carotid and vertebral arteries. The former terminate in the anterior and middle cerebral arteries, the latter in the basilar artery, which ends by forming the posterior cerebral arteries (Fig. 11.3). An anastomotic system at the base of the brain (the circle of Willis) connects these various components. The lateral surface of the cortex is supplied predominantly by the middle cerebral artery. The anterior cerebral artery supplies a strip of cortex spanning its superior margin, whereas the posterior cerebral artery supplies the occipital lobe and the inferior aspect of the temporal lobe (Fig. 11.4). Normal cerebral blood flow, at approximately 55 ml/100 g/min, represents approximately 15% of cardiac output. The level of blood flow is largely dependent on the P_{CO_2} of arterial blood. Vasodilatation and increased flow occur as P_{CO_2} rises. During a specific task orientated to speech, vision, hearing or motor activity, a focal increase in flow occurs in the appropriate part of the cortex.

The ventricular system contains cerebrospinal fluid (CSF) which originates predominantly in the choroid plexuses of the lateral ventricles, then circulates through the third ventricle and aqueduct before reaching the fourth ventricle. The CSF exits through the foramina of the fourth ventricle and is eventually reabsorbed through the arachnoid villae. The rate of CSF production is approximately 120 ml/24 h.

Acquisition of memory requires a number of stages. All data, whether visual or verbal, are recorded temporarily in a short-term pool. A selective and active process then passes some of the data into a long-term memory store. Finally, an active process of retrieval restores the memory to consciousness. Conventionally, memory is divided into immediate, recent and remote components, although these divisions are not absolute. Immediate or short-term memory lasts a few seconds; recent memory relates to activities or events occurring within a few hours or days and remote memory to events of the past, for example, the individual's youth. Structures particularly associated with learning storage include the hippocampi, the mamillary bodies and the dorso-medial nuclei of the thalami – the limbic system. Remote memory, however, can be retrieved even if these structures are damaged, suggesting that it is stored predominantly in the association cortex appropriate to the memory modality.

Visuospatial ability is dependent mainly on non-dominant parietal lobe function. Language function is located in the left hemisphere in over 95% of right-handed individuals. For left-handed individuals, some 60% have language dominance in the left hemisphere, with 40% in the right hemisphere. Something like 80% of all left-handed individuals have mixed dominance, with language represented in both hemispheres. Within the hemisphere, a posteriorly placed area (Wernicke) is concerned with the comprehension of spoken language and an anterior area (Broca) with language output. The two are connected by the arcuate fasciculus (Fig. 11.5). The integration of the auditory and visual data required for reading and writing is achieved by the angular gyrus (area 39) (Fig. 11.1).

Although certain functions can be localised to specific cortical areas, other aspects of higher cortical function are represented more diffusely.

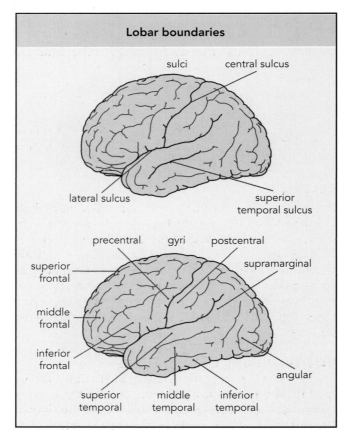

Fig. 11.2   Lateral surface of the cerebral hemisphere.

?   Questions to ask
Higher cortical function

- Has there been a change in your mood?
- Has your memory deteriorated?
- Do you have difficulty finding the right word in conversation?
- Have you ever become lost while travelling a familiar route?
- Do you have difficulty dressing?

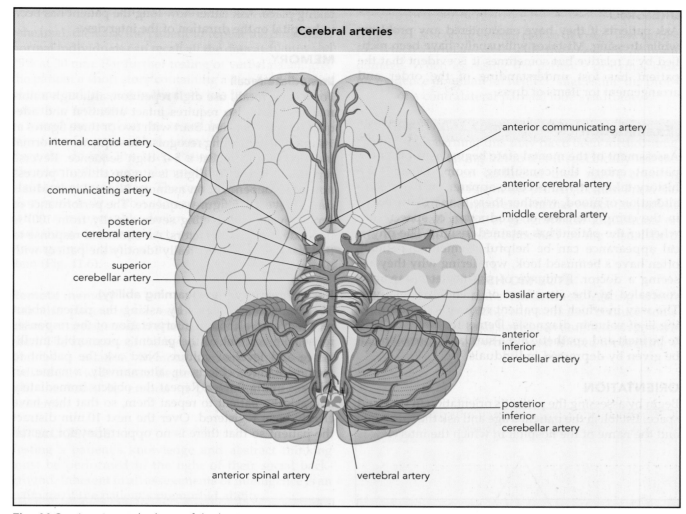

Cerebral arteries

internal carotid artery

posterior communicating artery

posterior cerebral artery

superior cerebellar artery

anterior communicating artery

anterior cerebral artery

middle cerebral artery

basilar artery

anterior inferior cerebellar artery

posterior inferior cerebellar artery

anterior spinal artery

vertebral artery

Fig. 11.3 Arteries at the base of the brain.

Symptoms

Many of the symptoms arising from a disorder of higher cortical function will be more evident to a close friend or relative than to the patient. Areas to cover, although some will be more evident during formal examination, are the following.

MOOD

This can be assessed by direct questioning but also by observation of the patient's behaviour. Is the mood appropriate to the setting of the interview? Is the patient passive, apparently disinterested or even denying disability? Is there evident anxiety or a heightened state of arousal, accompanied by restlessness and pressure of talk? Does the history suggest delusions or hallucinations?

MEMORY

The demented patient often denies loss of memory, particularly once the condition is established. In the early stages, however, patients can retain awareness of their difficulty, and sometimes volunteer that remote memory is partly spared.

SPEECH

Aphasic patients usually retain insight into their word-finding difficulty. At times the defect is so substantial that history-taking from the patient becomes impossible. Listening to the history allows estimation of the degree of fluency in speech production, an assessment that will continue during the course of the examination. Patients are likely to volunteer any associated difficulty with reading (dyslexia) or writing (dysgraphia).

GEOGRAPHICAL ORIENTATION

The first sign of geographical disorientation may be the inability to follow a familiar route. If the impairment is severe, patients can become lost in their own home but at this level of disability the problem will be volunteered by relatives rather than the patient.

Many symptoms are common to both physical and psychiatric illness but others are more specifically within the territory of psychiatry.

SPECIFIC SYMPTOMS

Mood

Enquire whether the patient, or a relative, has noticed any mood change. A particularly valuable question when screening for depression is whether the individual has lost pleasure in their normal activities (anhedonia). Supplementary to this will be enquiries regarding sleep pattern, loss of libido and suicidal ideation. Sometimes the patient denies flattening of mood, when that is all too evident from the interview. Such discrepancies should be carefully recorded.

Patients will usually complain of anxiety but sometimes its somatic manifestations, for example palpitations, sweating and tremulousness, predominate. The anxiety may be chronic and spontaneous or be triggered acutely by a specific stimulus – phobic anxiety.

Patients seldom complain of euphoria – a feeling of limitless physical and mental energy. There is likely to be a pressurised manic quality to the patient's conversation, coupled with physical restlessness.

Abnormal thoughts

These will only be elicited by sensitive questioning. The patient can be understandably reluctant to reveal certain abnormal thoughts. It may be apparent from the interview that the patient's thought pattern is difficult to follow or that abnormal thoughts have pervaded the conversation. Ask patients about paranoid ideas, in other words, whether they feel people are against them. Ask whether certain thoughts or ideas regularly intrude into their thinking, or whether they believe their thoughts are being interfered with or influenced by external agencies. Thought disorders include the following.

Delusions These are beliefs which can be demonstrated to be incorrect but to which the individual still adheres. Members of the Flat Earth Society are deluded. Often there is an element of reference, in other words that actions or words are directed specifically at that individual even if they appear on a global platform, for example television. Paranoid delusions contain a persecutory element. Delusions of worthlessness are particularly associated with depressive illness.

Obsessions These are recurrent thoughts which often result in the performance of repetitive acts (compulsions). The patient is aware that they are inappropriate but cannot resist returning to them or acting upon them. Examples of obsessional thought include convictions that a particular individual is antagonistic or that a spouse is unfaithful.

Questions to ask
Psychiatric assessment

- Do you feel unduly anxious or depressed?
- Do you repeat certain tasks over and over again?
- Do you feel people are against you?
- Have you heard or seen things that are not there?
- Do you ever lose the sense of yourself or your environment?

Abnormal perceptions

These are auditory or visual phenomena that other individuals are not aware of.

Hallucinations are experiences that have no objective equivalent to explain them. They are predominantly visual or auditory but can occur in other forms, for example of smell or taste in patients with complex partial seizures. Visual hallucinations can be unformed, for example an ill-defined pattern of lights, or formed, the individual then describing people or animals, often of a frightening aspect. Visual hallucinations are more often a feature of an organic brain syndrome (e.g. delirium tremens or adverse drug reaction) than a functional psychosis, e.g. schizophrenia. Auditory hallucinations are also either unformed or formed. They are found more often in the functional psychoses than in organic brain disease. The voices can take on a persecutory quality in schizophrenia and an accusatory element in depression. In déja and jamais vu, intense feelings of a relived experience or a sensation of strangeness in familiar surroundings occur, respectively. Both can be a feature of everyday life but when pathological are usually epileptic. Illusions are misinterpretations of an external reality: all of us have this when watching a magician at work. In deperson-

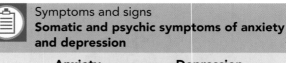

Symptoms and signs
Somatic and psychic symptoms of anxiety and depression

	Anxiety	Depression
Somatic	Palpitations	Altered appetite
	Tremor	Constipation
	Breathlessness	Headache
	Fatigue	Bodily fatigue
	Diarrhoea	Tiredness
	Sweating	
Psychic	Feelings of tension	Apathy
	Irritability	Poor concentration
	Difficulty sleeping	Early morning waking
	Fear	Diurnal mood swing
	Depersonalisation	Retardation
		Guilt

alisation, the individual feels a detachment from the normal sense of self; in derealisation, the individual feels a detachment from the external world. Both occur in neurotic illnesses but also, periodically, in normal individuals.

Cognition

The assessment of higher cortical function has already been discussed. It is necessary to distinguish cognitive impairment due to dementia from cognitive impairment due to delirium. In the latter there is clouding of consciousness, usually manifested as reduced awareness of, or response to, the environment.

THE FAMILY HISTORY

Begin by obtaining details of the patient's father and mother, in terms of their current age (or age at death), their own quality of health, whether they had any history of psychiatric disorder and the quality of the patient's relationship with them. Ask similar questions about the patient's siblings. Questions regarding the patient's own children are usually included in the personal history. Genetic factors are particularly strong in schizophrenia and manic-depressive psychosis.

THE PERSONAL HISTORY

Childhood

It is unlikely patients will have accurate details of their birth or early development unless there was a particular problem with them. A direct question to the patient regarding whether they were happy or unhappy in childhood is useful. Some 'happy' responses turn out to be rather less so with further delving. If there is an expression of remembered unhappiness, explore it further in terms of relationships with parents and any physical illness.

Schooling and further education

Establishing the details of this is helpful in forming an assessment of the patient's premorbid intelligence. At the same time, enquire about friendships or a tendency to isolation, and about teasing or bullying.

Sexual development

For female patients, enquire about the age of the menarche and how they attuned to adolescence in terms of menstruation and sexuality. For men, discussion should include whether their sexuality could be discussed in the home and how they acquired their sexual experience. Further issues relating to sexual development, for example homosexual experiences, are best left, at this stage, for the patient to raise.

Marital history

An overall outline includes the age of the spouse when the marriage occurred, the overall quality of the relationship, the state of the sexual relationship and details of any unease.

Occupational history

Ask how many jobs the patient has had, reasons for leaving previous posts, the quality of relationships in the workplace and the level of job satisfaction. If there has been one or more periods of unemployment, explore what effect this has had on the patient's overall welfare.

PAST MEDICAL HISTORY

This follows the usual pattern, and includes history of both physical and mental illness if these have occurred.

DRUG HISTORY

Determine alcohol consumption, but be aware of the possibility that the figure does not correspond to actual intake. Features suggesting alcohol dependency include early morning drinking, morning vomiting, taking a drink before an interview, erratic work attendance and drinking in isolation. Ask about narcotic exposure, the use of softer drugs such as cannabis and exposure to tranquillisers. If the patient is using codeine derivatives, ascertain for what purpose and the dosage.

PERSONALITY PROFILE

Evidence suggesting changing personality and mood is often better provided by colleagues, relatives or friends than by the patient. Questionnaires exist for the assessment of personality, but even without them the patient's attitude and behaviour, in terms of work and social relationships, personal drive, level of dependence, ambition and authority and response to stress will indicate the nature of the patient's personality.

Examination

The concept of the psychiatric examination needs to be interpreted broadly. A physical examination is necessary but the most telling diagnostic details will be revealed by an exploration of the patient's mental state, emerging as much from the history as from the answers to specific questions.

Clinical application

ORGANIC MENTAL STATES

In organic mental states, a specific pathological basis for the mental disorder has been established. Acute forms include the toxic confusional states, characterised by alteration of the conscious level, disordered perceptions (e.g. visual hallucinations), restlessness and thought disorder. Almost any structural or metabolic disorder can trigger the reaction. Examples include encephalitis, head injury and alcohol withdrawal. The principal chronic organic mental state is dementia.

FUNCTIONAL MENTAL STATES

In functional mental states, a specific underlying pathological or metabolic cause has not been identified. Psychotic states are those in which the individual has lost insight and neurotic states are those in which insight is preserved. The distinction is not absolute, however, and the terms are best avoided. In affective disorders, for example, anxiety, depression and mania, an alteration of mood is a major feature of the illness.

PHOBIAS

Phobias are a particular form of anxiety triggered by a specific environment or circumstance. Agoraphobia, for example, results in a fear of leaving the home, particularly if this involves entering crowded places.

DEPRESSIVE ILLNESS

Depressive illnesses include those triggered primarily by genetic or constitutional factors (endogenous) and those precipitated by adverse external events (reactive).

MANIA AND HYPOMANIA

In mania and hypomania (its lesser form), there is pressure of talk and physical activity. Patients lack insight and react adversely if their grandiose schemes are questioned. In manic-depressive illness, the mood fluctuates between two extremes.

SCHIZOPHRENIA

Schizophrenia has been classified into a number of types, although the entities defined are not absolutely distinct. It is characterised by thought disorder, blunting of emotional responses, paranoid tendencies and perceptual disorders. Thought disorder leads to irrational conversation, in which the development of ideas is either blocked or moves suddenly into unconnected channels. The emotions are blunted and the patient becomes increasingly withdrawn. Delusions are prominent and frequently contain paranoid elements. Auditory hallucinations are particularly characteristic of schizophrenia.

OBSESSIONAL STATES

In obsessional states, a preoccupation with mental or physical acts predominates. An obsessional personality displays these characteristics but not to the point where they interfere with the normal activities of life. In obsessional states, however, the relevant thought or action takes on a compulsive quality, ineffectively countered by the patient. Obsessional symptoms can feature in other psychiatric illnesses.

HYSTERIA (CONVERSION HYSTERIA)

Hysteria is a disorder in which physical symptoms or signs exist for which there is no objective counterpart

Differential diagnosis
Organic and functional mental states

- Acute anxiety state
- Chronic anxiety state
- Endogenous depression
- Reactive depression
- Manic depression
- Schizophrenia
- Obsessional states
- Conversion hysteria
- Drug and alcohol-related disorders
- Toxic confusional state
- Dementia

Questions to ask
Mental state

For anxiety
- Are the symptoms provoked by particular environments?

For depression
- Are there suicidal thoughts?

For schizophrenia
- Has the patient had auditory hallucinations?
- Does the patient believe his or her thoughts are controlled by others?

and which require, in the case of signs, an elaboration on the part of the patient of which he or she is unaware. Many of the symptoms are referred to the nervous system, for example, memory loss, paralysis, unsteadiness and visual impairment. Malingerers, on the other hand, consciously elaborate their disability.

HYSTERICAL PERSONALITY

Hysterical personality is distinct from hysteria, although individuals with this personality trait may develop conversion reactions. The hysterical personality is characterised by superficiality and shallow emotional responsiveness combined with a histrionic overwrought reaction to events.

Symptoms and signs
The psychiatric patient

A full examination is performed to exclude any physical disorder that may contribute to the patient's condition

THE CRANIAL NERVES THE OLFACTORY (FIRST) NERVE

STRUCTURE AND FUNCTION

The olfactory epithelium contains specialised receptor cells and free nerve endings, the latter derived from the first and second divisions of the trigeminal nerve. Unmyelinated axons from the receptor cells traverse the cribriform plate before synapsing in the olfactory bulb. From here, the olfactory tract passes backwards, dividing into lateral and medial roots in the region of the anterior perforated substance. The more important lateral root projects predominantly to the uncus of the ipsilateral temporal lobe.

Molecules derived from particular odours are absorbed into the mucus covering the olfactory epithelium. From here they diffuse via ciliary processes to the terminal processes of the receptor cells where they bind reversibly to receptor sites. This initiates an action potential in the olfactory nerve with a firing frequency related to the intensity of the stimulus.

Women have a more sensitive sense of smell than men. In both sexes, smell sensitivity declines with age. Many healthy individuals have difficulty naming or describing the quality of a particular odour even though they can distinguish it from others. The value of a particular odour for the testing of olfactory nerve function is determined principally by how selectively it stimulates the specialised receptor cells rather than the free trigeminal endings. Odours stimulating the latter include peppermint, camphor, ammonia, menthol and anisol. Highly selective stimulants of olfactory nerve endings include ß-phenyl ethyl alcohol, methyl cyclopentenolone and isovaleric acid. Coffee, cinnamon and chocolate are useful everyday odours for the bedside testing of smell.

	Symptoms and signs **Disturbance of smell**
Hyposmia	partial loss
Anosmia	total loss
Hyperosmia	exaggerated sensitivity
Dyosmia	distorted sense

Differential diagnosis
Disturbances of olfaction

- Post-traumatic anosmia
- Postinfective anosmia
- Olfactory hallucinations in complex partial seizures

SYMPTOMS

The disturbances of smell that occur are defined in the symptoms and signs box. For loss of smell, determine whether it is bilateral or unilateral.

Examination

The most convenient method for testing smell uses squeeze bottles bearing a nozzle that can be inserted into each nostril in turn. The patient is asked either to identify the smell or to describe its quality.

Clinical application

Olfaction is commonly disturbed by upper respiratory tract infection or local nasal pathology. Hyposmia can persist after an apparently banal viral illness and also after head injury. Smell sensitivity is diminished in dementia. Unilateral hyposmia is rarely the presenting symptom of a subfrontal meningioma. Olfactory hallucinations occur in complex partial seizures.

THE OPTIC (SECOND) NERVE

STRUCTURE AND FUNCTION

Two types of retinal photoreceptor, rods and cones, have been identified in humans. At the fovea only cones are found, with rods predominating in the periphery. Fibres from the nasal aspect of the fovea pass directly to the optic disc. Fibres from above and below the fovea pass almost directly but fibres from the temporal border pass almost vertically, both superiorly and inferiorly, before arching around the other foveal fibres on their way to the optic disc (Fig. 11.14). Axons in the papillomacular bundle originate in the cones of the fovea and occupy a substantial proportion of the temporal aspect of the optic disc. Fibres from the superior and inferior parts of the periphery of the retina occupy corresponding areas in the optic nerve. As the papillomacular bundle approaches the chiasm, it moves centrally. The crossing, nasal, macular fibres occupy the central and posterior part of the chiasm. The superior peripheral nasal fibres cross more posteriorly than the ventral fibres, which loop slightly into the terminal part of the opposite optic nerve (Fig. 11.15). Crossed and uncrossed fibres are arranged in alternate layers in the lateral geniculate body. The optic radiation extends from the lateral geniculate body to the visual (striate) cortex, area 17 (Fig. 11.1). The ventral fibres of the radiation loop forward towards the tip of the temporal lobe. The visual cortex is situated along the superior and inferior margins of the calcarine fissure, extending approximately 1.5 cm around the posterior pole. The macular representation lies posteriorly, with dorsal and ventral retina above and below the fissure, respectively. The unpaired outer 30° of the temporal field is represented in the contralateral hemisphere at the anterior limit of the striate cortex (Fig. 11.16).

Conditions of high (photopic) illumination activate cone photoreceptors, providing high spatial resolution and colour vision sense. Colour appreciation depends on three types of cone with spectral sensitivities spanning the range of colour vision. Low-illumination (scotopic) responses are mediated by rods.

SYMPTOMS

A number of questions are appropriate when assessing the patient's complaint of vision loss or alteration.

Examination

VISUAL ACUITY

Visual acuity is tested in conditions of high illumination, producing a measure of cone function. The Snellen chart is used for testing distance vision. With the patient at the distance shown above a particular line, the visual angle subtended by a letter in that line is 5′ and by individual components of the letter, 1′ (Fig. 11.17).

Seat or stand the patient 6 m from the card. Ask the patient to cover each eye in turn and find which is the smallest line of print that can be read comfortably. The visual acuity is then expressed as the ratio of the distance between the patient and the card (usually 6 m), to the figure on the chart immediately above the smallest visible line. An acuity of 6/18, therefore, indicates that, at 6 m from the chart, the patient is able to read down only to the 18 m line. Make sure the patient wears glasses if they contain a distance correction. If the patient's glasses are not available, reading through a pinhole will partly

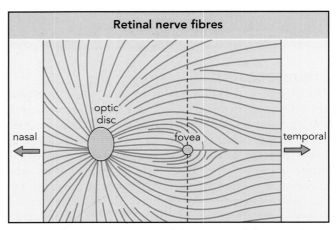

Fig. 11.14   Representation of the course of the retinal nerve fibres.

correct for any myopia. If unable to read the 60 m line at 6 m, the patient can move nearer the test type, say to 3 m. If the patient can then just read the 60 m line, the visual acuity, for that particular eye, is 3/60. A visual acuity of less than 1/60 can be recorded as counting fingers (CF), hand movements (HM), perception of light (PL) or no perception of light (NPL). Near vision is tested using reading test types, such as

> **? Questions to ask**
> **Visual disturbances**
>
> - Is the vision loss unilateral or bilateral?
> - Is it confined to one area of the visual field?
> - Are there positive as well as negative visual phenomena?
> - Do colours appear different?

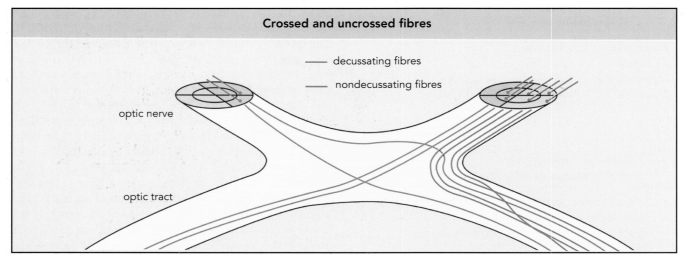

Fig. 11.15   Crossed and uncrossed fibres from the macula and the peripheral retina.

that produced by the UK Faculty of Ophthalmologists (Fig. 11.18). Near visual acuity does not necessarily correlate well with distance acuity.

COLOUR VISION

Bedside tests of colour vision are designed principally to detect congenital defects. In the Farnsworth Munsell test the patient grades the shading of 84 coloured tiles. Red–green deficiency can be assessed more rapidly using the Ishihara test plates (Fig. 11.19). With the plates at about 75 cm from the eyes, which are covered

in turn, ask the patient to read plates one to 15. If 13 or more plates are read correctly, colour vision can be regarded as normal.

VISUAL FIELDS

Retinal sensitivity diminishes with increasing distance from the fovea. Visual field mapping defines points in the visual field at which an object of a particular size or illumination is detected. The visual field is not symmetrical. It extends superiorly and medially for approximately 60°, temporally for about 100°, and

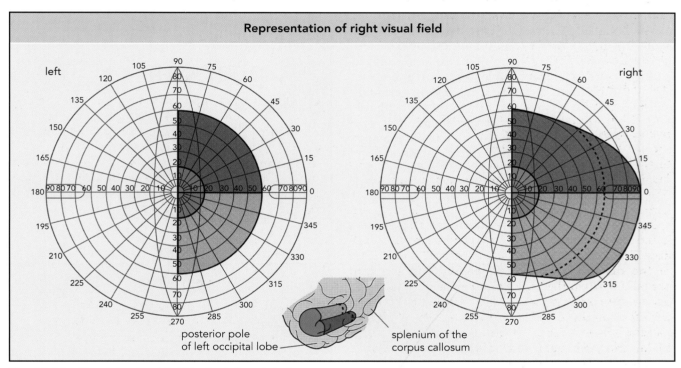

Fig. 11.16 The right visual field in the left occipital cortex.

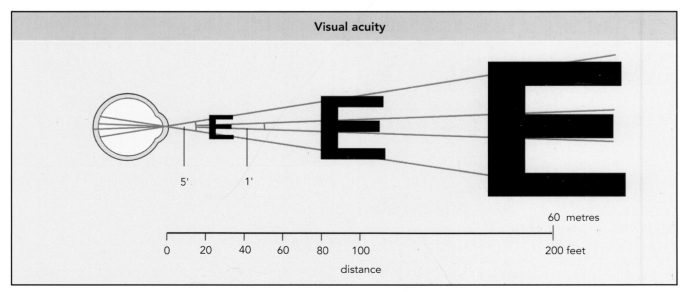

Fig. 11.17 The angles subtended by standard Snellen type.

inferiorly for approximately 75°. The blind spot, situated approximately 15° from fixation in the temporal field, marks the position of the optic disc. The field of vision to a coloured object, reflecting cone function, is more restricted than the field of a white object of the same size. Only the central portions of the two visual fields are binocular, the temporal margins being monocular (Fig. 11.20). Static perimetry involves the detection of a stationary target of varying brightness, whereas kinetic perimetry involves the detection of a moving target.

For bedside testing of the visual field sit approximately 1 m from the patient. In infants or poorly cooperating adults, a meaningful response may be impossible to elicit or may be obtained only by using visual threat, in other words, a sudden, unexpected hand movement. For cooperative adults and older children, either finger movements or coloured objects can be used. For testing the left visual field, ask the patient to close or cover the right eye with the right hand and you cover or close your left eye (Fig. 11.21). Ensure that the patient's left eye remains fixed on your right eye throughout the examination. The limits of the peripheral field can be determined by bringing the moving fingers of your right hand into the four quadrants of the patient's field. If individual half fields are full, then the target object,

usually your moving fingers, should be presented in both peripheral fields simultaneously. In parietal lobe lesions, particularly of the nondominant hemisphere, a visual target presented in isolation in the

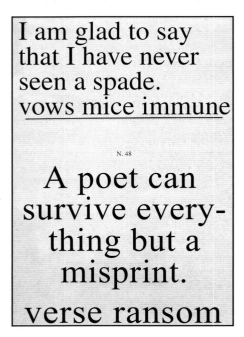

Fig. 11.18 Page from standard reading type.

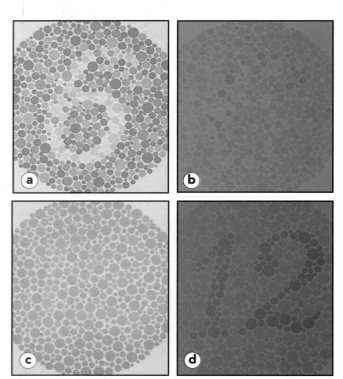

Fig. 11.19 Two plates from the Ishihara series. A patient with normal vision reads both (a) and (c) without difficulty; however, a patient with red–green deficiency is unable to read the figure 6 (b) but is able to read the figure 12 (d) correctly.

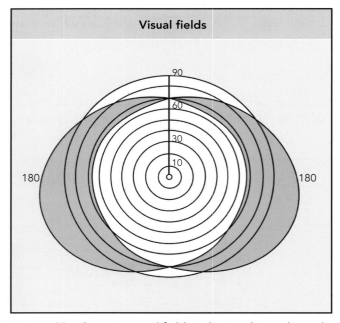

Fig. 11.20 Superimposed fields indicating binocular and monocular components.

contralateral field is perceived but is missed (visual suppression or inattention) when a comparable target is presented simultaneously in the ipsilateral half-field (Fig. 11.22). Peripheral field defects are sometimes detected only if a small target object (e.g. a 10 mm. red pin) is used rather than moving fingers.

Hand or finger movements are too crude a stimulus for assessing central field defects and here a small coloured object is used. It is useful to outline the blind spot first, partly because its successful identification increases confidence in one's own technique and partly because it indicates good fixation on the part of the patient. Move a red pin of some 10 mm in diameter into the temporal field along the horizontal meridian. First explain to the patient that the object will disappear briefly then reappear and that the patient should indicate when this happens. Once you have found the position of the blind spot its shape can be mapped. You will find that you map the position of your own and the patient's blind spot independently. Having identified the blind spot, assess the central visual field.

FUNDOSCOPY

Normally it is not necessary to dilate the pupils in order to examine the central fundus but if the patient has small pupils, or the background illumination is high, take the patient into a darkened room for the examination. If this fails to dilate the pupils sufficiently, then a mydriatic, for example, Mydrilate (1% cyclopentolate), can be instilled. This should never be done in the unconscious patient and must always be recorded in the patient's notes. Do not use mydriatics in a patient with glaucoma. Remember to reverse the effects of the mydriatic at the end of the examination by instilling 2% pilocarpine.

Ask the patient to fixate on a distant target (Fig. 11.24). If the patient wears glasses with a substantial correction, it sometimes facilitates the

Symptoms and signs
Types of field defect

Absolute central scotoma
- Area around fixation in which there is no appreciation of the visual stimulus

Relative central scotoma
- Area in which object is detected but its colour is diminished or desaturated (Fig. 11.23)

Centrocaecal scotoma
- Extends from fixation towards blind spot

Bitemporal hemianopia
- Temporal halves of both fields are affected

Homonymous hemianopia
- A field defect in which the left or right half field is affected. In a complete right homonymous hemianopia, therefore, the temporal field of the right eye and the nasal field of the left eye are lost

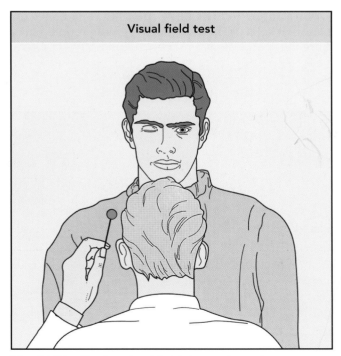

Fig. 11.21   Testing visual fields by confrontation.

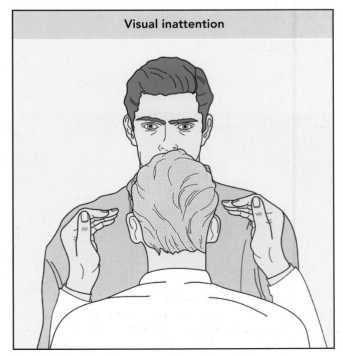

Fig. 11.22   Simultaneous presentation of finger movements in the two half fields.

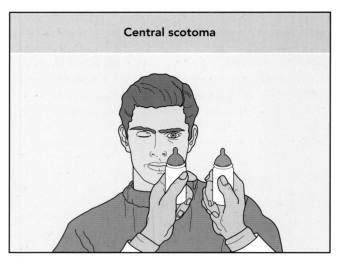

Central scotoma

Fig. 11.23 Comparison of colour sensitivity between central and peripheral field. In this patient with a central scotoma, the red object appears brown in the central field.

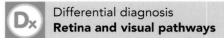

Differential diagnosis
Retina and visual pathways

- Anterior ischaemic optic neuropathy
- Optic neuritis
- Optic nerve compression
- Papilloedema
- Hypertensive retinopathy
- Diabetic retinopathy
- Glaucoma
- Chiasmatic compression due to pituitary tumour
- Optic tract, radiation or visual cortex lesions due to vascular disease

examination to perform it with the patient's glasses in place.

The optic disc is examined first to assess its shape, colour and clarity. The temporal margin of the disc is slightly paler than the nasal margin. The physiological cup varies in size but seldom extends to the temporal, and never to the nasal margins of the disc. The blood vessels are not obscured as they cross the disc margin, nor are they elevated (Fig. 11.25).

The vessels are examined next. The arteries are narrower than the veins and a brighter colour. They possess a longitudinal pale streak as a consequence of light reflecting from their walls. The retinal veins should be closely inspected where they enter the optic disc. In approximately 80% of normal individuals the veins pulsate. This pulsation ceases when CSF pressure exceeds 200 mm of water. Therefore the presence of retinal venous pulsation is a very sensitive index of normal intracranial pressure. Learn to identify this physical sign. It will save countless references to 'swollen optic discs?'. The fundus is examined for the presence of haemorrhages and exudates, the positions of which are best shown by a small diagram in the patient's notes, or by a description that uses the optic disc as a clock face for localisation purposes, for example, 'one large haemorrhage at 6 o'clock, one disc diameter from the disc'.

Clinical application

OPTIC ATROPHY

Optic atrophy follows any process that damages the ganglion cells or the axons between the retinal nerve fibre layer and the lateral geniculate body. It is asso-

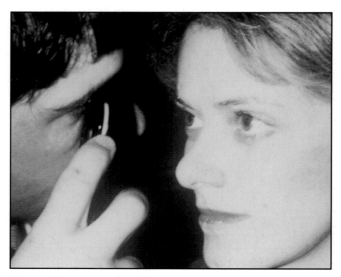

Fig. 11.24 Direct fundoscopy.

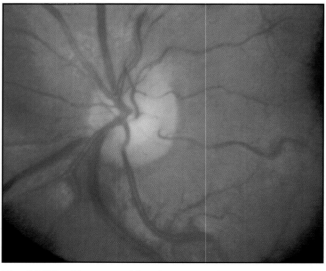

Fig. 11.25 The normal fundus.

ciated with loss of bulk of the nerve and pallor of the disc (Fig. 11.26). The pallor may be diffuse or segmental. Temporal pallor is the most common form of segmental atrophy, attributable to the susceptibility of the papillomacular bundle to degenerate after optic nerve damage by compression or metabolic disturbance.

The colour of the normal optic disc is variable and the ophthalmoscopic diagnosis of optic atrophy notoriously subjective. Additional features that may help the diagnosis include the number of capillaries visible on the optic disc, and the presence of retinal nerve fibre

atrophy. The former criterion has not been substantiated and detection of the latter requires considerable experience. Inspection of the retinal vessels is worthwhile. The presence of sheathing or attenuation of the retinal arterioles suggests that the optic atrophy is secondary to ischaemic optic neuropathy or central retinal artery occlusion.

PAPILLOEDEMA

Patients with papilloedema often have no visual complaints, although some describe transient obscurations of vision either occurring spontaneously or triggered by postural change. Papilloedema is usually bilateral, although sometimes asymmetrical. Its pathogenesis remains unsettled. The term papilloedema is best reserved for patients in whom the disc swelling is secondary to raised intracranial pressure. Transmission of the raised intracranial pressure, via the subarachnoid space of the optic nerve, results in venous stasis and also interrupts both fast and slow axoplasmic flow in the optic nerve.

As papilloedema develops, swelling of the nerve fibre layer appears (best seen with a red-free light), within which haemorrhages are visible. The disc becomes hyperaemic (as a result of capillary dilatation) with a loss of definition of its margins, and retinal venous pulsation disappears (Fig. 11.27). In fully developed papilloedema there is engorgement of retinal veins, obscuration of the disc margin, flame haemorrhages and cotton wool spots (the consequence of retinal infarction). The vessels are tortuous (Fig. 11.28). Often the only visual field change at this stage is an enlargement of the blind spot (Fig. 11.29). In the later stages of papilloedema, hard exudates appear on the disc, which becomes atrophic, and other visual field abnormalities appear, including arcuate fibre defects and peripheral constriction.

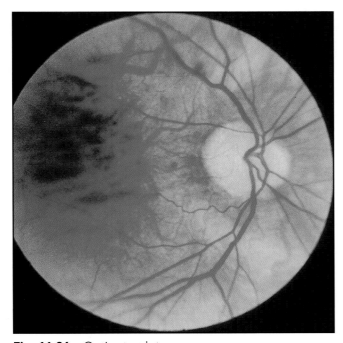

Fig. 11.26 Optic atrophy.

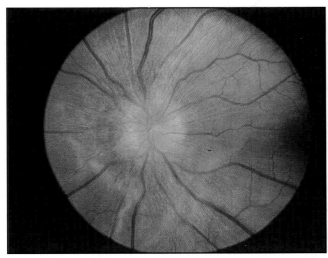

Fig. 11.27 Early papilloedema. Dilated nerve fibre bundles, superficial haemorrhages and disc hyperaemia.

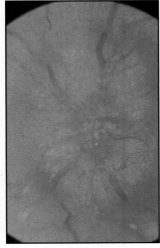

Fig. 11.28 Chronic papilloedema. Swollen optic discs, dilated capillaries, haemorrhages and cotton wool spots.

Papilloedema can probably appear within 4–5 h of the development of intracranial hypertension and may not resolve for some weeks after its reduction.

OTHER FUNDUS ABNORMALITIES

Myelinated nerve fibres
A congenital anomaly in which myelinated and therefore visible nerve fibres are found at, or adjacent to, the disc margin (Fig. 11.30).

Drusen (hyaline bodies)
Drusen are thought to be derived from axonal debris and are situated in the disc anterior to the lamina cribrosa, where they appear as yellow excrescences, often distorting the disc margin. They do not usually produce visual symptoms (Fig. 11.31).

RETINAL VASCULAR DISEASE

Retinal artery and vein occlusion
After occlusion of the central retinal artery, the retina becomes pale and opaque with a cherry-red spot at the macula. The optic disc, initially swollen, becomes atrophic (Fig. 11.32). The presence of microemboli, containing either cholesterol or a fibrin–platelet mixture, establishes that the occlusion is embolic (Fig. 11.33). A branch occlusion produces a corre-

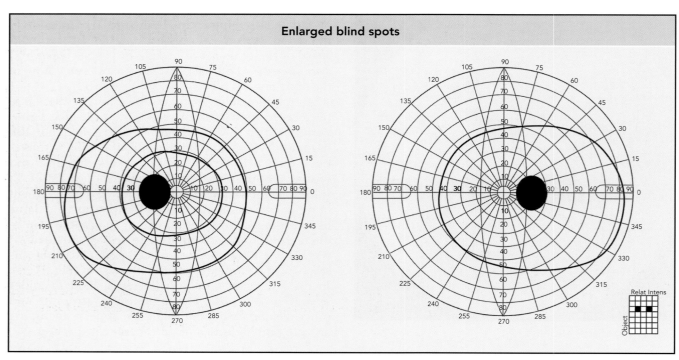

Enlarged blind spots

Fig. 11.29 Papilloedema. Visual fields showing bilaterally enlarged blind spots.

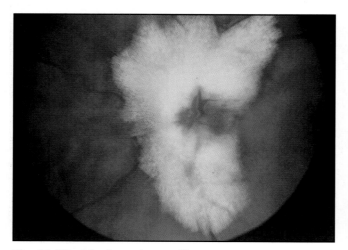

Fig. 11.30 Myelinated nerve fibres.

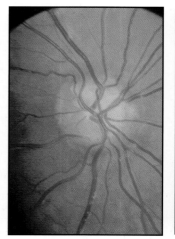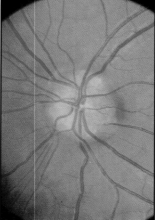

Fig. 11.31 Bilateral drusen (associated with peripapillary haemorrhage on right).

sponding sector-shaped visual defect. In central retinal vein occlusion there is swelling of the optic disc, dilatation of the retinal veins and fundal haemorrhages (Fig. 11.34).

Hypertensive retinopathy

In hypertensive retinopathy, the light reflex from the arteriolar wall is abnormal and constriction of the venous wall appears at sites of arteriovenous crossing. Both the former (silver or copper-wiring) and the latter (arteriovenous nipping) are encountered in normal older individuals. A more reliable sign of hypertensive retinopathy is variation in the calibre of the retinal arterioles. As the retinopathy advances,

haemorrhages and cotton wool spots appear (Fig. 11.35) and in malignant or accelerated hypertension disc swelling occurs.

Diabetic retinopathy

Diabetic retinopathy in its early stages principally affects the retinal microcirculation, producing the characteristic, although not pathognomonic, microaneurysm (Fig. 11.36). Subsequently small haemorrhages, exudates and cotton wool spots appear. Visual failure is usually due either to macular disease, in the form of oedema, infarction or lipid deposition (Fig. 11.37) or to the appearance of new vessel formation (proliferative diabetic retinopathy), leading to vitreous

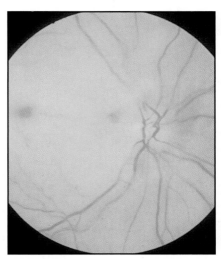

Fig. 11.32 Central retinal artery occlusion.

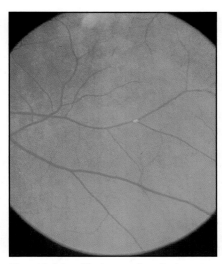

Fig. 11.33 Cholesterol embolus.

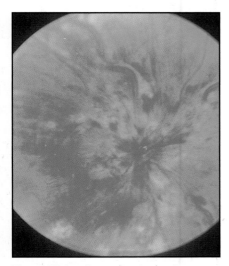

Fig. 11.34 Central retinal vein occlusion.

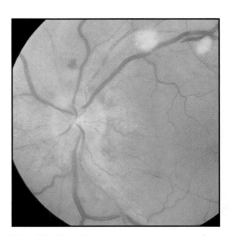

Fig. 11.35 Hypertensive retinopathy with haemorrhages, cotton wool spots and variation in arteriolar calibre.

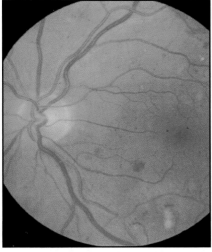

Fig. 11.36 Diabetic retinopathy. Microaneurysms, haemorrhages, exudates and cotton wool spots.

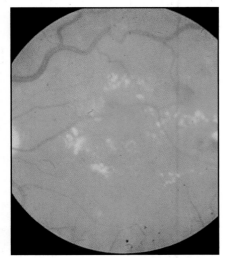

Fig. 11.37 Diabetic retinopathy. Hard exudates at the macula.

haemorrhage and retinal detachment caused by traction of fibrous tissue (Fig. 11.38).

GLAUCOMA

Glaucoma, characterised by raised intraocular pressure, can occur either secondarily to various ocular pathologies (e.g. uveitis) or in a primary form. The latter is far more common. Resulting changes in the optic disc include enlargement of the physiological cup (particularly significant if in the vertical axis), an increase in the ratio of cup size to vertical disc diameter beyond 0.6 and retinal nerve fibre atrophy. Arcuate field defects accompany these changes. With advanced glaucoma there is marked undermining of the disc margins and bowing of the blood vessels (Fig. 11.39).

OPTIC NERVE DISEASE

In lesions of the optic nerve, the visual defect is monocular. Visual acuity is usually reduced and colour perception is disturbed (particularly for red–green). There is a relative afferent pupillary defect (p. 324). The most likely visual field defect is a central scotoma (Fig. 11.40). Optic atrophy is a relatively late development in optic nerve compression. Proptosis is likely if the lesion is within the orbit.

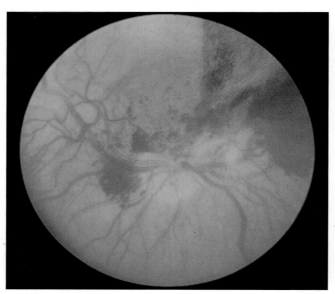

Fig. 11.38 Vitreous haemorrhage with evidence of new vessel formation at the disc margin.

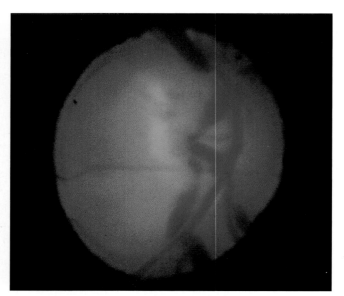

Fig. 11.39 Advanced chronic simple glaucoma.

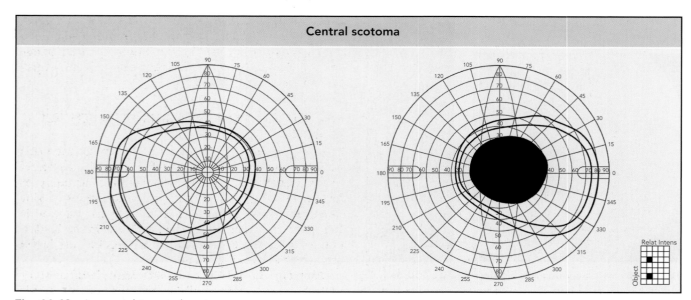

Fig. 11.40 Large right central scotoma.

CHIASMATIC LESIONS

Most chiasmatic syndromes are the result of compression by pituitary tumour, meningioma or craniopharyngioma. The result is a bitemporal hemianopia, although the type of defect relates to the position of the growth and its relation to the chiasm. Typically, the visual defect is asymmetrical (Fig. 11.41). In its earliest stages, the field defect can be detected only by moving a coloured target across the vertical meridian. (Fig. 11.42). Patients frequently complain of blurred or double vision, a conse-

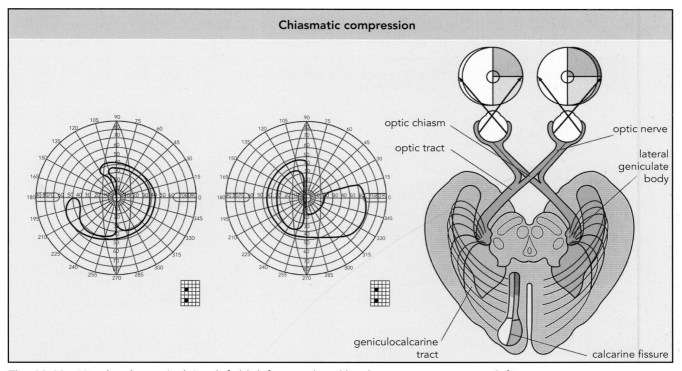

Fig. 11.41 Visual pathways (right) with field defect produced by chiasmatic compression (left).

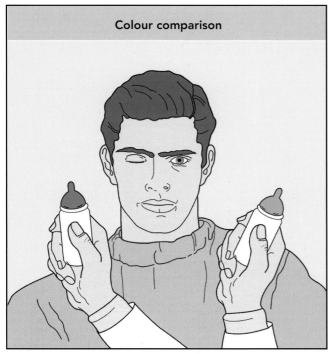

Fig. 11.42 Comparison of coloured targets in nasal and temporal fields.

quence of lost integration between independent nasal fields.

OPTIC TRACT AND LATERAL GENICULATE BODY LESIONS

These are uncommon. A lesion in the anterior part of the optic tract, before the homonymous fibres have joined, produces an incongruous homonymous hemianopia, that is, one in which the two half field losses are not equal (Fig. 11.43).

OPTIC RADIATION AND OCCIPITAL CORTEX LESIONS

The type of visual field loss from lesions of the optic radiation depends on their localisation. All the defects are homonymous but not necessarily congruous. In lesions affecting the temporal radiation, the superior quadrantic field is more affected than the inferior. If the defect is incongruous, the nasal loss in the ipsilateral eye is more extensive than the temporal loss in the contralateral eye (Fig. 11.44).

With parietal lobe lesions, the defect is often complete but rarely principally affects the inferior quadrants. Occipital lobe pathology produces congruous defects that can be total, quadrantic or scotomatous. In some instances there is macular sparing, probably because of a dual vascular supply to the macular area of the occipital cortex (Fig. 11.45). An isolated homonymous hemianopia is usually occipital in origin and almost always because of vascular disease. Temporal or parietal lobe pathology associated with visual field defects will usually produce additional symptoms and signs. Furthermore, the pathology is often neoplastic rather than vascular.

Bilateral occipital infarction results in cortical blindness. The pupillary responses are normal. In some instances there is denial of visual disability and confabulation of visual detail (Anton's syndrome).

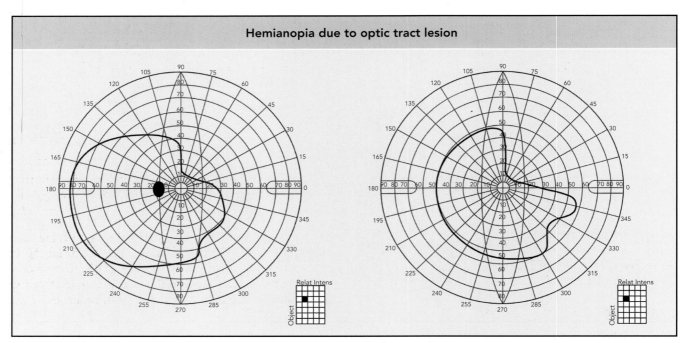

Fig. 11.43   Incongruous right homonymous hemianopia associated with a left optic tract lesion.

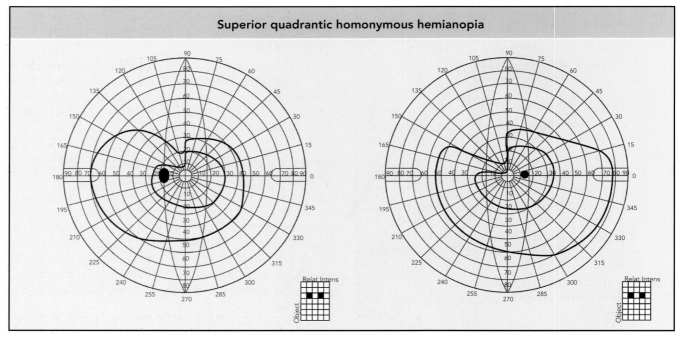

Fig. 11.44   Incongruous left superior quadrantic homonymous hemianopia associated with a lesion of the temporal part of the right optic radiation.

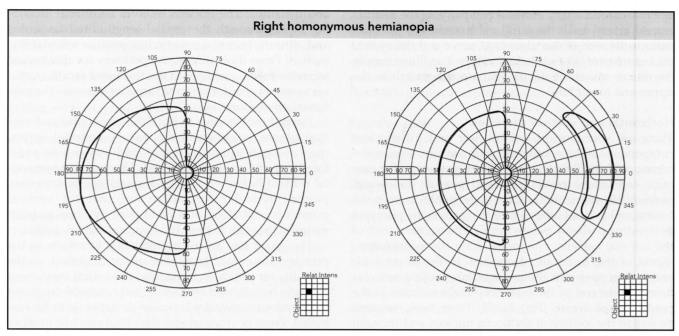

Fig. 11.45 A right homonymous hemianopia, sparing the macula and the peripheral temporal crescent of the right eye.

THE OCULOMOTOR, TROCHLEAR AND ABDUCENS (THIRD, FOURTH AND SIXTH) NERVES

STRUCTURE AND FUNCTION

Pupillary light response pathway

The pupillary light response pathway originates in the same rods and cones that register visual stimuli. Fibres from the receptors partly decussate in the chiasm, then leave the optic tract before the lateral geniculate body on their way to the brachium of the superior colliculus and, hence, the Edinger–Westphal nucleus, via the pretectal nuclear complex (Fig. 11.46). A light stimulus to one eye triggers a bilateral, symmetrical, pupillary response. The pupillomotor fibres lie superficially in the oculomotor nerve before joining the inferior division of the nerve on their way to the ciliary ganglion. After synapsing, the fibres enter the short ciliary nerve.

Near reaction

The near reaction comprises pupillary constriction, ocular convergence and increased accommodation of the lens. The accommodation reaction is controlled by the rostral and midportion of the Edinger–Westphal nucleus. The efferent pathway passes through the oculomotor nerve, ciliary ganglion and short ciliary nerve.

Ocular sympathetic fibres

The ocular sympathetic fibres originate in the hypothalamus and remain uncrossed. The first-order neurons terminate in the spinal cord in the intermediolateral cell column between the spinal segments of C8 and T2. Second-order neurons exit from the cord, principally in the first ventral thoracic root, and pass through the inferior and middle cervical ganglia before terminating in the superior cervical ganglion (Fig. 11.47). Sudomotor and vasoconstrictor fibres to the face, except for those to a small area on the forehead, run with branches of the

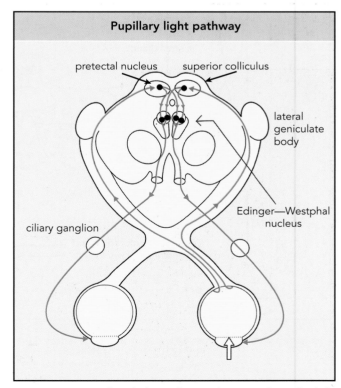

Fig. 11.46 Pupillary light pathway. The input from the left eye decussates at the chiasm and reaches both third nerve nuclei.

Nystagmus

Nystagmus is a repetitive to-and-fro movement of the eyes. In pendular nystagmus, the phases are of equal velocity, in phasic (jerk) nystagmus they differ. The slow phase of jerk nystagmus may show a linear or nonlinear time course. Vestibular dysfunction, either centrally or peripherally, is the usual cause of a jerk nystagmus in which the slow-phase is linear. In gaze-evoked nystagmus the eyes drift back from an eccentric position with a nonlinear velocity, followed by a saccadic correction. This type of nystagmus is thought to result from dysfunction of the neural integrater, the mechanism that sustains a tonic discharge of neuronal activity during eccentric gaze.

SYMPTOMS

If the patient complains of ptosis, find out whether the problem is bilateral or unilateral and whether it fluctuates. If necessary obtain old photographs to make a comparison.

For diplopia, a number of questions may help to suggest the underlying mechanism. Weakness of the lateral or medial rectus muscles produces a horizontal diplopia. Weakness of the other eye muscles produces a vertical or oblique diplopia. The diplopia increases as the patient looks in the direction of action of the paralysed muscle.

Examination

INSPECTION OF THE EYELIDS AND PUPILS

Note the position of the eyelids. If there is a ptosis, assess its fatiguability by asking the patient to sustain upward gaze. Next examine the pupils, which normally are circular and symmetrical, although a slight difference in size (anisocoria) of up to 2 mm is seen in some 20% of the population. If there is a slight size difference, take the

Questions to ask
Diplopia

- Is the diplopia relieved by covering one or other eye?
- Is the diplopia horizontal, vertical or oblique?
- Does the diplopia increase in one particular direction of gaze?
- Does the diplopia fluctuate or is it constant?

patient into a darkened room. A physiological anisocoria will remain unchanged. An irregular pupil is most commonly the consequence of iris disease. Ask the patient about previous ocular trauma or infection. If the pupils are markedly different in size, make sure that the patient is not using a mydriatic or meiotic in one eye alone.

Pupillary light response

Now examine the pupillary light response using a bright pencil torch. The background illumination should be low, and to prevent a near reaction the patient should fixate on a distant object. Observe the direct (ipsilateral) and consensual (contralateral) responses. A unilateral depression of the light response may be obvious but a defect of the afferent pupillary pathway is best appreciated by swinging the torch from one eye to the other. As the torch swings from, say, the right eye to the left, the pupil of the latter, which has just started to dilate because of the loss of its consensual reaction, immediately constricts.

Near reaction

If the light response is normal there is little point in testing the near reaction. If the light response is depressed, test the near reaction by asking the patient to fixate on a target (e.g. your forefinger) as it approaches

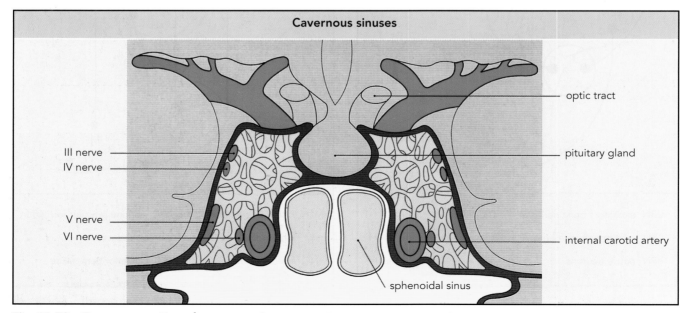

Fig. 11.50 Transverse section of cavernous sinuses.

the eyes. Many patients, especially elderly people, have difficulty sustaining convergence. If there is no immediate reaction, maintain convergence for a minute or so to see if a delayed reaction appears. The near reaction is additive to the pupillary light response, in other words, it can be tested in bright light.

INSPECTION OF EYE MOVEMENTS

Conjugate eye movements

Next assess conjugate eye movements. To test pursuit, ask the patient to follow a slowly moving target, first in the horizontal then in the vertical plane. If pursuit movements are slowed, brief saccades must be superimposed to allow the eyes to catch their target. The resulting movement is jerky rather than smooth. The slowing may be in one or more directions. To assess saccadic movements, ask the patient to rapidly fixate between two targets, for example, two fingers in the same plane. Saccades may be abnormal in terms of their velocity, accuracy or persistence. An overshoot or undershoot is readily detected during refixation movements. Slowing, in either initiation or performance, can occur in the horizontal or vertical plane. Inappropriate saccades will disrupt fixation. When continuous, they are described as ocular flutter if confined to the horizontal plane or opsoclonus if multidirectional.

Doll's head manoeuvre (oculocephalic reflex)

If the eyes fail to respond to a saccadic or pursuit stimulus, perform the doll's head manoeuvre. Ask the patient to fixate on your eyes, grasp the head and rotate it, first in the horizontal then in the vertical plane. An intact response (a measure of vestibular eye function) allows the patient's eyes to remain fixed on your own (Fig. 11.51).

TESTING THE ACTION OF INDIVIDUAL EYE MUSCLES

The action of the individual eye muscles can now be assessed. This is particularly relevant if the patient complains of double vision (diplopia).

In a strabismus, or squint, the axes of the eyes are no longer parallel, esodeviation indicates that the axes are convergent and exodeviation that they are divergent. The strabismus is concomitant if the angle of deviation remains constant throughout the range of eye movement and incomitant if the angle of deviation varies. The latter is usually caused by paresis of one or more of the extraocular muscles. Now perform a cover test.

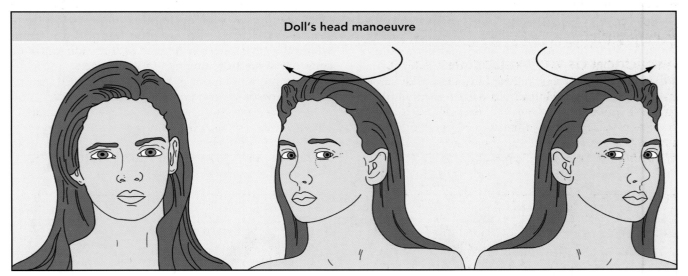

Fig. 11.51 Performing the doll's head manoeuvre in the horizontal plane.

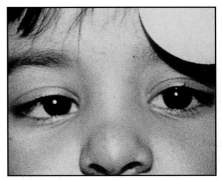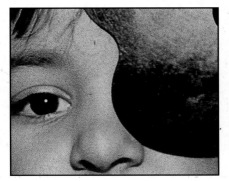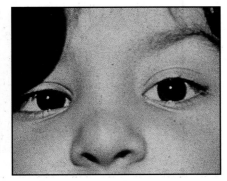

Fig. 11.52 Cover testing. There is a right esotropia that corrects temporarily when the left eye is covered.

In the presence of a concomitant squint, covering the fixating eye produces a movement in the squinting eye that allows it to take up fixation (unless the vision in that eye is severely depressed) (Fig. 11.52). Most patients with concomitant squint do not complain of diplopia, a symptom that suggests a disorder of one or more of the extraocular muscles or their nerve supply. After a recent oculomotor nerve paresis, altered patterns of contraction in the yoke and antagonist muscles produce characteristic deviations when alternate cover testing is performed. In the presence of a right lateral rectus weakness, the patient fixates with the left eye, the right eye tending to turn inwards because of the unopposed action of medial rectus (the primary deviation). If the left eye is now covered, increased innervation attempts are made in order to achieve fixation with the paretic eye. This abnormal stimulus spills over to the yoke muscle, the medial rectus of the left eye, which accordingly overadducts that eye (secondary deviation). In a paralytic strabismus, secondary deviation is greater than primary (Fig. 11.53).

Having confirmed that the diplopia is binocular (in other words, that it disappears when one or other eye is covered) ask the patient to look in the six directions illustrated in Figure 11.54. The false image (which often appears indistinct or blurred) is peripheral to the true image and belongs to the affected eye. Having elicited the diplopia, cover first one eye, then the other, to establish to which eye the false image belongs. Observe if the patient has an abnormal head tilt as a compensation for the diplopia. To establish whether the head tilt is longstanding, examine old photographs. Finally, remember that a pattern of diplopia

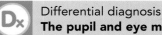

Differential diagnosis
The pupil and eye movements

Pupillary syndromes
- Horner's
- Tonic pupil
- Argyll Robertson pupil
- Relative afferent pupillary defect

Eye movement disorders
- Gaze paresis
- Internuclear ophthalmoplegia
- One-and-a-half syndrome
- Abducens, trochlear and oculomotor nerve palsies

Nystagmus
- Congenital
- Vestibular
- Gaze-evoked
- Downbeat
- Convergence-retractory

that is variable and difficult to interpret suggests the possibility of myasthenia gravis.

Nystagmus
Note the presence of nystagmus and whether it is pendular or jerk. Record the amplitude (fine, medium or coarse), persistence and the direction of gaze in which it occurs. Additionally, indicate whether the movement is horizontal, vertical, rotary or a mixture of several types. First-degree nystagmus

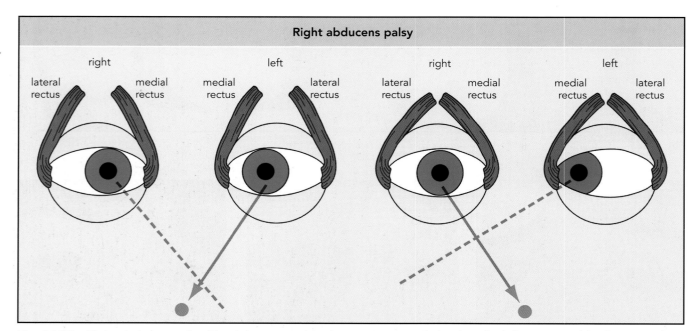

Fig. 11.53 Right abducens palsy. The right eye tends to converge, particularly when the left eye is used for fixation. When the right eye tries to fixate, overaction of the left medial rectus occurs.

to the left is a fast beating nystagmus to the left on left lateral gaze. In second- and third-degree nystagmus to the left, the same nystagmus is present on forward and right lateral gaze, respectively.

Optokinetic nystagmus

Optokinetic responses are assessed using a drum painted with vertical lines, which is rotated first in the horizontal and then in the vertical plane. As the patient looks at the drum a pursuit movement is seen in the direction of its rotation, followed by a saccade returning the eyes to the midposition (Fig. 11.55). Both movements are generated by the hemisphere towards which the drum is rotating. Thus, with the drum rotating to the right, pursuit is controlled by the right parieto-occipital cortex and the correcting saccade by the right frontal cortex.

Clinical application

THE PUPIL

Horner's syndrome

Horner's syndrome results from interruption of the sympathetic fibres to the eye. The pupil is miosed and the palpebral fissure is narrowed because of mild ptosis of the upper lid and elevation of the lower lid. The pupillary asymmetry is often slight but can be accentuated by taking the patient into a darkened room. Although enophthalmos is suggested by the appearance of the eye,

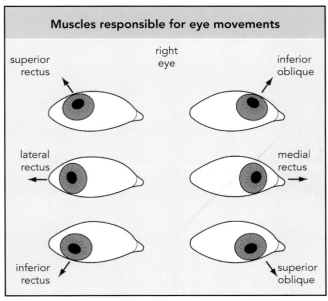

Fig. 11.54   The muscles responsible for eye movements in particular directions.

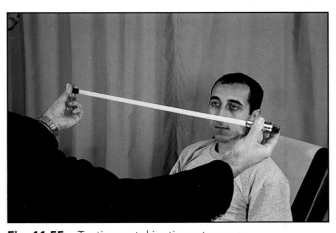

Fig. 11.55   Testing optokinetic nystagmus.

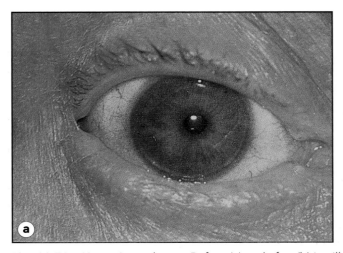

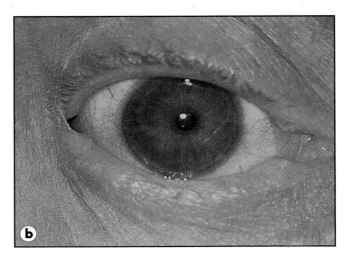

Fig. 11.56   Horner's syndrome. Before (a) and after (b) instillation of cocaine.

this is not confirmed by formal measurement. The distribution of sweating loss on the ipsilateral face depends on the site of the lesion. If there is uncertainty regarding the diagnosis, instil 4% cocaine into each eye. The normal pupil dilates, the affected pupil fails to do so (Fig. 11.56) irrespective of the site of the lesion.

Tonic pupil syndrome

The tonic pupil syndrome is usually unilateral. The affected pupil is dilated, although in longstanding cases it becomes progressively smaller. The light response is absent or markedly depressed and, consequently, in a darkened room, the affected pupil becomes smaller than its fellow because of a failure of reflex dilatation. The near reaction is delayed but sometimes is then more marked than that of the normal pupil. On relaxing the near effort, dilatation is delayed so that for a period the previously larger pupil is the smaller one (Fig. 11.57). The accommodation reaction is often sustained, resulting in blurred vision when switching from a distant to a near target or vice versa. The iris contains areas of focal atrophy and, characteristically, the pupils are hypersensitive to dilute parasympathomimetic agents (e.g. 0.125% pilocarpine). Tonic pupil syndrome is sometimes associated with depression of the deep tendon reflexes (Holmes–Adie syndrome).

Argyll Robertson pupil

The Argyll Robertson pupil is miosed, with a light response that is diminished compared with the near reaction (light–near dissociation). When the defect is fully developed, the pupil is fixed to light and fails to dilate in the dark. The pupil is often irregular with evidence of iris atrophy (Fig. 11.58). When complete, the syndrome is pathognomonic of neurosyphilis. The lesion responsible is thought to lie in the midbrain immediately above the Edinger–Westphal nucleus. A pupil of normal size with light–near dissociation can occur in other circumstances (e.g. in a blind eye).

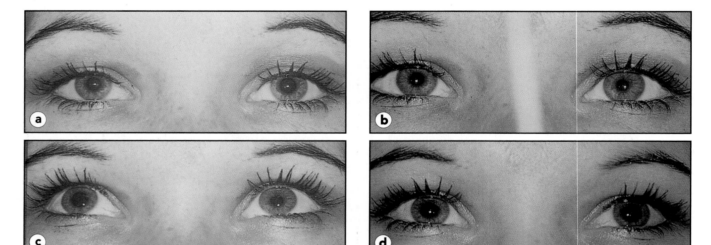

Fig. 11.57   Tonic pupil syndrome. (a) Left pupil is dilated. (b) After 1 min near effort. (c) Partial dilatation 15 s after release. (d) Virtually complete at 60 s.

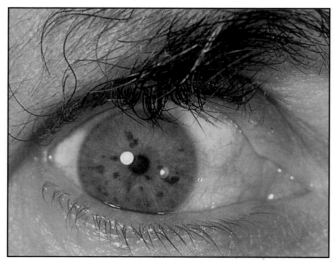

Fig. 11.58   Argyll Robertson pupil.

Relative afferent pupillary defect

This results from a lesion of the afferent light reflex pathway between the retina and the optic tract. It is not found with disease of the lens or vitreous. The conducting systems of the two optic nerves are best compared by performing the swinging light test. In the presence of a unilateral optic nerve lesion, for example, caused by optic neuritis, the affected pupil dilates as the torch is swung onto it from the sound eye.

DISORDERS OF EYE MOVEMENTS

Gaze paresis

In an acute frontal lobe lesion, contralateral saccadic eye movements in the horizontal plane are depressed or absent and there is limb paresis ipsilateral to the gaze palsy (Fig. 11.59). Both pursuit movements and the oculocephalic responses are spared. Saccades return later but now initiated by the contralateral frontal lobe. Subsequent damage to that frontal lobe will result in a complete horizontal saccadic palsy. A lesion at the level of the paramedian pontine reticular formation produces an ipsilateral gaze paresis for both saccadic and pursuit movement (Fig. 11.60). The limb

paresis is contralateral. An ipsilateral pursuit paresis occurs with posterior hemisphere disease and is associated with a contralateral homonymous field defect.

A paresis of upward saccades, initially with relative preservation of pursuit, is a feature of the dorsal-midbrain (Parinaud's) syndrome (Fig. 11.61). Other

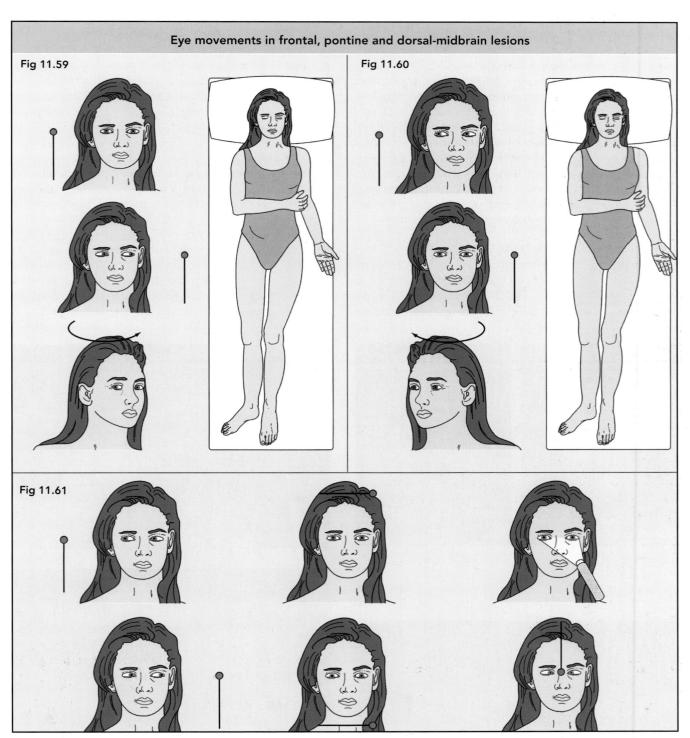

Eye movements in frontal, pontine and dorsal-midbrain lesions

Fig 11.59

Fig 11.60

Fig 11.61

Fig. 11.59 Left frontal lobe lesion. Absent sacccades to right, intact to left, preserved doll's head manoeuvre, right hemiparesis.

Fig. 11.60 Left pontine lesion. Absent saccades, pursuit and doll's head movements to the left. Right hemiparesis.

Fig. 11.61 Dorsal-midbrain syndrome. Full horizontal and downward saccades, absent upward saccades. Light–near dissociation.

findings include impaired convergence and dilated, light–near dissociated pupils. At a later stage upward pursuit and down gaze become affected. Causes include vascular disease and pinealoma.

OTHER SACCADIC AND PURSUIT MOVEMENT DISORDERS

Saccadic slowing, accompanied by disorganised pursuit movements, is found in both Huntington's and Parkinson's disease. In progressive supranuclear palsy, downward saccades and pursuit fail first, followed by involvement of upward and, finally, horizontal movements. Doll's head movements are spared, at least initially (Fig. 11.62). A delay in the initiation of saccades occurs in many extrapyramidal disorders. Overshooting or undershooting saccades (hypermetria and hypometria, respectively) occur with cerebellar disease. Large or small inappropriate saccades can interrupt fixation. Causes include multiple sclerosis and cerebellar disease. Slowing of pursuit movement is most commonly caused by sedative medication.

INTERNUCLEAR OPHTHALMOPLEGIA

A lesion of the medial longitudinal fasciculus leads to slowing, or total failure of medial rectus contraction during lateral gaze (Fig. 11.63). The slowing affects all movement, whether saccadic, pursuit or reflex. To assess subtle slowing, observe the relative velocity of the two eyes while the patient rapidly fixates between two targets. There is usually an accompanying nystagmus in the abducting eye. Bilateral internuclear ophthalmoplegia is accompanied by upbeat vertical nystagmus. Multiple sclerosis is the most common cause in younger patients, vascular disease in elderly patients.

THE 'ONE-AND-A-HALF' SYNDROME

If the lesion responsible for a unilateral internuclear ophthalmoplegia spreads into the pontine gaze centre, a more profound loss of ocular motility results. The only normal horizontal movement possible is abduction of the opposite eye (Fig. 11.64). The finding is usually the consequence of vascular disease.

ABDUCENS PALSY

A lesion of the sixth nerve nucleus produces a gaze paresis rather than an isolated lateral rectus weakness. The latter is usually due to a lesion of the central or peripheral course of the sixth nerve but it can be caused by myasthenia or orbital disease. The eye fails to abduct. When the defect is complete, there may be a convergent strabismus because of unopposed action of the ipsilateral medial rectus (Fig. 11.65). Unilateral or bilateral sixth nerve palsies sometimes result from the effects of raised intracranial pressure (Fig. 11.66).

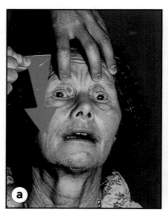 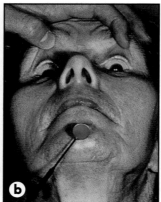

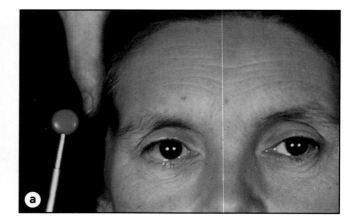

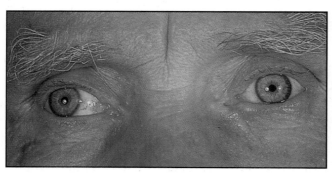

Fig. 11.63 Left internuclear ophthalmoplegia. Failure of adduction of the left eye on right lateral gaze.

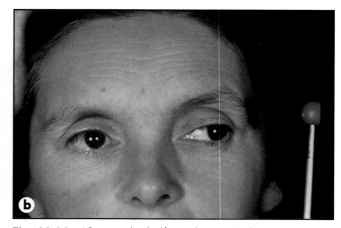

Fig. 11.64 'One-and-a-half' syndrome. Right gaze paresis with right internuclear ophthalmoplegia.

TROCHLEAR PALSY

Although normally a result of trochlear nerve palsy, weakness of the superior oblique muscle can occur with myasthenia or dysthyroid eye disease. An isolated trochlear nerve palsy sometimes follows a closed head injury. The head tilts to the side opposite the affected eye and the patient complains of diplopia, particularly on downward gaze. There is defective depression of the adducted eye (Fig. 11.67).

OCULOMOTOR PALSY

Nuclear oculomotor palsies tend to be either incomplete or complete but with pupillary sparing. A complete third nerve palsy cannot be nuclear unless there is involvement of the contralateral superior rectus muscle. Peripheral third nerve lesions are commonly caused by diabetes. The paresis is typically painful and pupil-sparing in about 50% of patients (Fig. 11.68). In a complete third nerve palsy there is a substantial ptosis and the eye is deviated laterally and slightly downwards. Compression of the oculomotor nerve, for example by a posterior communicating aneurysm, almost always results in pupillary dilatation (Fig. 11.69). To assess whether the fourth nerve is intact in the presence of a

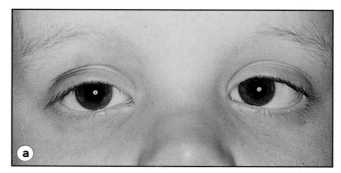
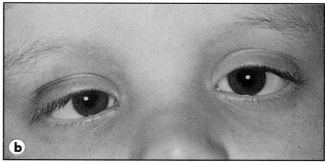

Fig. 11.65   Left sixth nerve palsy. Left esotropia on forward gaze (a). Failure of abduction of left eye (b).

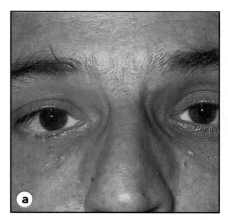
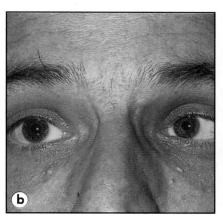
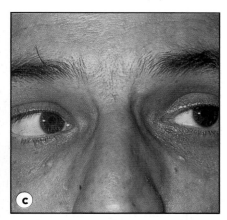

Fig. 11.66   Bilateral sixth nerve palsies. There is a tendency for the eyes to converge on forward gaze (a), with partial failure of abduction to right (b) and to left (c).

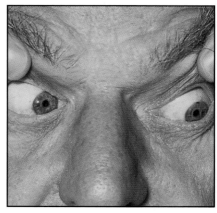

Fig. 11.67   Right superior oblique palsy.

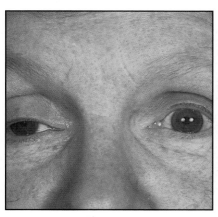

Fig. 11.68   Pupil-sparing right oculomotor palsy caused by diabetes.

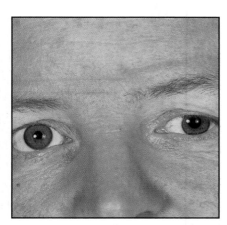

Fig. 11.69   Left third nerve paresis. The pupil is dilated.

complete third nerve palsy, ask the patient to look down. If the superior oblique muscle is still functioning, the abducted eye shows an inwardly rotating twitch.

COMBINED PALSIES

A lesion within the cavernous sinus, for example a cavernous aneurysm, is liable to affect the oculomotor nerves in combination rather than individually. At risk are the third, fourth and sixth nerves, the first and second divisions of the trigeminal nerve and the ocular sympathetic fibres. A complex, mixed ophthalmoplegia without pupillary involvement raises the possibility of myasthenia or dysthyroid eye disease (Fig. 11.70).

NYSTAGMUS

Certain types of nystagmus suggest disease at particular sites of the nervous system.

Pendular – usually congential but sometimes found in brainstem vascular disease or multiple sclerosis.

Vestibular – if peripheral, usually both horizontal and rotary components and is suppressed by visual fixation. The slow phase is to the side of the lesion. If central, more variable and unaffected by fixation.

Gaze-evoked – often drug-induced but also seen with disease of the cerebellum or brainstem. Vertical components indicate brainstem or cerebellar disease.

Down-beat – when present on down and out gaze, very suggestive of a lesion at the foramen magnum, for example Chiari malformation.

Convergence-retractory – occurs in the dorsal-midbrain syndrome. Attempts at upwards saccades produce retractory movements of the globes.

End-point – physiological. Occurs at extremes of lateral gaze and can affect one eye more than the other.

THE TRIGEMINAL (FIFTH) NERVE

STRUCTURE AND FUNCTION

The motor nucleus of the nerve lies in the floor of the upper part of the fourth ventricle and receives fibres from both hemispheres, but principally the contralateral one. Initially, the motor root remains separate, running below the gasserian ganglion before joining the mandibular division of the nerve to emerge through the foramen ovale. The principal muscles supplied by the nerve are the medial and lateral pterygoids, temporalis and masseter. Smaller muscles supplied include tensor tympani and tensor palati. Jaw closure is achieved by contraction of temporalis and masseter. Jaw opening and lateral movements are performed by the pterygoids.

There are three sensory nuclei: the main nucleus, the mesencephalic nucleus and the nucleus of the spinal tract (Fig. 11.71). Tactile stimuli are relayed through the main nucleus. From here, ascending fibres, most of which decussate, terminate in the thalamus. The spinal nucleus, continuous above with the main nucleus,

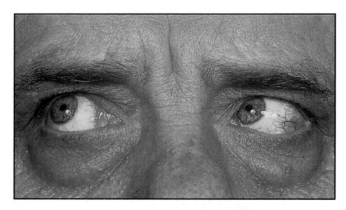

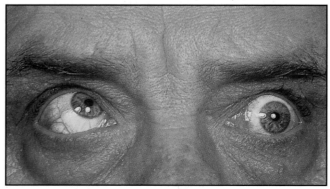

Fig. 11.70 Dysthyroid eye disease. Failure of laevoelevation of the left eye.

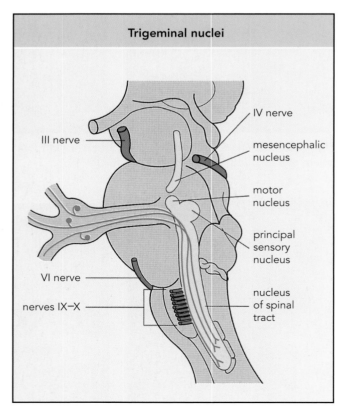

Fig. 11.71 Organisation of trigeminal nuclei within the brainstem.

extends caudally to the second cervical segment where it lies in the posterior horn continuous with the substantia gelatinosa. A rostrocaudal organisation of fibres from concentric segments over the face and head has been suggested, based on the pattern of facial sensory loss sometimes seen with lesions of the spinal tract (Fig. 11.72). Terminating in close proximity to the nucleus of the spinal tract are fibres from the seventh, ninth and tenth cranial nerves that supply cutaneous fibres to the region of the ear. The nucleus contains fibres concerned principally with pain and temperature sensation. Fibres from the nucleus decussate then ascend to the thalamus. The mesencephalic nucleus receives proprioceptive fibres from the muscles of mastication. Collaterals from the afferent fibres synapse on cells in the motor nucleus.

The sensory root accompanies the motor root through the pontine cistern before entering the gasserian ganglion, which is situated in a depression in the petrous temporal bone (Fig. 11.73). From here the ophthalmic division enters the orbit through the superior orbital fissure and the maxillary and mandibular divisions leave the skull through the foramina rotundum and ovale, respectively. The facial and scalp innervation of the three divisions is shown in Figure 11.74. In addition, the trigeminal nerve innervates the mucous membranes of the nose and mouth, certain sinuses, part of the external auditory meatus and most of the dura.

The jaw jerk

The afferent part of this reflex is formed by large afferents from muscle spindles in masseter and temporalis, which pass to the mesencephalic nucleus in the motor rather than the sensory root. Collaterals from the axons of the unipolar mesencephalic neurons synapse with cells in the motor nucleus, producing a monosynaptic reflex arc, the efferent pathway being within the motor root.

The corneal reflex

The afferent limb of the corneal reflex is contained in the ophthalmic division of the trigeminal nerve. The efferent pathway is within the seventh nerve. Stimulation of the cornea produces both an ipsilateral and a contralateral blink response, the latter being approximately 5 ms slower than the former. The central conduction time for the reflex, approximately 40 ms, indicates it is polysynaptic. Scleral, rather than corneal, stimulation results in a reflex with a considerably longer latency.

Examination

SENSORY

Details of the techniques for sensory examination are given on pp 362–364. Convenient sites for testing are the forehead, the medial aspect of the cheek and the chin. Normally, it suffices to test light touch and pinprick

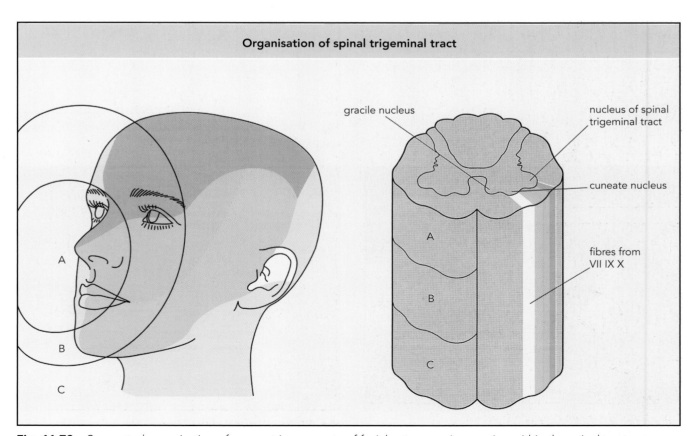

Fig. 11.72 Suggested organisation of concentric segments of facial cutaneous innervation within the spinal tract.

alone but occasionally it is necessary to assess temperature appreciation.

With the patient's eyes closed, test light touch by touching the appropriate areas of the face with a wisp of cotton wool. Avoid dragging the stimulus across the skin. A partial loss of sensation is more likely than total anaesthesia, so ask the patient to compare the stimulus with sites in other divisions of the nerve on that side, then with comparable areas on the other side of the face. Now test pinprick sensation at the same sites. If there is sensory loss confined to the trigeminal nerve distribution, the response to this stimulus becomes normal at the level of the vertex but well above the angle of the jaw (Fig. 11.74). Again, variations in the response at different

sites should be noted. As it is difficult to repeat the stimulus with equal force, minor differences of sensitivity should be ignored unless they are consistent.

THE CORNEAL RESPONSE

The corneal response is elicited by lightly touching the cornea with cotton wool. Carefully explain the procedure to the patient before proceeding. The patient's subjective reaction is assessed and the ipsilateral and contralateral blink reaction noted. Corneal sensitivity varies considerably. Patients who wear contact lenses will need to remove them first; even then dulling of the response is likely but will be symmetrical. If the response is substantially depressed, the cotton wool can be held

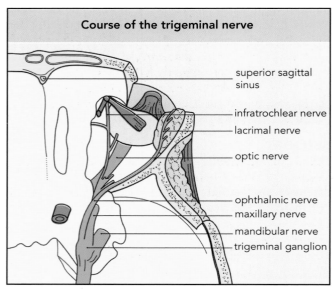

Fig. 11.73   The peripheral course of the trigeminal nerve.

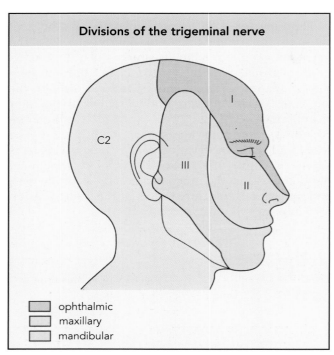

Fig. 11.74   Cutaneous distribution of the three divisions of the trigeminal nerve.

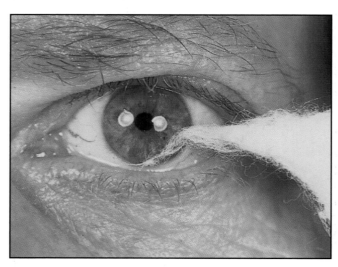

Fig. 11.75   A depressed left corneal response.

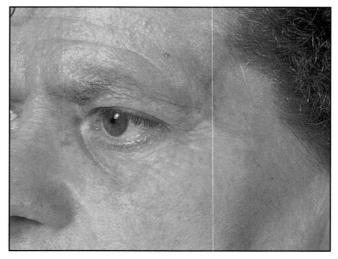

Fig. 11.76   Wasting of the temporalis producing hollowing above the zygoma.

against the cornea without provoking a reaction (Fig. 11.75). Testing the response in an unconscious patient must be done with great care. Repeated stimulation can easily traumatise the cornea.

MOTOR

Look for muscle wasting before testing the muscles of mastication. Wasting of temporalis produces hollowing above the zygoma (Fig. 11.76). Wasting of the masseter is more difficult to detect but both masseter and temporalis

can be palpated while the teeth are clenched (Fig. 11.77). The power of pterygoids and of masseter and temporalis can be assessed by resisting the patient's attempts at opening and closing the jaw, respectively. Ask the patient to open the jaw first without, then with, resistance. In a unilateral trigeminal lesion, the jaw deviates to the paralysed side (Fig. 11.78).

THE JAW JERK

Ask the patient to open the mouth slightly. Rest your index finger on the apex of the jaw and tap it with the patella hammer (Fig. 11.79). The response, a

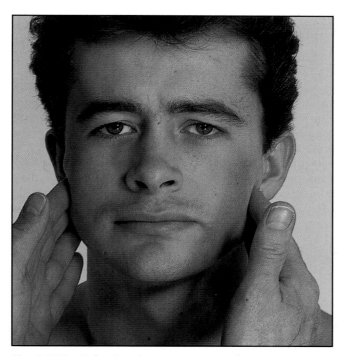

Fig. 11.77 Palpating the masseter muscles.

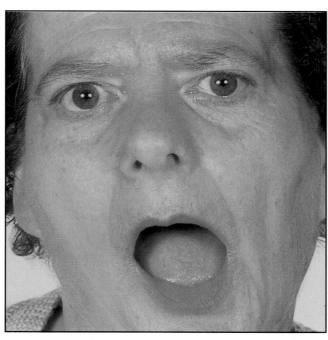

Fig. 11.78 Left trigeminal nerve lesion. Jaw deviation to the left.

> **Dx** Differential diagnosis
> **Facial numbness**
>
> - Malignant invasion of the trigeminal nerve
> - Isolated trigeminal neuropathy
> - Involvement in the lateral medullary syndrome
> - Involvement with cerebellopontine angle tumours
> - Sensory involvement with thalamic, capsular or cortical infarction

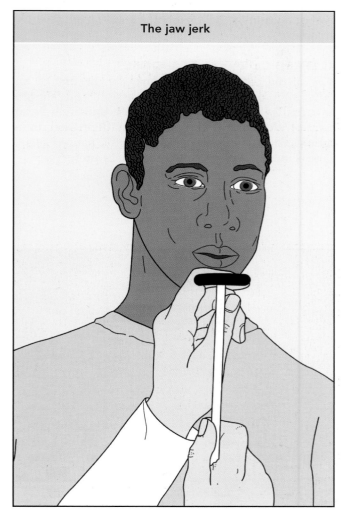

The jaw jerk

Fig. 11.79 Testing the jaw jerk.

contraction of the pterygoid muscles, varies widely in normal individuals.

Clinical application

MOTOR INVOLVEMENT

In a unilateral upper motor neuron syndrome, motor involvement of the trigeminal distribution is not usually clinically detectable. In a bilateral upper motor neuron syndrome, the jaw jerk is exaggerated.

SENSORY INVOLVEMENT

Malignant invasion of the nerve or its ganglion results in both sensory and motor deficit, although the latter is spared initially if the ganglion is invaded. In isolated trigeminal neuropathy, motor function is spared but there is progressive loss of facial sensation. Inadvertent self-injury can result in tissue necrosis (Fig. 11.80). In spinal lesions above C2, selective loss of facial pain and temperature sense is possible, sometimes with an 'onion ring' distribution (Fig. 11.72). Loss of facial pain and temperature sense occurs ipsilaterally in the lateral medullary syndrome. Depression of light touch alone occurs with damage to the main sensory nucleus, whereas thalamic infarction is liable to affect all facial sensory modalities.

ALTERED CORNEAL RESPONSE

Loss of the corneal response may be the first or an early sign of trigeminal compression and should be carefully assessed in patients with unilateral facial pain or deafness. The response is depressed in a patient with a unilateral lower motor neuron facial paresis but the contralateral response is preserved.

THE FACIAL (SEVENTH) NERVE

STRUCTURE AND FUNCTION

Fibres from the seventh nerve nucleus loop around the lower end of the abducens nucleus before leaving the pons in close proximity to the acoustic nerve. Having crossed the cerebellopontine angle, the nerve enters the internal auditory meatus along with the acoustic nerve and the internal auditory artery and vein. Shortly afterwards, the facial nerve enters its own canal, passing forwards above the cochlea before bending sharply backwards, at which point the nerve expands to form the geniculate ganglion. Here, the greater superficial petrosal nerve leaves, eventually to reach the lacrimal gland via the sphenopalatine ganglion (Fig. 11.81). The nerve to stapedius and the chorda tympani leave the facial nerve before its exit from the stylomastoid foramen. Parasympathetic fibres in the chorda tympani supply the submandibular and sublingual glands. Special afferent fibres in the nerve supply taste sensation to the anterior two-thirds of the tongue. After leaving the stylomastoid foramen, the nerve courses through the parotid gland on its way to the muscles of facial expression. Of these, frontalis elevates the eyebrow, orbicularis oculi closes the eye and orbicularis oris the mouth, whereas platysma depresses the angle of the mouth. The buccinator muscle, also supplied by the facial nerve, assists in mastication.

Frontalis receives an innervation from both cortices but the muscles of the lower face are innervated solely by the contralateral hemisphere. Emotional movements receive an additional supply from other sources, including the thalamus and globus pallidus.

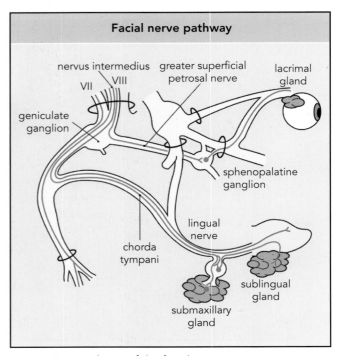

Fig. 11.81   Pathway of the facial nerve.

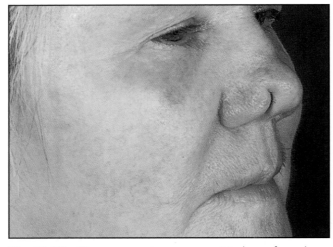

Fig. 11.80   Tissue necrosis consequent to loss of nasal sensation.

The sensory component of the nerve innervates the external auditory meatus, the tympanic membrane and a small area of skin behind the ear. The taste fibres, having entered the pons, terminate in the nucleus of the tractus solitarius. From here, fibres project to the thalamus and hence the cortical gustatory area.

The intensity of a taste experience is determined by the size of the neural response. Taste buds are found in the tongue, soft palate, pharynx, larynx and oesophagus. A particular taste represents an amalgam of four primary taste functions, sweet, sour, bitter and salt, combined with any olfactory stimulating effect that the food or beverage possesses. There is some decline in taste acuity with age but to a lesser extent than occurs with olfaction.

SYMPTOMS

In a patient with a lower motor neuron facial weakness, certain questions may help to define the site of the lesion.

Examination

Facial asymmetry is common, as is an asymmetry of movement of the lower face during conversation.

Questions to ask
Facial weakness of lower motor neuron type

- Have you noticed any loss of taste on the front part of the tongue?
- Have you noticed that noises appear excessively loud in the ear on the same side?
- Does the eye on that side still water?

Carefully observe the movements of the patient's face while you are taking the history. An asymmetry of blinking is a useful indicator of mild weakness of orbicularis oculi. Decide whether the nasolabial folds are equally well defined. Note any difference in the position of the angles of the mouth but remember that in a long-standing facial weakness fibrotic contracture of the muscles can elevate the angle of the mouth, suggesting that the facial weakness is on the other side. Bilateral facial weakness is easily overlooked. The face lacks expression and appears to sag (Fig. 11.82).

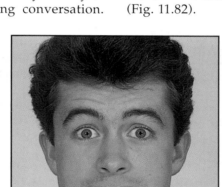

Fig. 11.82   Bilateral facial weakness.

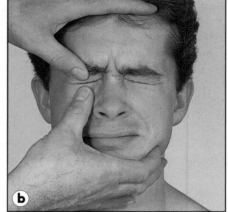

Fig. 11.83   The patient has been asked to elevate the eyebrows, then to close the eyes tightly.

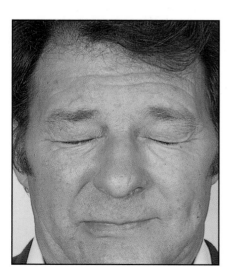

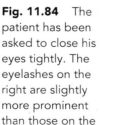

Fig. 11.84   The patient has been asked to close his eyes tightly. The eyelashes on the right are slightly more prominent than those on the left.

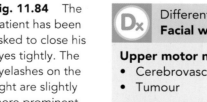

Differential diagnosis
Facial weakness

Upper motor neuron facial weakness
- Cerebrovascular disease
- Tumour

Lower motor neuron facial weakness
- Bell's palsy
- Ramsay Hunt syndrome
- Trauma
- Parotid tumour
- Sarcoid
- Multiple sclerosis

Ask the patient to elevate the eyebrows (Fig. 11.83) then close the eyes tightly. Normally, the eyelashes virtually disappear. A useful sign of a mild weakness is a more marked protrusion of the eyelashes on the affected side (Fig. 11.84). Try to open the eyes by pressing the eyelids apart with your thumbs. If there is no weakness, the patient can prevent the eyelids separating. Now ask the patient to blow out the cheeks, then purse the lips tightly together (Fig. 11.85). Finally, ask the patient to tighten the neck muscles in order to assess platysma. Weakness of stapedius is suggested if the patient complains of an undue sensitivity (hyperacusis) to noise in the affected ear.

Many patients who complain of an altered sensation of taste are found to have a disturbance of olfaction. Taste is difficult to test. Simply applying drops of a test solution on the protruded tongue seldom produces a consistent response. For assessing seventh nerve function, the stimulus should be confined to the anterior two-thirds of the tongue, each side of which is tested separately. Sweet (sugar), salt, bitter (quinine) and sour (vinegar) solutions are applied in turn, the mouth being washed out with distilled water between testing. Taste assessment is seldom justified for routine diagnostic purposes. Ask the patient if there has been any loss of lacrimation.

The area of skin around the ear that is supplied by the seventh nerve receives overlapping innervation from the fifth and ninth nerves. Nothing is gained, therefore, by testing sensation in this area.

Clinical application

UPPER MOTOR NEURON FACIAL WEAKNESS

An upper motor neuron facial weakness results from interruption of descending fibres passing from the contralateral motor cortex to the ipsilateral facial nerve nucleus. There is minimal asymmetry of frontalis contraction on the two sides but substantial asymmetry of the lower face (Fig. 11.86). Causes include cerebrovascular disease, tumour and head injury.

LOWER MOTOR NEURON FACIAL WEAKNESS

In a lower motor neuron facial weakness, all the facial muscles are equally affected unless the lesion lies so distally that it involves individual branches of the nerve. The site of the lesion can be deduced from the presence or absence of certain symptoms and signs. If it lies at or beyond the stylomastoid foramen, there will be no disturbance of taste, hearing or lacrimation. Involvement of the nerve immediately proximal to the origin of chorda tympani will result in loss of taste over the anterior two-thirds of the tongue; involvement proximal to the departure of the nerve to stapedius will result in hyperacusis. Loss of lacrimation is added to these other symptoms if the nerve is damaged at or proximal to the gasserian ganglion.

BELL'S PALSY

Bell's palsy is an idiopathic paralysis of the facial nerve. When the resulting facial weakness is substantial, there is loss of forehead furrowing, eye closure and mouth elevation (Fig. 11.87). If denervation occurs, regrowth of fibres may extend to muscles not originally part of their innervation (aberrant reinnervation). In such patients blinking can result in synkinetic contraction of muscles in the lower face (Fig. 11.88) and misdirection to the lacrimal gland of fibres originally destined for the salivary glands results in eye watering when a food stimulus appears (crocodile tears).

RAMSAY HUNT SYNDROME

The Ramsay Hunt syndrome is the consequence of herpetic involvement of the geniculate ganglion. A vesicular eruption can occur at a number of sites, including the pinna (Fig. 11.89).

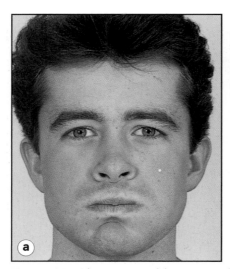
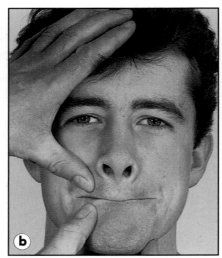
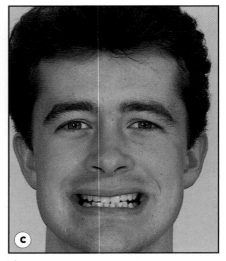

Fig. 11.85   The patient is blowing out the cheeks, pursing his lips and baring his teeth.

FACIAL MOVEMENT DISORDERS

Fasciculation – virtually confined to patients with motor neuron disease.

Myokymia – produces a fine, more or less continuous, shimmering contraction of some or all of the muscles supplied by the facial nerve. Multiple sclerosis is the most common cause.

Hemifacial spasm – involuntary, haphazard contraction of facial muscle, often initially confined to orbicularis oculi (Fig. 11.90). Eventually a mild facial weakness appears.

Blepharospasm – forced involuntary repetitive blinking.

Tics – stereotyped repetitive movements, at least in part under voluntary control.

Orofacial dyskinesia – involuntary semirepetitive contraction of muscles round the mouth, often with abnormal movements of the tongue. Occurs spontaneously and with certain drugs, particularly phenothiazines.

THE ACOUSTIC (EIGHTH) NERVE

STRUCTURE AND FUNCTION

Vibration of the tympanic membrane, triggered by a sound stimulus, is transmitted through a chain of three ossicles (the malleus, incus and stapes) situated in the middle ear (Fig. 11.91). The movements of the ossicles are also influenced by the tensor tympani and stapedius muscles. The base of the stapes is attached to the oval window. Vibration of the oval window sets up movement in the perilymph which occupies the bony labyrinth, comprising the cochlea, the vestibule and the semicircular canals. Lying within the bony labyrinth and containing endolymph is the

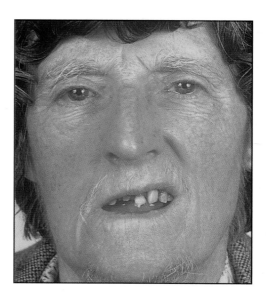

Fig. 11.86 Upper motor neuron facial weakness. The patient has been asked to bare her teeth.

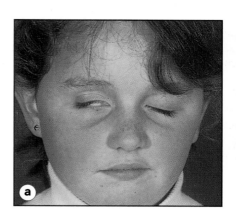

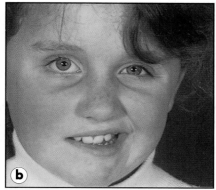

Fig. 11.87 A right Bell's palsy in a girl aged 11 years.

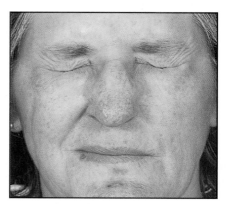

Fig. 11.88 Aberrant reinnervation. The right angle of the mouth elevates during eye closure. Previous right Bell's palsy.

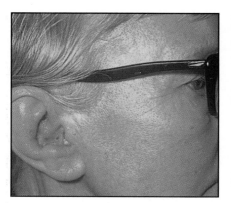

Fig. 11.89 Vesicular eruption in a case of the Ramsay Hunt syndrome.

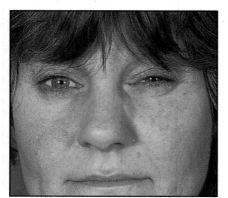

Fig. 11.90 Left hemifacial spasm. The left palpebral fissure has narrowed during the contraction.

membranous labyrinth comprising the cochlear duct, the saccule, the utricle and three semicircular ducts. The semicircular canals, each surrounding a semicircular duct, are arranged in planes roughly at right angles to each other. The canals open into the vestibule which contains the saccule and utricle. Specialised receptor areas (maculae) are found in the saccule and utricle. At one end of each semicircular canal is a receptor organ (crista ampullaris).

The inferior part of the bony labyrinth contains the osseous canal of the cochlea. A bony spur, the osseous spiral lamina, projects into the canal, dividing it into two corridors: the scala vestibuli and the scala tympani (Fig. 11.92). In the wall of the cochlear duct, resting on the basilar membrane, is the spiral organ of Corti, which is innervated by the cochlear component of the auditory nerve. The vestibular component innervates the specialised receptor areas of the utricle and the semicircular canals. The saccule and part of the posterior semicircular canal receive fibres from the cochlear division.

The vestibular and cochlear components unite within the internal auditory canal. The nerve then crosses the subarachnoid space and enters the brainstem at the junction of pons and medulla, lateral to the facial nerve. In the brainstem the acoustic nerve projects predominantly to the contralateral inferior colliculus. From here, fibres pass to the medial geniculate body and then in the auditory radiation to the auditory cortex in the upper aspect of the temporal lobe (Heschl's gyrus). The fibres of the vestibular nerve terminate in four separate nuclei. A projection from the lateral vestibular nucleus forms the vestibulospinal tract, which descends, mainly ipsilaterally, to the cervical and lumbar motor neurons. The medial vestibular nucleus has connections to the contralateral abducens nucleus and the cerebellum. These pathways are important in gaze-holding and for the control of smooth pursuit eye movements.

Sound waves, transmitted through the perilymph, reach the organ of Corti via the ossicular chain, by vibration of the round window or by bony transmission. High-frequency waves produce a maximal response in the basal part of the cochlea; low-frequency waves at its apex. Activity in the components of the auditory brainstem pathway is reflected in a succession of negative potentials recorded from mastoid and scalp electrodes following a click stimulus. Seven potentials occurring within the first 10 ms of the stimulus are thought to relate to specific anatomical sites.

The nerve endings in the cristae and maculae are triggered by movements of the endolymph, either from stimulation of the hair processes of the cristae or by movements of small calcific particles (the otoliths) embedded in a membrane of the maculae of the utricle and saccule. Head position is coded by the receptors of the utricle and saccule. Head tilt shifts the otoliths, displaces the hair cells and initiates an action potential in the fibres of the vestibular nerve. The semicircular canals are responsible for the detection of rotational head movements, via patterns of flow produced in the endolymphatic system.

Overall, the vestibular system provides information on head posture and movement, integrated with visual data and proprioceptive information arising from neck muscle receptors.

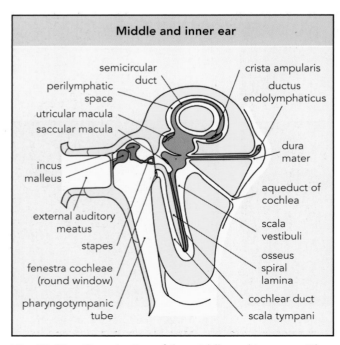

Fig. 11.91 Organisation of the middle and inner ear. The endolymphatic system is coloured.

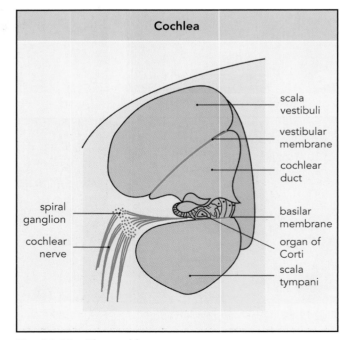

Fig. 11.92 The cochlea.

SYMPTOMS

Deafness

If the patient complains of deafness, determine the mode of onset, whether progressive or static, and whether unilateral or bilateral. Other important factors include the family history and noise exposure.

Vertigo

If the patient has vertigo, ascertain whether symptoms can be induced by certain postures or movements.

Questions to ask
Dizziness

- Does the patient describe dizziness or giddiness or is there an experience of rotation, either of the patient or of the environment (vertigo)?
- Is the dizziness accompanied by an unsteadiness when walking?
- Is any vertigo triggered only by a certain movement or head posture?

Examination

AUDITORY FUNCTION

Each ear is tested separately. Ask the patient to occlude the ear not being tested by pressing on the tragus. Hearing sensitivity can be assessed by the capacity to hear a whispered sound (normally possible at least 0.8 m away), a wristwatch (possible at approximately 0.75 m) or the sound of the fingers being rubbed together. Further tests are required to differentiate the result of damage to the cochlea or cochlear nerve (perceptive or nerve deafness) from damage to the conducting system leading to the cochlea (conductive deafness).

Rinne's test

Place a 512 Hz tuning fork on the mastoid process, then hold it adjacent to the pinna (Fig. 11.93a, b). Ask the patient which sound appears louder. Normally, air conduction is better perceived than bone conduction (Rinne positive). In perceptive deafness, this discrep-

ancy remains but in conductive deafness it is reversed (Fig. 11.93c, d).

Weber's test

Place a 512 Hz tuning fork at the midline over the vertex or on the forehead and ask the patient whether the sound appears equally loud in each ear or more so in one than the other. Normally, the sound is perceived equally by the two ears but it is heard better by the intact ear in perceptive deafness and by the affected ear in conductive deafness (Fig. 11.94).

VESTIBULAR FUNCTION

Peripheral vestibular function can be assessed using the head impulse test (Fig. 11.95). The head is turned rapidly through about 15°, first to one side then to the other, while the patient fixates on a distant target. In the presence of, say, a right peripheral vestibular lesion with loss of lateral semicircular canal function, when the head is

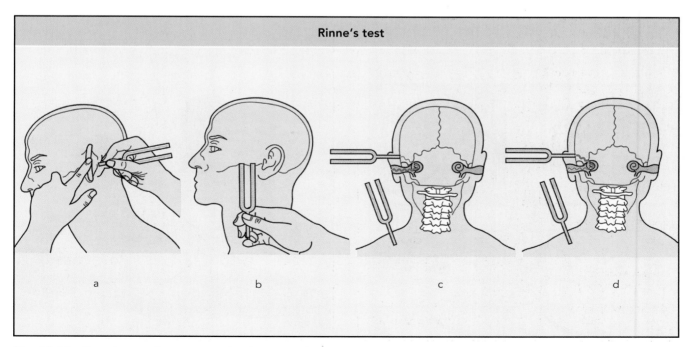

Rinne's test

a   b   c   d

Fig. 11.93   Rinne's test. Comparison of (a) bone conduction and (b) air conduction. (c) Perceptive deafness, (d) conductive deafness.

rotated to the right, the vestibular ocular reflex fails and the eyes fail to remain fixed on the target. A saccadic correction is then made to bring the eyes back to the target, a movement which can be detected by the examiner. If a patient complains of positional vertigo, then the effect of posture should be included in the examination. Position the patient at the edge of the examination couch, facing away from the edge, then depress the head and trunk so that the head is almost 30° below the horizontal but turned first to one side then the other (Fig. 11.96). If nys-

tagmus appears, record whether it begins immediately or after an interval, whether it persists or fatigues and if it then reappears when the patient returns to the sitting position. Warn the patient that vertigo may be experienced and explain that the eyes should be kept open during the manoeuvre. If the test proves positive, ask the patient whether the symptoms resembled those of the presenting disorder.

Clinical application

DEAFNESS

Conductive deafness is usually caused by either debris or wax in the external auditory meatus, loss of elasticity of the ossicular chain (otosclerosis) or disease of the middle ear. Nerve deafness occurs with end-organ change (e.g. in Ménière's disease) or consequent to a disturbance of the auditory nerve itself (e.g. after occlusion of the internal auditory artery). Lesions of the central nervous system rarely cause deafness because of the bilateral projections of the central auditory pathways at multiple levels.

TINNITUS

Patients with tinnitus complain of noise in one or both ears. The noise may be continuous or intermittent and of varying pitch. The symptom occurs with cochlear disease or damage, or with compression of the auditory nerve. Some patients with abnormal intracranial blood flow, for example through an arteriovenous malformation, are able to hear the flow and describe it as a form of pulsatile tinnitus. In these patients, a bruit is usually audible over the skull.

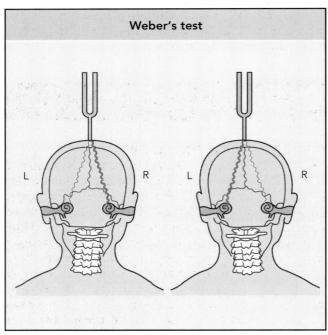

Fig. 11.94   Weber's test. Left-sided perceptive deafness (left) and left-sided conductive deafness (right).

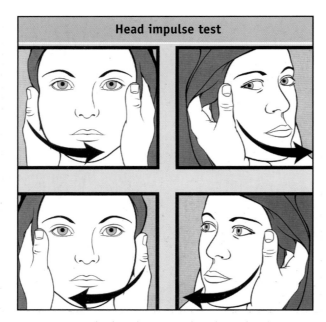

Fig. 11.95   As the head is rotated to the right, the eyes fail to remain fixed on the target.

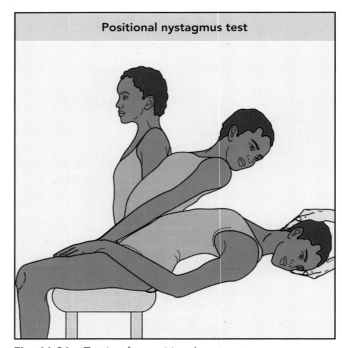

Fig. 11.96   Testing for positional nystagmus.

Differential diagnosis
Deafness and vertigo

Conductive deafness
- Wax
- Otosclerosis
- Middle ear disease

Perceptive deafness
- Ménière's disease
- Vascular event
- Acoustic neurinoma

Peripheral vertigo
- Vestibular neuronitis
- Benign positional vertigo
- Ménière's disease

Central vertigo
- Cerebrovascular disease
- Multiple sclerosis

VERTIGO

Vertigo is a sense of rotation either of the individual or of the environment. Patients rarely complain of persistent vertigo, although many describe a persistent dizziness or giddiness, much less clear-cut symptoms that commonly elude diagnosis. Vertigo is usually a result of disruption of either the labyrinthine system (peripheral vertigo) or the central connections of the vestibular nerve (central vertigo).

An acute peripheral vestibular disturbance causes a unidirectional jerk or rotatory nystagmus, with the slow component to the affected side. With the eyes closed, the patient tends to fall to the side of the slow phase and to point to that side of a stationary target. A sense of rotation of the environment is experienced in the direction of the fast phase. If the findings are less clear-cut, then a disorder of the central vestibular pathway is likely.

Patients with peripheral vestibular disorders are ataxic while the vertigo persists but not at other times.

Epidemic labyrinthitis and acute vestibular neuronitis

These diagnoses have been applied to patients who give a history of acute vertigo, often with vomiting, together with ataxia and malaise, on the assumption that an acute disruption of the labyrinth or the vestibular nerve has occurred.

Benign positional vertigo

Benign positional vertigo is a more specific, peripheral, vestibular dysfunction. Patients complain of attacks of vertigo, typically triggered by lying down in bed on one particular side. Tests for positional nystagmus are positive. The condition, sometimes triggered by head injury but often spontaneous, remits within a few weeks but is liable to relapse briefly over subsequent years.

Ménière's disease

In Ménière's disease, thought to be the consequence of a distention of the endolymphatic space, paroxysms of vertigo occur together with a persistent unilateral tinnitus and progressive sensorineural deafness.

Central vertigo

Central vertigo is likely to persist longer than peripheral vertigo and, if posture related, is less likely to be delayed in onset or to fatigue after posture change than benign positional vertigo. Both cerebrovascular disease and multiple sclerosis are common causes of a central vestibular disturbance. Usually, other signs of brainstem disease are evident.

THE GLOSSOPHARYNGEAL (NINTH) NERVE

STRUCTURE AND FUNCTION

The ninth, tenth and eleventh cranial nerves share a motor nucleus (nucleus ambiguus) that innervates the striated muscle of the pharynx, larynx and upper oesophagus (Fig. 11.97). Corticobulbar fibres destined for each nucleus ambiguus originate in both cerebral hemispheres. The glossopharyngeal nerve emerges from the upper part of the medulla, bounded above and below by the facial nerve and the vagus. It leaves the skull through the jugular foramen in company with the vagus and the accessory nerves. The general visceral efferent and special visceral afferent fibres are

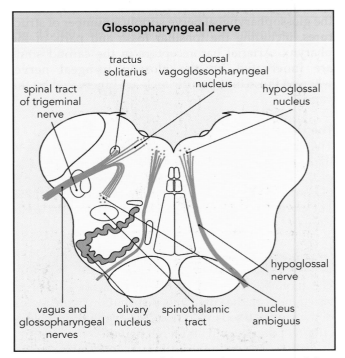

Fig. 11.97 Relationship of the central components of the glossopharyngeal nerve.

the lateral aspect of the cervical spinal cord down to the fifth segment. The rootlets form a single trunk that ascends alongside the cord, passes through the foramen magnum and unites with the cranial component. The combined nerve leaves the skull through the jugular foramen.

The cranial root joins the vagus, whereas the spinal root receives contributions from the second, third and fourth cervical roots (Fig. 11.100) before innervating sternomastoid and the upper fibres of trapezius. The fibres from the second and third cervical roots passing to the sternomastoid are probably proprioceptive, whereas the fibres from the third and fourth roots to the lower part of trapezius are purely motor.

The spinal accessory nucleus receives innervation from both cerebral hemispheres. The fibres concerned with the innervation of sternomastoid possibly undergo a double decussation within the brainstem.

Examination

There is no way of assessing the innervation of the cranial component of the accessory nerve but that of the spinal component can be assessed by examining trapezius and sternomastoid. The function of trapezius is assessed by asking the patient to elevate the shoulder, first without, then with, resistance (Fig. 11.101). The strength of contraction of sterno-

---

Dx Differential diagnosis
Accessory nerve disorders

- Involvement in jugular foramen tumours
- Accessory palsy of unknown cause
- Spasmodic torticollis

---

mastoid can be gauged by asking the patient to rotate the head to the relevant side against resistance (Fig. 11.102).

Clinical application

Isolated lesions of the eleventh cranial nerve are rare. Tumours in the region of the jugular foramen are likely to produce a combined palsy of the ninth, tenth and eleventh nerves (Fig. 11.103). In the presence of a hemiplegia, the trapezius muscle on the hemiplegic side is affected. A delay in shoulder shrug may be an early sign. The same hemiplegia, however, will affect the contralateral sternomastoid, that is the muscle rotating the neck towards the hemiplegic limbs. The weakness in such patients is incomplete. Spasmodic torticollis is a focal dystonia particularly affecting the sternomastoid muscle. Typically, there are repetitive rotatory movements of the head and neck, which lead to to hypertrophy of the relevant muscles in long-standing cases (Fig. 11.104).

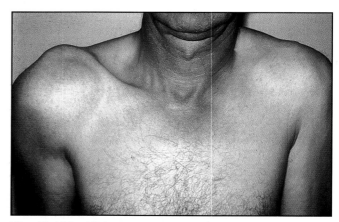

Fig. 11.103 Right accessory nerve lesion.

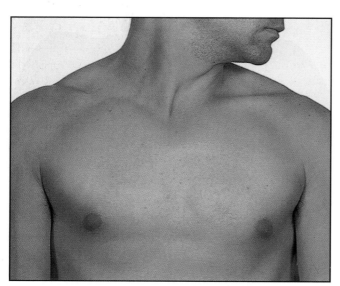

Fig. 11.102 Testing head rotation.

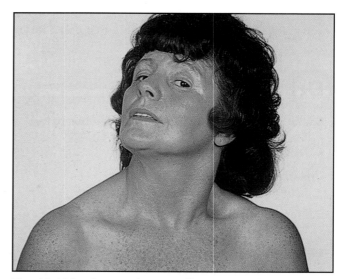

Fig. 11.104 Spasmodic torticollis associated with contraction of the left sternomastoid.

THE HYPOGLOSSAL (TWELFTH) NERVE

STRUCTURE AND FUNCTION

The hypoglossal nucleus lies close to the midline in the floor of the fourth ventricle and receives supranuclear fibres from both but principally the contralateral hemisphere. The hypoglossal nerve leaves the skull through the anterior condylar canal and supplies all the intrinsic muscles of the tongue, and all its extrinsic muscles except palatoglossus.

Examination

First inspect the tongue as it lies in the base of the oral cavity. In many patients there are tremulous movements that are often hard to distinguish from fasciculation or true involuntary movements. Fasciculation imparts a shimmering motion to the surface of the tongue. Involuntary movements include a coarse tremor, for example in Parkinson's disease, and complex, unpredictable movements found in such conditions as Huntington's disease

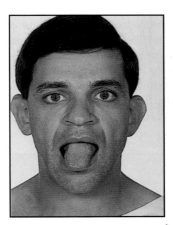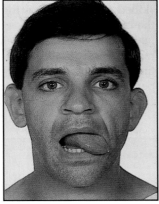

Fig. 11.105 Examination of the tongue. Protrusion (a) and lateral movements (b).

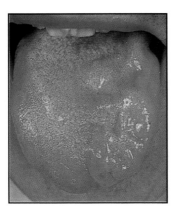

Fig. 11.106 Left hypoglossal nerve lesion.

 Differential diagnosis
Tongue paralysis

- Malignant invasion of the skull base
- Chiari malformation
- Pseudobulbar palsy with cerebrovascular disease or motor neuron disease

and orofacial dyskinesia. While assessing the tongue for spontaneous contractions, observe its bulk. As the tongue wastes it becomes thinner and more wrinkled. Now ask the patient to protrude the tongue. Minor deviations from the midline are sometimes seen in normal individuals. Finally, ask the patient to move the tongue rapidly from side to side and assess its power by instructing the patient to push the tongue against the side of the cheek (Fig. 11.105). A disturbance of the speed of tongue movement occurs in extrapyramidal diseases, including Parkinson's disease.

Clinical application

UNILATERAL AND BILATERAL LOWER MOTOR NEURON LESIONS

In a unilateral hypoglossal nerve lesion, there is focal atrophy, fasciculation and deviation to the paralysed side (Fig. 11.106). Such a lesion can occur in isolation or as the consequence of malignant invasion of the skull base. Bilateral involvement of the lower motor neuron projections to the tongue is usually part of a bulbar

 Review
Cranial nerve examination

I	Examine smell in each nostril
II	Examine visual acuity, visual field, fundus and pupillary light response
III, IV, VI	Examine eye movements and near reaction. Check for nystagmus
V	Examine motor and sensory innervation plus the jaw jerk and the corneal response
VII	Examine the muscles of facial expression (plus buccinator) and taste over the anterior two-thirds of the tongue
VIII	Examine hearing and perform Rinne's and Weber's tests
IX	Examine pain sensation in the tonsillar fossae
X	Examine palatal movement plus the gag reflex
XI	Examine sternomastoid and the upper fibres of the trapezius
XII	Examine tongue movements and appearance

DEEP TENDON REFLEXES

Testing the reflexes assesses the reflex arc and the supraspinal influences that operate on it. Each reflex is graded according to strength of response, as shown in the symptoms and signs box.

Reflexes are remarkably variable in normal individuals. Some patients have very brisk reflexes, although unaccompanied by clonus. Others have very depressed responses that often appear better preserved at the ankle than elsewhere, the opposite of what one would find if a neuropathy was the cause of the hyporeflexia.

THE UPPER LIMB

The reflexes of the upper limb routinely tested are the biceps, triceps and supinator (the roots subserving each reflex are shown in brackets). The biceps and supinator reflexes are tested first, with the patient in the posture shown in Figure 11.116.

Biceps (C5/6)

The whole arm must be exposed when testing this reflex. Place the thumb or index finger of your left hand on the biceps tendon then strike it with the patella hammer using a pendular motion by extending then flexing your wrist. Grasp the hammer at the end rather than halfway down the shaft (Fig. 11.117). The response consists of contraction of the biceps muscle. If there is no response, ask the patient to clench the teeth or grip the fingers of the other hand shortly before testing (Jendrassik manoeuvre). Now examine the reflex in the left arm. Lean over and use your inverted thumb to mark the position of the tendon.

Supinator (C5/6)

With the patient's arm in the semipronated position, strike the radial margin of the forearm approximately 5 cm above the wrist (Fig. 11.118). You can if you wish interpose your finger. The response is a contraction of brachioradialis and biceps. When eliciting the biceps and supinator reflexes, observe also the fingers of the hand. A brisk reflex is accompanied by finger flexion. In certain instances, despite a depression of the direct reflex, flexion of the fingers still occurs (inversion). This physical finding, usually due to cervical spondylosis, suggests the combination of a depression of the

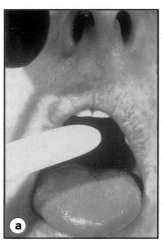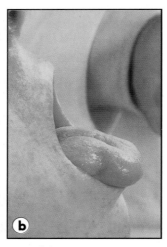

Fig. 11.115 Percussion myotonia of the tongue.

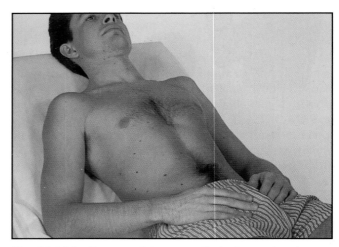

Fig. 11.116 Posture of the upper limbs for testing the biceps and supinator reflexes.

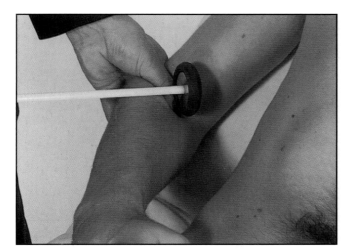

Fig. 11.117 Testing the right biceps reflex.

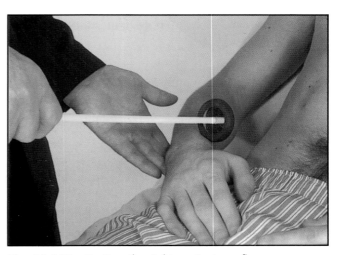

Fig. 11.118 Testing the right supinator reflex.

reflex arc at the C5/C6 level, together with an exaggeration of reflexes at a lower level due to a coexistent pyramidal tract disorder.

Triceps (C6/7)

To test the right triceps jerk, bring the patient's right arm well across the body, with the elbow flexed at approximately 90° so that the triceps tendon is adequately exposed (Fig. 11.119). Strike the tendon with the patella hammer. A normal response is contraction of the triceps. Having tested the reflex on the right, bring the left arm over and test the reflex on that side.

Finger (C8)

The finger jerk is usually present only when there is a pathological exaggeration of the reflexes. With the patient's arm pronated, exert slight pressure on the flexed fingers with the fingers of your left hand. Now strike the back of your own fingers with the hammer. A positive response leads to a brief flexion of the fingertips (Fig. 11.120).

LOWER LIMB

Knee (L2/3/4)

To test the knee jerks insert your left arm underneath the patient's knees and flex them to approximately 60° (Fig. 11.121). If the patient is properly relaxed, the legs will sag when you remove your arm. Tap first the right patella tendon and then the left. If one or both reflexes is particularly brisk, test for knee clonus by fitting your thumb and index finger along the upper border of the patella with the knee extended (Fig. 11.122). Exert a sudden, downward stretch and maintain it. Any repetitive contraction of the quadriceps (i.e. clonus) even if only two or three beats, is strongly suggestive of a pyramidal tract disorder.

Ankle (S1)

The patient's leg is abducted and externally rotated at the hip, flexed at the knee and flexed at the ankle. If hip abduction is limited, rest the leg on its fellow to allow adequate access to the Achilles tendon (Fig. 11.123). If the reflex is brisk, look for clonus. With the limb in the same

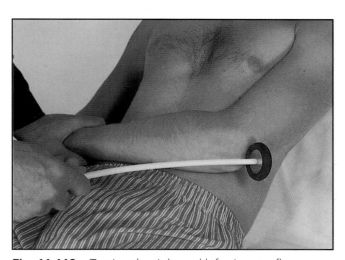

Fig. 11.119 Testing the right and left triceps reflexes.

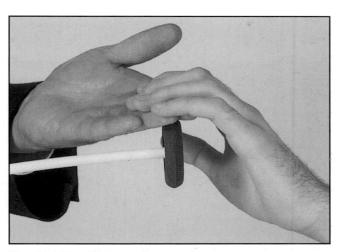

Fig. 11.120 Eliciting a finger jerk.

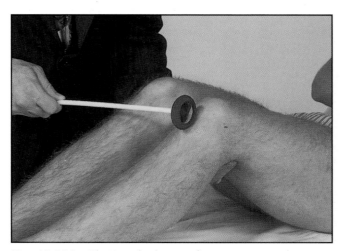

Fig. 11.121 Eliciting the knee reflexes.

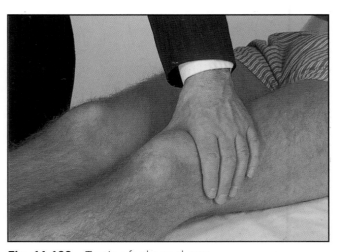

Fig. 11.122 Testing for knee clonus.

position, forcibly dorsiflex the ankle and maintain that position (Fig. 11.124). Three to four beats of symmetrical ankle clonus is acceptable in normal individuals but asymmetric or more sustained clonus is pathological.

OTHER REFLEXES

Abdominal responses

The abdominal responses diminish with age and are more difficult to elicit in the obese or in women who have had children. They are cutaneous reflexes whose latency suggests mediation through a spinal reflex arc. Before you can assess the abdominal reflexes, the patient must be relaxed and lying flat. Lightly draw the end of an orange stick across the four segments of the abdomen around the umbilicus (Fig. 11.125). Normally there is a reflex contraction in each segment. To summarise the findings in your notes draw a cross with an o, ± or + in each segment according to response.

Cremasteric reflex

The cremasteric reflex is elicited by stroking the upper inner aspect of the thigh. It is mediated through segments L1 and L2 and leads to retraction of the ipsilateral testicle.

Plantar response

The plantar response is elicited by applying firm pressure (use an orange stick) to the lateral aspect of the sole of the foot, moving from the heel to the base of the fifth toe, then, if necessary, across the base of the toes (Fig. 11.126). While you do this observe the metatarsophalangeal joint of the big toe. In the normal adult, the toe plantar flexes. In the presence of a pyramidal tract lesion, the toe dorsiflexes. The same dorsiflexion appears in normal individuals if a sharp stimulus is applied to the big toe and in infants if the stimulus is applied over a wider area. The reflex is considered to be part of a flexor withdrawal response to a noxious stimulus. With the development of the upright posture, descending pathways, one of which is the pyramidal tract, inhibit the reaction except when stimulation is applied directly to the big toe. Damage to descending pathways, particularly the corticospinal system, releases the inhibition and allows the appearance of the pathological response. In certain spinal cord disorders, in which the flexor withdrawal response is totally disinhibited, minor stimulation of the foot or other part of the leg results in flexion at hip, knee, ankle and toe. There is no point in testing the plantar response if the big toe is immobile or if there

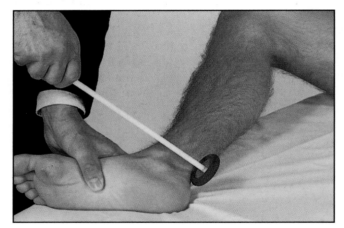

Fig. 11.123 Eliciting the ankle reflex.

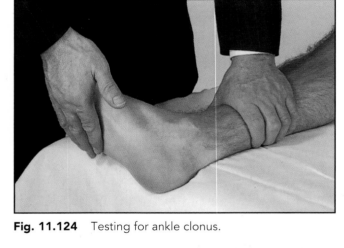

Fig. 11.124 Testing for ankle clonus.

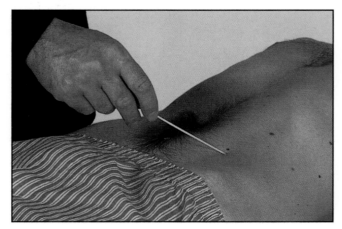

Fig. 11.125 Testing the abdominal responses.

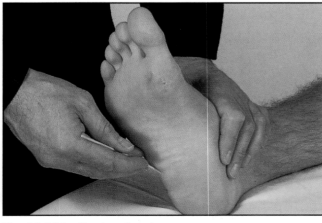

Fig. 11.126 Testing the plantar response.

is severe loss of S1 cutaneous innervation. Summarise your findings with arrows: for flexor↓, for extensor↑and for equivocal↑↓.

Anal reflex

The anal reflex is assessed by pricking the skin at the anal margin. Normally, there is a brisk contraction of the anal sphincter. The tone of the anal sphincter can be assessed by inserting a finger into the anus and asking the patient to bear down.

THE EXTRAPYRAMIDAL SYSTEM

Examination of tone has already been considered and the interpretation of abnormal movements including tremor will be considered later.

Bradykinesia

Bradykinesia is particularly associated with Parkinson's disease. The problem may be confined to one limb, at least initially, or it may be generalised. Initiation of movement is delayed, the actual movement slowed and its adjustment insensitive. Muscle power remains intact. To look for bradykinesia in the upper limbs, ask the patient to tap repetitively the back of one hand with the other. Ask the patient to use such force that the tapping is audible. Typically, if the movement is bradykinetic, its sound diminishes and falters. Now ask the patient to 'polish' the back of one hand with the other. In brady-kinesia, a movement of reduced amplitude is seen that eventually may cease completely. To assess brady-kinesia in the lower limbs, ask the patient to tap your hand repetitively, first with one foot, then the other. Many individuals find it difficult to sustain a rhythm but with bradykinesia the movement will again fade away. There are many ways of assessing bradykinesia without recourse to formal examination. Watch the patient dressing or using a knife and fork. Ask them to write and examine the size of the script and its legibility. See how easily they stand from a sitting posture and time how long they take to walk a set distance.

Involuntary movement

Begin by detailing the characteristics of the movement. Is it present at rest, with the limb completely supported or when the limb takes up a particular posture or only when the patient carries out a skilled activity? Ascertain the frequency of the movement and its distribution. Is the problem mainly proximal or distal? Are the movements brief or sufficiently prolonged to cause an abnormal posture?

Questions to ask
Tremor

- Is the tremor mainly present at rest, when the hands are held out, or when they are used?
- Is the tremor relieved by alcohol?
- Is there a family history of tremor?

Tremor

Tremor is a rhythmic movement that, at a particular joint, is usually confined to a single plane. Physiological tremor is a normal finding, usually detectable only with electromyograph recording. Enhanced physiological tremor is triggered by agitation, the use of sympathomimetic agents and thyrotoxicosis. Its frequency is around 9 Hz in younger people. Stimulation of β_2-adrenergic receptors in muscle accounts for enhanced physiological tremor.

Myoclonus

Myoclonus is characterised by rapid, recurring muscle jerks. The movement is similar to the startle reaction described as 'jumping out of one's skin'. The movements are either generalised or confined to one part of the body. In some patients they appear only when the limb is activated.

Chorea

Patients with chorea appear to fidget. They show brief, random movements that do not have the shock-like quality of myoclonus. Typical movements include furrowing of the eyebrows, pursing of the lips, elevation of a shoulder and random contraction of the fingers. Both proximal and distal limb muscles can be affected. As the movements are short-lived, sustained postures do not occur. Ask the patient to grip your hand: you will find that the grip waxes and wanes with the fluctuations of the chorea. The tendon reflexes may be prolonged because of the superimposition of a late, sustained contraction on the phasic reflex. The choreiform movements tend to be accentuated by a skilled action.

Athetosis

Athetoid movements are slower still than chorea and become prominent during the performance of voluntary activity. The distal parts of the limbs are predominantly affected. In the hand, the posture oscillates between hyperextension of the fingers and

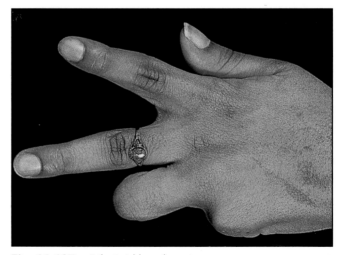

Fig. 11.127   Athetoid hand posture.

will be evident from the patient's history or imaging. Identification of drug-induced or metabolic coma is likely to take longer.

There are certain spinal reflexes that can persist in the presence of brainstem death. These include the stretch reflexes, plantar responses or withdrawal and flexion of the upper or lower limb triggered by neck flexion. The United Kingdom criteria for brain death no longer include the presence of an isoelectric electroencephalogram recording, although this criterion still receives support in other countries, for instance the United States of America.

 Examination of elderly people
The nervous system

Primitive reflexes
- Glabellar tap
  – found with increasing frequency with age
- Palmomental reflex
  – bilateral responses found with increasing frequency with age
- Snout and suckling reflexes
  – seldom, particularly the latter, found in normal, elderly, individuals
- Grasp reflex
  – the presence of grasp reflexes correlates with evidence of cognitive impairment

Cranial nerve function
- Smell
  – sensitivity declines after the age of 65 years
- Eyes
  – mild ptosis common in elderly people
  – upgaze declines with age
  – the light and accommodation responses decline with age and the pupils become more miosed
- Taste
  – sensitivity declines with age, with a higher threshold
- Hearing
  – declines with age

Motor system
- Reflexes
  – contrary to established teaching, the ankle jerks are preserved in old age
  – the abdominal responses diminish and their latency increases with age
- Movements
  – lingual–facial–buccal dyskinesias are found in elderly people without a history of neuroleptic drug exposure

Sensation
- Vibration
  – threshold for appreciation increases with age
- Two-point discrimination
  – threshold increases with age

Gait
- Becomes increasingly cautious with increasing age

12.
Infants and Children

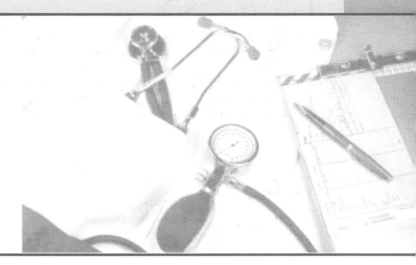

One of the challenges of paediatric medicine and child health is dealing with a range of patients, from the preterm newborn weighing under 1 kg to the postpubertal 15-year-old weighing 55 kg. The younger the child, the more often he or she is brought to see the doctor, and the younger the child, the more different the consultation is from that described in previous chapters.

> *Children are not just small adults – their needs are different and have to be recognised.*
> Professor James Spence, 1943

When examining children, the general principles of history-taking and examination also apply, although the manner and order in which they are approached differ: the convention of taking a history, inspecting, palpating, percussing and auscultating remain the cornerstones of all consultations but the emphasis is different in children.

Trainee doctors need basic skills to begin to feel confident in dealing with the child patient and their families.

For convenience, this chapter divides the child patient into five age categories, although these groups tend to merge into one another:

- Newborn and very young baby (0–8 weeks)
- Older baby and toddler (2–24 months)
- Preschool child (2–5 years)
- School child (5–10+ years)
- Adolescent (10+ to approximately 16 years).

In each section of this chapter, the discussion of growth, development, history-taking and examination of systems will take into account important age-related differences.

TAKING A HISTORY

History-taking is the key part of an assessment of a child's condition. The diagnosis is often revealed by a well-taken history, with the examination findings confirming or refuting the working diagnosis revealed during the history. In previous chapters, advice was given on how to approach patients who provide their own histories of complaints and symptoms; children come to the doctor with their parents and it is the parents who usually supply these details, although older children will often make important contributions.

Listen to the parents: they know their child best and, generally, if they describe a problem then there is a diagnosis to be made. The younger the child the more reliant you will be on the parents' account of the problem. Sometimes acute anxiety about a child's well-being, coupled with parental exhaustion, leads to difficulties in effective communication between parent and doctor but if you can empathise with the parents' perspective it will help you to be a more understanding and compassionate doctor.

The older the children, the more you can communicate with them. The challenges lie in communicating effectively with children of different ages and abilities. This skill takes time to acquire; some will acquire it faster than others.

It is important to establish a rapport with the child and his or her parents and siblings. Introduce yourself to the child and other family members as you welcome them into the consulting area. Try and allow the children (including the siblings) to feel relaxed and comfortable during the consultation; this is more likely if there are a variety of toys and games lying about the room. Children up to and including school age may well prefer to be on a parent's lap, eventually feeling confident enough to explore the room during the history-taking.

After the presenting complaint has been defined, information about the child's previous well-being and that of the family and their circumstances need to be recorded.

In the very young child, history-taking should include information about the pregnancy, labour and delivery as well as the condition at birth and early feeding progress, details of immunisations and a developmental history. These details may become less relevant in the older child. Previous illnesses, hospital or doctor attendances as well as recent and previous medications are required in any child's history.

The family history is important and can be clearly presented by using a two-generation family tree. Include details about parents' and siblings' medical histories and make direct queries in line with the presenting problems (Fig. 12.1). If an autosomally recessive condition is being considered, it may be necessary to ask if the parents are consanguineously related. Although a large proportion of the world's families involve cousin marriages, this is a delicate subject that should be dealt with in a tactful way. One approach is to enquire if the parents have any relatives in common (e.g. grandparents or cousins) (Fig. 12.2).

At first it can seem intrusive to ask about the child's family and any surrounding issues. One approach is to tell the child and family that you are going to ask a number of routine questions about the child's background after hearing about the presenting complaints. The initial history-taking is the most 'natural' opportunity to collect this information, as having to go back and ask more questions out of the context of history-taking is more awkward.

The social history is separate from but allied to the family history. It is important to understand the composition of the household in which the child lives. The two-generation family tree can be further annotated with names, occupations and other details, helping to fill in details of the child's social

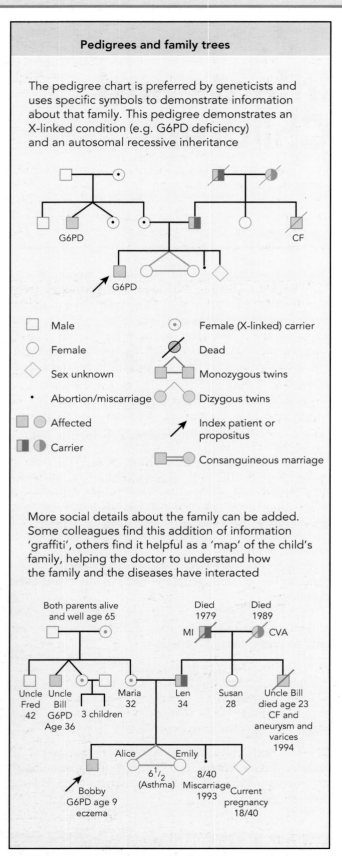

Pedigrees and family trees

The pedigree chart is preferred by geneticists and uses specific symbols to demonstrate information about that family. This pedigree demonstrates an X-linked condition (e.g. G6PD deficiency) and an autosomal recessive inheritance

More social details about the family can be added. Some colleagues find this addition of information 'graffiti', others find it helpful as a 'map' of the child's family, helping the doctor to understand how the family and the diseases have interacted

Fig. 12.2 The three-generation family tree.

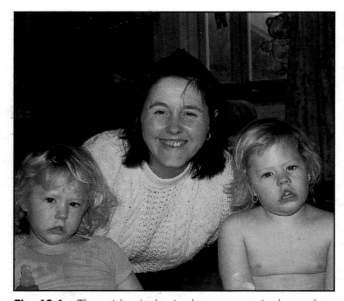

Fig. 12.1 These identical twins have myotonic dystrophy, as does their mother. This picture shows the phenomenon of 'anticipation', in which the condition is worse in each successive affected generation.

history. It should include details about the parents' occupations and whoever else is helping with child care. Children old enough to be attending nursery or school should be asked the name of the establishment as well as how they are getting on.

Child abuse is a common problem. Children can be harmed by adults in a number of different ways: emotionally, physically, neglected, sexually or, rarely, by induced illnesses and poisoning. The nature of any injury or illness in any child, from any background, must be explained satisfactorily in the history and be a plausible cause of the findings seen on examination. If you have any such concerns about a child or family you must share them with colleagues and social services.

THE EXAMINATION

Inspection and observation are the most important skills to be developed if you are going to arrive at the right diagnosis. The younger the child, the more important it is to be able to observe the child's well-being and any physical signs from a distance. This process should start from the moment the child and family appear in front of you. Do not wake up sleeping children to examine them until you have observed them carefully first (Figs 12.3, 12.4).

How one approaches a child to be examined is determined by the child's age, level of development and understanding. The younger the child (except in the youngest of infants), the more imaginative one may have to be to ensure a satisfactory consultation but remember it is easy to make older children and adolescents feel patronised.

Whenever possible try not to allow your eye level to be higher than that of your patient. If necessary, get down on the floor; this may be very basic psychology but it works. If you are approaching a child seated on its parent's lap or on a bed or couch, when you are within 1 m of the patient the child should see you are coming down to eye level. This is especially important when several doctors congregate around a bed, for example, on ward rounds. Always remember what it is like from the child's perspective, especially when being surrounded by a group of unfamiliar adults.

It may take some time to win the confidence of young children. Sometimes the pyrexial, irritable child may not allow you any physical contact without crying and, despite a friendly approach, it may also be impossible to observe the child at rest. Once a child starts crying it may be difficult to continue with the examination.

Palpation and auscultation may be important parts of the physical assessment. The order in which you perform them depends on where the problem is, what the problem is likely to be and how ill and how cooperative your young patient is. Whenever possible start peripherally with the hands or feet, making it clear to the child that you are a friendly doctor. Percussion is rarely a rewarding process in the very young.

Young patients should think the examination is fun: if you present yourself as playing a game, they will be relaxed and you will gain more information; if a child

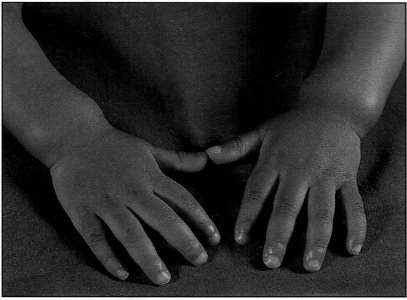

Fig. 12.3

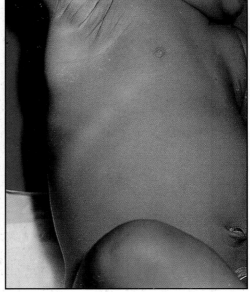

Fig. 12.4

Figs 12.3 and 12.4   Swollen wrists and rib ends seen in rickets. Observation may be all that is needed to notice these signs of rickets. Sometimes these findings are coincidental to the presenting problem.

is frightened or in pain, then this can be impossible to achieve. Make the child comfortable first. Ensure your hands are clean and warm and that your stethoscope will not be too cold on the child's skin.

Avoid unpleasant procedures if at all possible (e.g. rectal examinations). Think of what implications your actions may have in the future: if your examination and care of a child does not cause upset, and you relieve pain and discomfort effectively, that child is more likely to tolerate future examinations. It is better to have a limited but tolerable examination than to try and complete a full examination that results in an inconsolable child because the child is more likely to be uncooperative next time.

GROWTH AND DEVELOPMENT

Growth involves an increase in size and concludes when an individual has acquired full size and reproductive capabilities. Development parallels growth and leads to individuals acquiring all the skills and attributes that enable them to achieve full independence from their parents and to raise their own children.

GROWTH

Compared with other mammals and primates, humans give birth to very immature and dependent offspring. A human newborn will be completely dependent for most of its first year until weaned and walking. Our newborns have a head that is only just small enough to be delivered through the average woman's pelvis. The cerebral neuronal network is almost completed at birth, but is more or less devoid of myelin, whereas most other species have completed this essential 'wiring' before the end of gestation, hence the more advanced abilities of their newborns. Examine the growth in head circumference (or occipital frontal circumference) (Fig. 12.5) of a child in the first year of life and extrapolate this into the volume of brain growth. You can see why human beings cannot have more developed newborns – this is the price *Homo sapiens* pays for being bipedal with a narrow pelvis and large brain.

The continuum of growth from baby to adult has been described by three main phases (Fig. 12.6):

- The infant phase: a continuation of the exponential fetal growth rate that slows down into the second

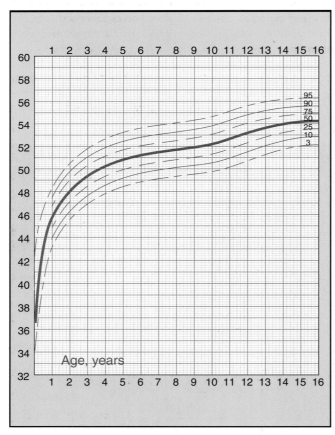

Fig. 12.5 Head circumference chart. The phenomenal growth in head circumference seen during the first years of life is as a result of brain myelination, without which the infant's development cannot advance. (© Child Growth Foundation, adapted with permission.)

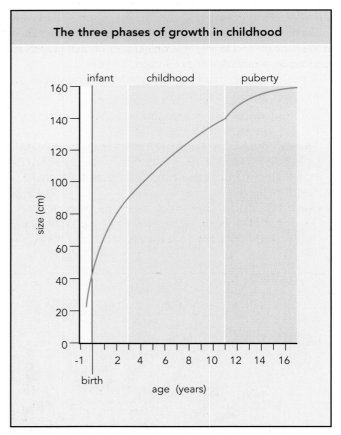

Fig. 12.6 Three phases of growth in childhood (after Professor J. Karlberg). The growth velocity varies at different ages, this is as result of many variable influences. Karlberg summarised the continuum into three phases, each with their own principal factors.

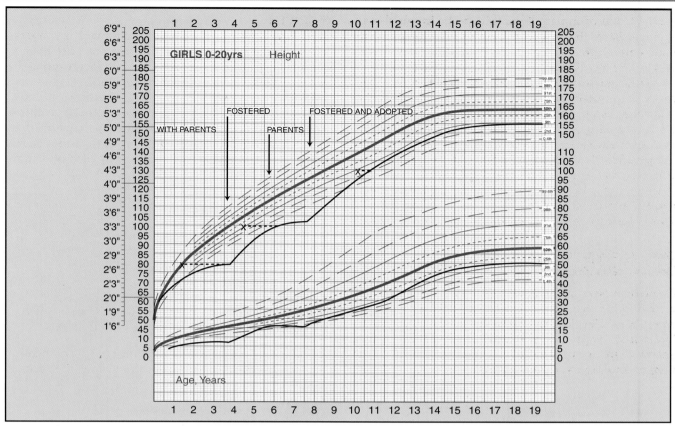

Fig. 12.7 Nonorganic failure to thrive. For some children who are not growing as well as expected, no organic cause can be identified. If they are removed from their home environment, their growth velocities may accelerate. The importance of an affectionate and loving environment for normal growth and development cannot be over estimated. (© Child Growth Foundation, adapted with permission.)

year of life. The critical factors in this phase are nutrition and hormones controlling metabolism, such as insulin-like growth factors (IGF) such as IGF_1.

- The childhood phase: this extends from the second to beyond the 10th year. The critical factors in this phase are the pituitary hormones (especially growth hormone).

- The adolescent (pubertal) phase: this extends from the onset of puberty until the achievement of final adult stature and fully mature reproductive capabi-

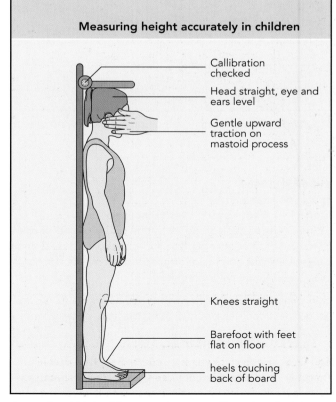

Measuring height accurately in children

Callibration checked

Head straight, eye and ears level

Gentle upward traction on mastoid process

Knees straight

Barefoot with feet flat on floor

heels touching back of board

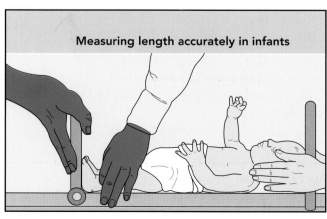

Measuring length accurately in infants

Figs 12.8 (left)/12.9 (right) Measurement of supine length and standing height. The measurement of length or height can be misleading and inaccurate unless done correctly, especially in infants.

lities. The critical factors in this phase are the sex steroids (androgens and oestrogens).

Each of these phases is interdependent on a large number of factors such as genetics, nutrition, hormones and the environment (including love and affection) (Fig. 12.7).

Any examination of a child is incomplete without an assessment of growth and development. It is usual to assess weight in all ages, supine length (Fig. 12.8) and head circumference in infants (under the age of 2 years), and standing height (Fig. 12.9) in older children. Growth charts are used to help to determine the expected range at any given age; there are standards derived for most developed nations and by the World Health Organization. Either the standard deviation scores either side of the mean, or centiles, are used to recognise the different normal variations in growth and growth velocity. The more serial measurements there are available to plot, the more

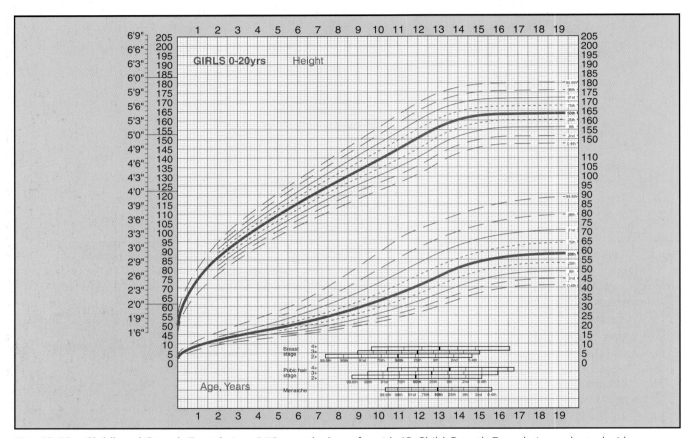

Fig. 12.10 Childhood Growth Foundation. (UK) growth charts for girls (© Child Growth Foundation, adapted with permission.)

Pubertal stages

Breast development
Stage 1 – Preadolescent: elevation of papilla only
Stage 2 – Breast bud stage: elevation of breast and papilla as small mound. Enlargement of areola diameter
Stage 3 – Further enlargement and elevation of breast and areola, with no separation of their contours
Stage 4 – Projection of areola and papilla to form a secondary mound above the level of the breast
Stage 5 – Mature stage: projection of papilla only, due to the general contour of the breast

Pubic hair
Stage 1 – Preadolescent: the vellus over the pubes is not further developed than that over the abdominal wall, i.e. no pubic hair
Stage 2 – Sparse growth of long slightly pigmented downy hair, straight or slightly curled, chiefly along labia
Stage 3 – considerably darker, coarser and more curled. The hair spreads sparsely over the junction of the pubes
Stage 4 – Hair now adult in type, but the area covered is still considerably smaller than in the adult. No spread to the medial surface of the thigh
Stage 5 – Adult in quantity and type

certain one can be about whether the pattern of growth falls within an expected range (Figs 12.10, 12.11).

DEVELOPMENT

The evaluation of a child's development is more complicated than an assessment of growth. This is because there is a large variation in the normal patterns of development. Furthermore, an individual child's rate of development can vary, and there are also confounding transcultural and transracial differences.

Although newborn babies are dependent, they can hear, smell, taste, feel and see. By the end of their development they will be able to think and solve problems, be mobile and agile, develop innumerable skills and be capable of rearing their own children.

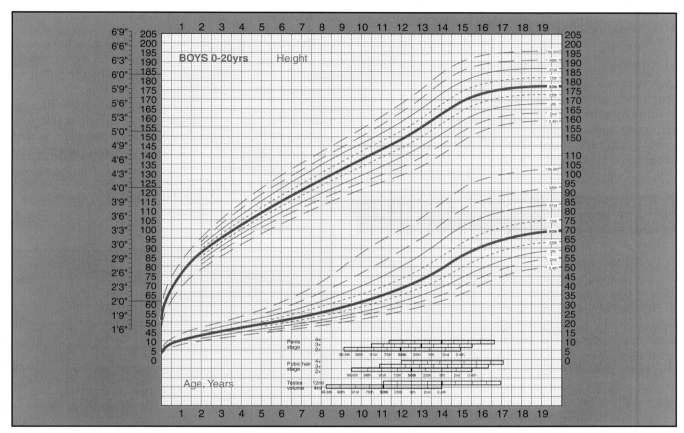

Fig. 12.11 Childhood Growth Foundation (UK) growth charts for boys. The charts for boys and girls are British standards derived from longitudinal data observed in cohorts of British children with cross-sectional observations used in updating them. (© Child Growth Foundation, adapted with permission.)

Pubertal stages

Genital (penis) development

Stage 1 – Preadolescent: testes, scrotum and penis are of about the same size and proportion as in early childhood

Stage 2 – Enlargement of scrotum and testes. Skin of scrotum reddens and changes in texture. Little or no enlargement of the penis at this stage

Stage 3 – Enlargement of the penis, which occurs at first mainly in length. Further growth of testes and scrotum

Stage 4 – Increased size of penis with growth and breadth and development of glans. Testes and scrotum larger; scrotal skin darkened

Stage 5 – Genitalia adult in size and shape

Pubic hair

Stage 1 – Preadolescent: the vellus over the pubes is not further developed than that over the abdominal wall, i.e. no pubic hair

Stage 2 – Sparse growth of long slightly pigmented downy hair, straight or slightly curled, chiefly at the base of the penis

Stage 3 – Considerably darker, coarser and more curled. The hair spreads sparsely over the junction of the pubes

Stage 4 – Hair now adult in type, but the area covered is still considerably smaller than in the adult. No spread to the medial surface of the thighs

Stage 5 – Adult in quantity and type

parents) is a very important milestone of higher cortical function. Most behaviour observed in newborns before this event is the result of responses initiated by the brainstem and spinal cord, for example, startling to sound and the primitive reflexes.

HISTORY

The feeding history is important because feeding is the most strenuous action the newborn has to do. Any compromise in cardiorespiratory function is revealed in difficulty in taking or completing feeds. In breastfed babies, it is difficult to be certain how well the feeding is progressing because the quantities of feed are unknown. Mothers breastfeeding for the first time may not be sure how well they (both) are doing. Ask the mother how often and for how long her baby breast feeds, how she feels the feeds are progressing, and whether she has any subjective feelings of let down of milk. Documented weight gain in the baby and the mother feeling that her breasts empty are helpful indicators. With bottlefed babies it should be easy to ask about quantities of infant formula taken.

Details about maternal health, the pregnancy and delivery, as well as the baby's condition and birth weight, are important to record. Apart from any parental concerns, ask about vitamin K administration, jaundice, stools and how the baby responds to handling. Pay close attention to what an experienced mother's observations have to say about her baby: she will have spent a great deal of time observing the baby closely; if she perceives something different about this baby then it may be an important diagnostic clue.

EXAMINATION

Newborns and young babies are examined when they are acutely ill or, more commonly, during routine checks. The observation and skills used are common to both the acute and routine situations. You should plot the progress of weight and head circumference on a centile chart. The baby must be undressed to be fully examined.

Specific aspects about the 'routine neonatal examination' are discussed at the end of this section.

Review
Gestation and weight of gestation

- Term
  - born before 37 and 42 completed weeks gestation from last menstrual period (LMP)
- Preterm
  - born before 37 completed weeks (259 days) gestation from LMP
  - note that a preterm baby's age can be expressed as either a chronological (uncorrected) age or an age postconception (corrected); the latter is important when considering growth and development in the first 2 years
- Post-term
  - born after 42 completed weeks (294 days) gestation from LMP
- Small for gestational age or 'small for dates'
  - birth weight below 10th centile for gestational age
- Large for gestational age or 'large for dates'
  - birth weight greater than 90th centile for gestational age

Review
Low birth weight (LBW) babies

- Important because of the increased morbidity and mortality seen in the affected infants
- You must differentiate between babies who are preterm, normal for gestation or small for gestational age
- LBW defined as < 2.5 kg birth weight; about 7% of UK births
- Babies > 2.5 kg birth weight may be at risk of similar complications because of antenatal growth retardation such babies appear emaciated.
- Very low birth weight (VLBW) defined as < 1.5 kg; about 1% of UK births (mostly all preterm)
- Extreme low birth weight (ELBW) defined as < 1.0 kg; about 0.5% of UK births (almost exclusively very preterm)

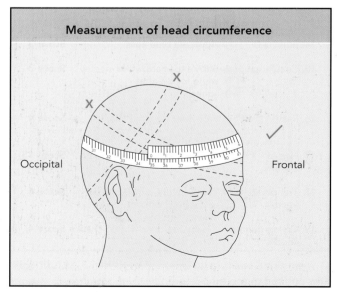

Measurement of head circumference

Occipital   Frontal

Fig. 12.15 Measurement of head circumference. The simplest 'investigation' in paediatric neurology.

Circulation and cardiovascular

The order of examination will depend on the condition of the baby. Auscultation of the heart sounds and listening for murmurs may be the priority before the baby cries. Inspection of the newborn's colour and perfusion is crucial. Peripheral cyanosis is common in the first days of the newborn period (acrocyanosis) because of vasoconstriction and relative polycythaemia (haemoglobin range 14.9–23.7 g/dl at birth): capillary refill time may therefore be more sluggish. Central cyanosis is best observed in the tongue and mucous membranes; these may be the only sites that are noticeably blue in cyanosed nonwhite babies. On inspection, the only signs of congenital heart disease, may be respiratory distress at rest. A pale baby may be anaemic or even hypoxic.

The rate, rhythm and character of the brachial and femoral pulses (Fig. 12.16) need to be assessed. Weak or absent femoral pulses may suggest coarctation of the aorta, as would four-limb blood pressure measurements demonstrating an upper limb to lower limb gradient in blood pressure. Large volume pulses are found with a patent ductus arteriosus. The precordium should be palpated and the presence of an apex beat (usually on the left) and heaves or thrills noted (Fig. 12.17).

The separation of the two components of the second heart sound on auscultation may be difficult because of the baby's fast heart rate (Fig. 12.18). A single second heart sound may indicate pulmonary outflow obstruction. Innocent (nonpathological) systolic murmurs are common in the newborn and may be heard on day 1 in over 20% babies who have structurally normal hearts. Pansystolic and continuous murmurs are suspicious, as are ejection systolic murmurs that radiate to the back or neck. Many babies with structural congenital heart disease may not have a murmur, although they may have symptoms and other signs of cardiovascular disease.

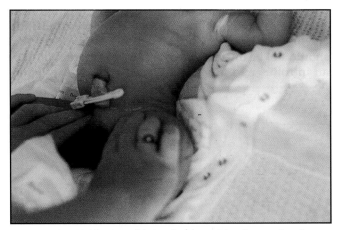

Fig. 12.16 Palpating femoral pulses. The femoral pulse can be difficult to feel; use a point halfway from pubic tubercle to anterior superior iliac spine as a guide and do not press so firmly as to occlude the pulsation.

> **Review**
> **Normal range for newborns**
>
> - Heart rate: 110–160 beats/min (>180 tachycardia)
> - Systolic blood pressure: 50–85 mmHg (very variable, depending on age, gestation and weight)
> - Respiratory rate: 30–50 breaths/min (>60 tachypnoea)

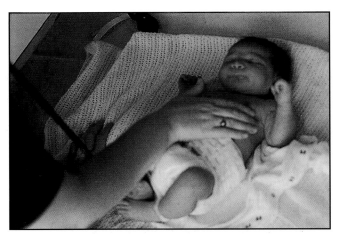

Fig. 12.17 Palpating the apex beat. Palpate the whole precordium, left and right. The apex beat is usually palpated in the left fifth intercostal space in the midclavicular line.

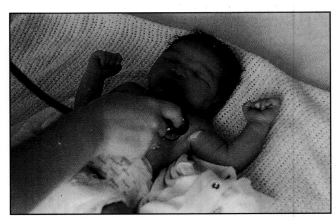

Fig. 12.18 Auscultating the heart sounds and listening for murmurs. Even when the baby is asleep, it can be hard at first to differentiate the first and second heart sound; palpating a brachial or femoral pulse simultaneously may help you.

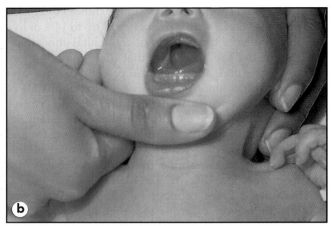

Fig. 12.30b Cleft palate. Inspect the palate and palpate for any clefts.

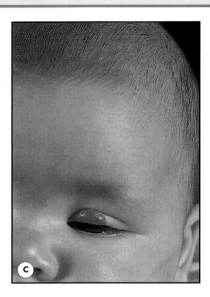

Fig. 12.30c
Cavernous haemangioma. Cavernous haemangiomas ('strawberry naevus') can occur anywhere, are more common in preterm babies; they get bigger during the first year and eventually regress. Treatment is only indicated if the naevus interferes with breathing, feeding or vision or if otherwise problematic.

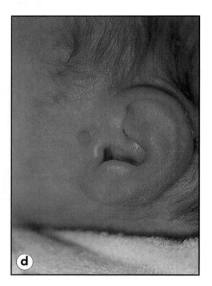

Fig. 12.30d
Preauricular tags. Preauricular tags are common and often there is a family history. They may represent a cosmetic problem requiring plastic surgery or they may be associated with other otological abnormalities.

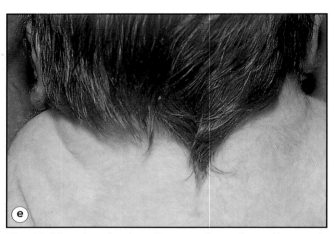

Fig. 12.30e Low hairline. Examine the scalp and hair and hairline. This may be indicative of a syndrome, a low hairline is seen in Turner's syndrome.

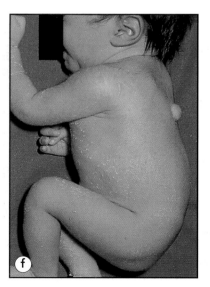

Fig. 12.30f
Thoracic myelocele. Neural tube defects are now less prevalent in developed countries. Examine the back carefully by inspection and palpation from occiput to coccyx. If a neural tube defect is detected, remember to examine for signs of hydrocephalus and bladder and bowel function as well as dislocated hips.

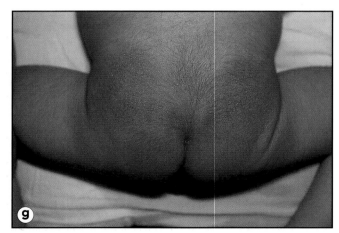

Fig. 12.30g Blue spots. These 'Mongolian' blue spots are common in all racial groups (except those of Northern White European origin). They are present from birth and may persist beyond the third year.

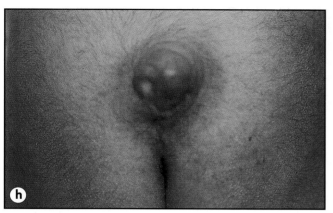

Fig. 12.30h Lumbar meningomyelocele. Lumbosacral neural tube defects are the most common. Folic acid supplements before conception and in early pregnancy have helped to reduce the incidence of these serious malformations.

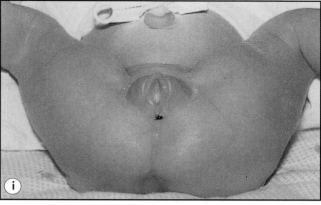

Fig. 12.30i Imperforate anus. Anogenital abnormalities need to be excluded by careful history and inspection. Meconium can be passed via a fistula into any other cloacal structure (e.g. the vagina). These abnormalities are seen associated with other congenital abnormalities.

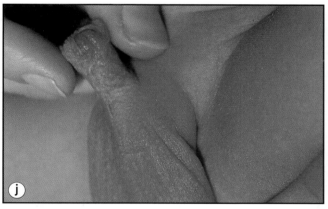

Fig. 12.30j Hypospadias. Check that the foreskin has fused normally on the ventral surface of the glans. If it has not, then note where the external urethral meatus is sited. Hypospadias occurs when the urethral meatus is not at the tip of the glans; commonly it is mild and on the glans, or rarely, more severe and on the shaft of the penis or perineum. Check for fixed flexion of the penis (chordee).

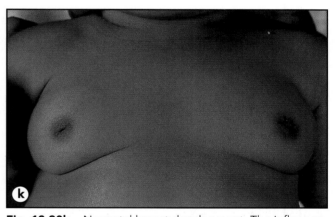

Fig. 12.30k Neonatal breast development. The influence of maternal hormones may result in palpable breast tissue of babies of either sex. No action is required and this resolves spontaneously.

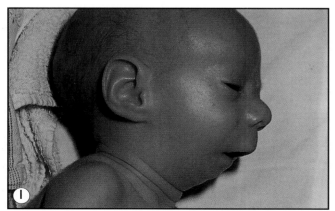

Fig. 12.30l Micrognathia. A small mandible with a normal-sized tongue represents a potential hazard to this baby's airway. A cleft palate can be associated. Breathing and feeding may need some assistance.

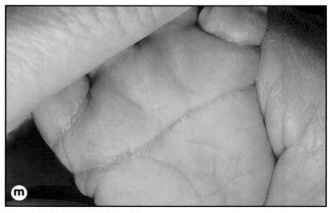

Fig. 12.30m Single palmar crease. A single palmar crease can be a normal finding. However, it can be part of a series of minor observations which can add up to a more important diagnosis, such as Down's syndrome.

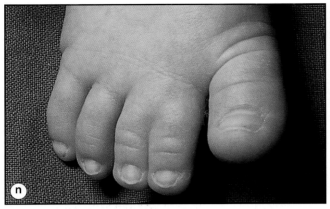

Fig. 12.30n Syndactyly of the second and third toes. Minor congenital abnormalities like this, when isolated, are common and often familial. Noticing one minor finding should prompt you to ensure there is not another to be observed.

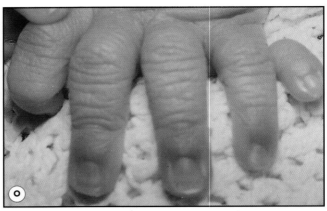

Fig. 12.30o Postaxial extra digit. Also very common and often familial. Refer for a plastic surgery consultation, rather than having them 'tied off'.

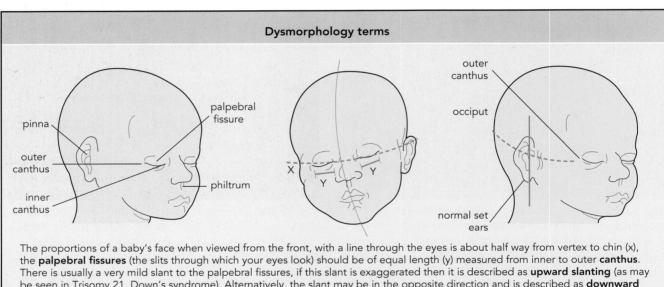

Dysmorphology terms

The proportions of a baby's face when viewed from the front, with a line through the eyes is about half way from vertex to chin (x), the **palpebral fissures** (the slits through which your eyes look) should be of equal length (y) measured from inner to outer **canthus**. There is usually a very mild slant to the palpebral fissures, if this slant is exaggerated then it is described as **upward slanting** (as may be seen in Trisomy 21, Down's syndrome). Alternatively, the slant may be in the opposite direction and is described as **downward slanting** (as may be seen in many syndromes).

The distance between the eyes is approximately that of the palpebral fissures (y).

Hypotelorism is when this distance is too short and **hypertelorism** is when this distance is too long and the eyes appear too far apart. The **philtrum** leads from the nostrils to the edge of the upper lip.

A line from the outer canthus towards the occiput should cross the attachment of the upper helix of the **pinna** (ear lobe) to the side of the head. Where this does not occur then the ear is described as **low set** and may appear **simple** (poorly formed helix) and **rotated** as well.

upward slanting palpebral fissures

downward slanting palpebral fissures

low set and rotated ear

Fig. 12.31 Facial dysmorhology vocabulary explained. A few of the commonly referred to anatomical terms used in describing facial features are demonstrated.

Differential diagnosis
Baby rashes

Newborns have to adapt from an aqueous, thermally-regulated environment to the outside world. They have to keep their skin moist and stay warm. There are a variety of cutaneous phenomena that are benign and self-limiting.

Confusion can occur when trying to differentiate between staphylococcal septic spots (not common but serious) (Fig. 12.32) and erythema toxicum, a transient eosinophilic infiltration of the skin (very common and completely benign) (Fig. 12.33). The former spots are often in skin creases and get bigger and 'more angry', the latter look red but are transient and appear anywhere on the baby.

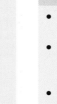

Review
Examination of newborns and young babies

- Babies are routinely seen by doctors for checks at birth and at 6–8 weeks old
- All newly qualified doctors should be able to perform a routine neonatal examination and define a baby as normal or otherwise
- Babies can become ill at an alarming rate and all healthcare professionals seeing them can benefit from scoring systems to help them to evaluate symptoms and signs
- Observation is the most important skill that paediatricians and children's nurses use to assess babies

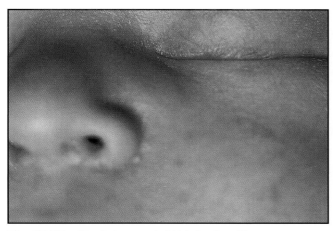

Fig. 12.32 Staphylococcal skin infection. The appearance of pustules in moist skin creases that do not spontaneously go away may herald the collapse of the baby with staphylococcal sepsis.

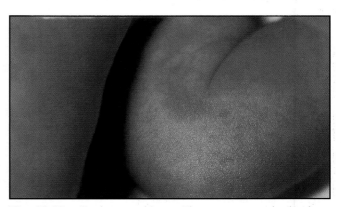

Fig. 12.33 Erythema toxicum. These spots can look a lot like staphylococcal pustules except that they spontaneously disappear and reappear in another area of skin. The rash is caused by eosinophilic infiltrates that are of no serious significance.

OLDER BABIES AND TODDLERS

The term 'infant' has been used previously to describe children under 2 years of age. We prefer to think of 'older babies' as being infants that are not yet walking and 'toddlers' as babies who have only recently acquired this skill. These children are frequently brought to their doctor. They attend for routine immunisations and developmental checks and are most likely to be seen by doctors in various settings (e.g. primary care, accident and emergency departments, community clinics, paediatric departments).

This period involves very rapid changes in growth and especially in development. During this period, the child progresses from being primarily supine and unable to move around, to becoming a toddler who is able to run and talk.

At the beginning of this period the effects of passively acquired maternal immunity (transplacental immunoglobulin G) mean that babies are not as prone to inter-current viral illnesses as they will be later (Fig. 12.34). From the age of 3 or 4 months this passive immunity is diminishing and immunologically the baby is now on his or her own. On average, the healthy older baby and toddler will have to deal with eight self-limiting viral illnesses per year. Sometimes two or three of these illnesses will occur 'back to back', causing a great deal of anxiety in the parents, and the infant may temporarily fail to thrive. This acquisition of active immunity to the common viruses prevalent in the child's community is a part of normal growth and development.

In many developed countries, a comprehensive immunisation programme from birth to 2 years aims to prevent up to nine or more important infectious diseases (e.g. diphtheria, tetanus, pertussis, polio, *Haemophilus* type B infections, meningococcal group C infections, measles, mumps and rubella). Visits for primary immunisation provide an opportunity for the infant's primary care physician to observe an infant's growth, development and general health.

GROWTH

Babies in this phase are still growing rapidly. There is a distinct deceleration in their growth velocity in the latter part of the first year and into the second year. The 'average infant' will have doubled birth weight by approximately 5 months and trebled it by just after a year.

The most dramatic changes are seen in head growth. This is as a result of myelination of cortical tracts and pathways leading to rapid brain growth, which are crucial in enabling developmental advances in this period.

DEVELOPMENT

At the beginning of this phase, a baby's cortical function has only recently demonstrated the important milestone of social smiling (6–8 weeks age). By the end of this phase (aged 2 years) the child will be walking, communicating wants and needs verbally and nonverbally and have developed sophisticated hand function and coordination.

The key question in this age group is: *Are the parents concerned about their child's developmental progress?* Only occasionally do parents seem truly unaware of their child's significant developmental problem.

The first areas to develop rapidly are vision and the control of hand movements and the next are the gross locomotor skills needed to roll over and sit without support. During this time visual acuity and hand dexterity are continuing to improve. Fine and gross motor development rely heavily on the progression of visual development. The child listens to adults and siblings intently. He or she starts to babble and to understand more and more of what is said. Once confidence is gained when prone with hips flexed, the baby finds himself or herself teetering on hands and knees and then begins to crawl. Soon after that, the toddler is pulling up to stand and cruising around the furniture: the prelude to solo walking. Fine motor skills include the continued refinement of grasp until the pincer grip (Fig. 12.35) is achieved. At around the same time, vocalisations have become more and more specific and 'dada' and 'mama' are said with meaning. Comprehension of language now includes following some instructions and commands. This is all usually achieved in the first year.

In the following year, continued improvements in walking (with the feet less far apart) are followed by running at speed, kicking a ball and rapid changes in direction. Fine motor skills are seen in manual dexterity (tower of six cubes) and improved self-help abilities (feeding with a spoon, drinking from a cup and beginning to undress themselves). Communication continues to advance with the increase in vocabulary and the combination of words to make short phrases. Comprehension of language is still greater than expressive language abilities.

HISTORY-TAKING

During a consultation the parents are the usual historians. The baby or toddler will often arrive with siblings in tow. By involving the whole family in the consultation, the child may be put at ease and a more satisfactory result obtained.

The history should cover the same areas as with the newborn and very young baby and include points particularly relevant to this period, for example, current feeding, weaning, developmental abilities, immunisations received.

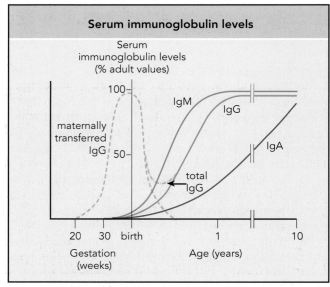

Fig. 12.34 Immunoglobulin levels vary with age. At birth babies have had a transplacental transfusion of maternal IgG that wears off by the end of the first 6 months. This provides passive immunity to the newborn baby; afterwards the child must develop his or her own active immunity after infection or immunisation.

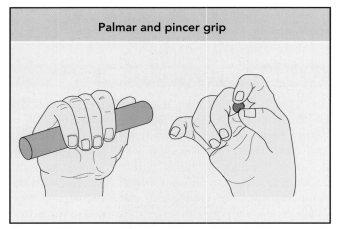

Fig. 12.35 Palmar and pincer grasp. The development of palmar and then pincer grasp represents a great step forward in fine motor skills and relies heavily on visual feedback.

EXAMINATION

During the history it is often best to keep the child on the parent's lap and play with them. Depending on how well you are getting on, you may be able to start examining the child. If the child is wary, it may be necessary to demonstrate your intentions by examining an elder sibling, teddy or parent. Try and show the child that whatever you are going to do is more of a game, rather than anything threatening to them.

It is important, as with newborns, to examine the most relevant system indicated by the history first because this may be your only chance. Make sure that you have examined the whole child undressed by the end of your examination. This should be done in stages. Save the more unpleasant parts of the examination (e.g. looking at the ears and throat) until last.

Circulation and cardiovascular system

Look at the child's colour and ask if there have been any dramatic changes in this. Infants are now no longer polycythaemic; indeed they are likely to be 'physiologically' anaemic (lower end of expected range for haemoglobin is 9.4 g/dl at 2 months and 11.1 g/dl at 6 months).

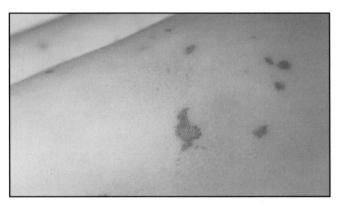

Fig. 12.36 Purpuric rashes: meningococcal septicaemia. All purpuric rashes in childhood need careful evaluation. The lives of patients with meningococcal disease depend on their doctor recognising this purpuric rash as early as possible. Note that the rash may start off as erythematous and then progress to nonblanching purpura. It is the speed of the rash's progression and the patient's degree of illness that are the hallmark of this infection. Treat immediately with an appropriate parenteral antibiotic.

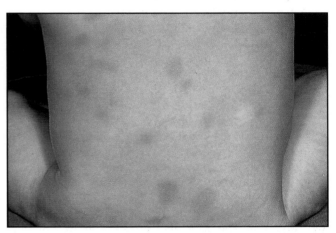

Fig. 12.38 Purpuric rashes: fingertip bruising; nonaccidental injury. All children have falls and minor injuries that result in bruises. Most bruises occur in areas of likely accidental impact (e.g. shins and elbows). Any bruise in a usually protected site is a worry. Ask how it happened. Is the injury consistent with the history? If you are worried, discuss immediately with senior staff.

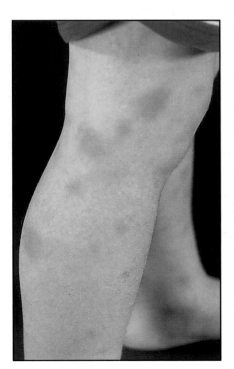

Fig. 12.37 Purpuric rashes: idiopathic thrombocytopenic purpura (ITP). ITP in childhood differs from the adult condition by being more benign and is self-limiting. Acute leukaemia is a very important differential diagnosis to be rapidly excluded by a full blood count and blood film.

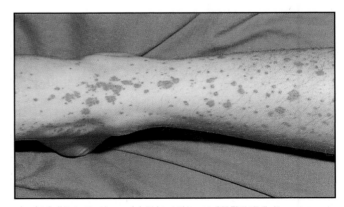

Fig. 12.39 Purpuric rashes: Henoch–Schönlein purpura (HSP). HSP is an 'allergic' vasculitis that has a characteristic distribution along the back of the legs, extending up to the buttocks. It is associated with many systemic symptoms, such as joint swelling and (uncommonly) may result in permanent renal impairment.

Rashes in childhood are very common and all you need is a simple and logical approach to make a diagnosis most of the time.

- The most clinically important rashes to recognise promptly are ones that are purpuric (nonblanching), for example, meningococcal septicaemia (Fig. 12.36), idiopathic thrombocytopenic purpura (Fig. 12.37), fingertip bruises in nonaccidental injury (Fig. 12.38) and Henoch–Schönlein purpura (Fig. 12.39).
- If the rash is erythematous (blanching) and is associated with an intercurrent illness, then it is most probably related to an infection: often viral and self-limiting
- Any chronically itchy rash is likely to be eczema and should be treated with emollients

Central cyanosis can be missed if a 'dummy' (or pacifier) is not removed from the mouth.

Capillary refill time is a very sensitive sign and should be the same as for adults (less than 2–3 s). Environmental cold stress can prolong the capillary refill time in otherwise well babies. As in newborns, the cardiac output is mostly regulated by rate rather than stroke volume. Tachycardia is an important physical sign that needs evaluation, e.g. febrile, unwell, upset and crying?

Blood pressure should be measured in any sick infant or when cardiovascular, renal, endocrine or neurological diagnoses are being considered. The interpretation of a single blood pressure measurement requires knowledge of three factors: what size of cuff was used relative to the child's upper arm; the size of the child; and what emotional state the child was in at the time of measurement. The cuff size is critical, as blood pressure measurements may be spuriously high if too small a cuff is used or the infant is crying. Normal ranges are published according to size and age.

Palpation of the apex beat is helpful because some murmurs may be palpable as heaves or thrills. During auscultation of the heart sounds, normal splitting of the second heart sound may be difficult to hear in a tachycardic child.

Nearly one-third of children will have a murmur heard at some point of their lives. Less than 1% of children will have a structural heart lesion. Innocent murmurs have particular characteristics: ejection systolic flow murmurs are either 'short and buzzing' (caused by turbulent aortic flow) or 'soft and blowing' (caused by turbulent pulmonary flow); venous hums are low pitched and more noticeable after exertion or inspiration and they are abolished by lying supine.

True pathological murmurs are usually louder, harsher and longer and may radiate or have a diastolic

Children's blood pressure measurements can be obtained using:
- Oscillometry (dynamap)
- Sphygmomanometry (using a stethoscope or Doppler probe or by palpation)
- Direct (invasive) measurement (in intensive care)

Remember the two-thirds rule:
- Cuff width must be at least two-thirds of the distance from shoulder to elbow
- Cuff (bladder) length must be at least two-thirds of the limb circumference

component to them. Look for other symptoms and signs of cardiovascular disease.

Breathing and respiration

Watching and listening to the child's respiratory pattern is the most useful part of the examination of the respiratory system. Auscultation may add some more information, but is frequently 'drowned' by loud transmitted upper respiratory tract breath sounds.

Look at the upper respiratory tract (in the ears, nose and throat) at the end of the examination. Coryza (profuse discharge) and pink inflamed mucous membranes in the throat and ears are most likely to be caused by a viral upper respiratory infection. Antibiotics are not required unless a true secondary bacterial infection is suspected.

Lymphadenopathy (localised or generalised) is common in association with frequent upper respiratory tract infections and viral illnesses. It may appear to persist if there is little or no interval between these infections. Acutely tender lymphadenopathy can be associated with bacterial infections. Persisting, asymmetrical large and nontender lymphadenopathy in association with constitutional symptoms needs accurate diagnosis and prompt treatment.

Abdomen

Bile-stained vomiting, pallor, excessive inconsolable crying, a distended abdomen, lumps in the groin and blood in the stool are all indicators of an acute abdo-

- Heart rate: 110–150 beats/min (>160 tachycardia)
- Systolic blood pressure: 80–95 mmHg (depends on age and height)
- Respiratory rate: 25–35 breaths/min (>40 tachypnoea)

minal problem. Children with peritonitis will lie very still, with their knees flexed, and breathe without moving the diaphragm. A diagnosis needs to be established and the child treated promptly.

After careful inspection, palpation can be attempted with warm hands. This will be a fruitless exercise if the infant is crying. Patience is needed and more than one attempt at palpation may be required, perhaps when the child is sleeping on a parent's lap.

Examine the anogenital area. In boys, always check that the testes are in the scrotum (a visual check will do, if they are obviously present). Do not attempt to retract the foreskin (it is physiologically adherent to the glans). In girls the external genitalia are less visible than when they are newborn. The labia majora are fleshy and obscure the introitus, clitoris and urethral opening. The vulval area in young girls is consequently infrequently observed by doctors. It is often preferable to ask someone more used to examining girls' perineums when this area is the focus of the presenting problem in young girls.

The hip joint is a frequent causes for concern (in many age groups) because of an acquired limp. As in abdominal palpation, if the child is not relaxed then the chances of a meaningful examination are limited. With the child on the parent's lap, gently explore the passive range of movements the child will tolerate. Look at the child's expression, to know when to stop. Internal and external rotation of the hip (with the hip and knee both in 90° of flexion) is one of the most reproducible and sensitive ways to pick up hip joint pathology.

Neurology and development

The neurological assessment of infants relies heavily on history (for developmental skills) and inspection and observation for confirmation of the reported abilities and the presence of any focal signs. The history is the key in many neurological diagnoses. When dealing with possible fits or 'funny turns', a first-hand account is best of all; a parent's video of the episode may be most valuable. Observation is more important than testing reflexes. Flexibility and improvisation are needed to extract whatever physical sign you are trying to elicit. Save the cranial nerve examination until last and check behaviour, movement, gait and coordination by observation while the child plays.

Observation of gross motor skills will enable posture, power and, when the child is picked up, tone to be assessed. In younger babies antigravity power should be demonstrable by lifting the limbs or, when prone, the head off the bed. Assessment of truncal tone is important in the youngest of babies upwards. The limbs can be inspected and palpated in play to ascertain tone, muscle bulk, power and sensation (by gently tickling). Deep tendon reflexes can be elicited with patience. In an easily distracted child, reinforcement can be employed in play (squeeze the toy) if necessary. Coordination is hard to test formally in this age group and the observation of fine motor skills and gait are the most one can rely on.

The cranial nerves can be assessed by observation of behaviour and facial expression.

The olfactory (first) nerve This is rarely tested but smell can be assessed by asking the toddler to find a mint hidden in a handkerchief.

The optic (second) nerve In babies and toddlers visual acuity can be checked formally by a variety of techniques in a visual laboratory. Examining the visual fields and employing fundoscopy is often difficult in this age group. However, in the older (preschool age) child this is more straightforward and acuity can be checked beyond the age of 2 years with shape or letter matching.

The oculomotor, trochlear and abducens (third, fourth and sixth) nerves For assessing these nerves, eye movements can be observed when the child follows a toy or light in the vertical and horizontal plane. Nystagmus is normally seen in extremes of lateral gaze or may be pendular in a severely visually impaired child.

The trigeminal (fifth) and facial (seventh) nerves
The trigeminal nerve can be tested when the jaws are clenched on a bottle or biscuit, and the facial nerve by encouraging the child to smile or shut their eyes.

The acoustic (eighth) nerve In some places hearing is still routinely screened in children from 7 to 8 months of age. Many places have now introduced universal Oto-Acoustic Emission (OAE) Hearing Screening in the neonatal period.

 Differential diagnosis
Cranial nerve lesions in children

Cranial nerve lesions are not very common. Here are three important ones:
- Probably the most common cranial nerve to malfunction is the eighth nerve. Sensorineural hearing impairment occurs in approximately 0.1% live births and has a variety of congenital and acquired causes
- A lower motor seventh nerve lesion, as seen in a Bell's palsy, or after birth injury (forceps), is reasonably common. Remember that there are a number of causes, some more benign than others. With Bell palsy check blood pressure and perform an audiogram
- A sixth nerve palsy may be a sign of raised intracranial pressure. (The affected eye looks medially or convergently.) Most childhood squints are convergent (or alternating) and are due to refraction differences or ocular muscle imbalances

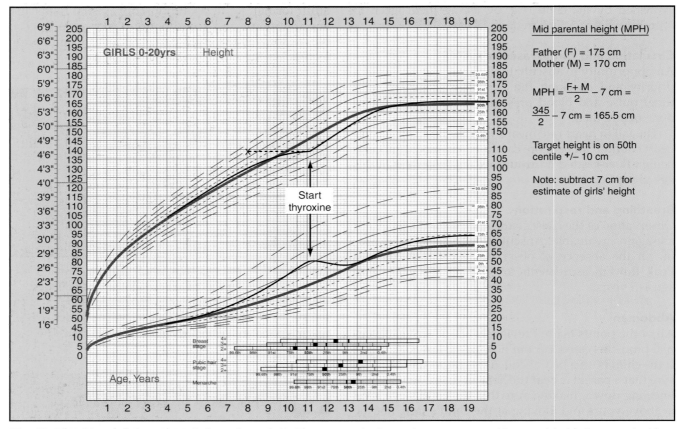

Fig. 12.41 Growth failure: juvenile hypothyroidism. These growth charts demonstrate an 11-year-old girl diagnosed with hypothyroidism. Note how her height velocity has decelerated with a retarded bone age. After starting thyroxine she looses weight, her height catches up and her puberty progresses rapidly (see Fig. 12.10 for pubertal stages). (© Child Growth Foundation, adapted with permission.)

tions may be due to inadequately managed or unrecognised chronic illness (e.g. asthma or coeliac disease) or endocrine problems (Fig. 12.41, 12.42).

DEVELOPMENT

These children are spending the majority of the day away from home, at school. They will become more independent from their parents and carers but more dependent on their peer group. Social and behavioural aspects of development are now more important. Language and cognitive skills, literacy and numeracy are further developed in class and at home. Vision, hearing and motor skills are approaching adult abilities.

HISTORY

It is a good idea to invite the child to be the historian and rely on the parent for back-up. Some will want their parents to give all the history, whereas others may be very capable historians. This will depend on the child's character, previous (good or bad) experience of a doctor and how ill they are. Children with chronic diseases are often poor at the long-term history but more reliable with the acute story. It is important to pitch the questions in terms the child understands and which are not patronising (e.g. using the family's terms for faeces, penis, bottom and so on).

Background information about the home and especially school is important. Establish how much the presenting complaint affects the child's life at school and at home. It only school time is affected then the problem may not be an organic one. Hobbies, sports and pastimes give other clues to the seriousness of the illness and its impact on the child's life.

EXAMINATION

The sequence of the examination is now more or less dictated by you. There are very few differences in technique from examining adults, except that the examination should continue to be fun. Peak flow can be used as a reproducible way of monitoring asthma (Fig. 12.43).

ADOLESCENTS

The adolescent group of patients is not usually very well served by the medical profession, particularly in the latter half of adolescence.

Paediatricians and general practitioners usually feel confident with the initial part of adolescence but this wanes towards the middle and end of adolescence. There are many reasons for this:

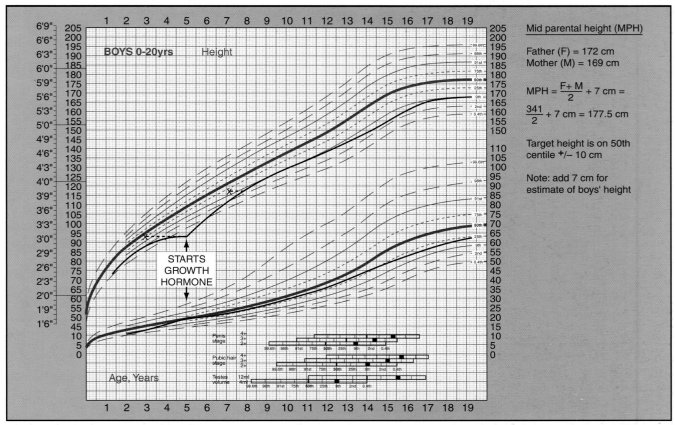

Fig. 12.42 Growth failure: early idiopathic growth hormone deficiency. This boy's infant growth appears reasonably normal, although perhaps less than his midparental height may suggest. His height velocity decelerates drastically by the age of 5 years and the diagnosis is made. Growth hormone supplementation through the rest of childhood and adolescence provides catch-up growth and a reasonable final adult height. His puberty is a little later than average (see Fig. 12.11 for pubertal stages). (© Child Growth Foundation, adapted with permission.)

Review
Normal ranges for school-age children

- Heart rate: 80–120 beats/min (>120 tachycardia)
- Systolic blood pressure: 90–110 mmHg (depends on age and height)
- Respiratory rate: 20–25 breaths/min (>25 tachypnoea)

Review
Examination of school-age children

- School-age children are usually very healthy and do not see their doctors much
- Examination is in a manner similar to adults, as long as everything is explained adequately
- Psychological factors are becoming increasingly relevant

- Adolescents seldom consult their doctor, so neither is very familiar with each other.

- Adolescents are in the transition from childhood to adulthood and are uncertain as to how to behave as adults, but do not want to behave as children.
- Doctors need to allow them to be adolescent and accept that the adolescent is easily embarrassed and often anxious.
- The presenting problems can have a psychological basis.
- Adolescents with a chronic illness (e.g. diabetes, cystic fibrosis, sickle cell disease) will demonstrate normal adolescent rebellion, which can have serious long-term health consequences.
- Risk-taking behaviour (cigarettes, alcohol, drugs, sex, etc.) is normal and when it does go wrong, in health terms, it is hard not to appear judgemental and authoritative as the doctor.
- Deliberate self-harm (overdoses especially) in adolescents is becoming more prevalent. Understanding the reasons for this behaviour can be challenging.
- Confidentiality and consent are sometimes a source of conflict between patient, parent and doctor.

The adolescent's doctor needs to be aware of, and open-minded about, the nature and cause of the com-

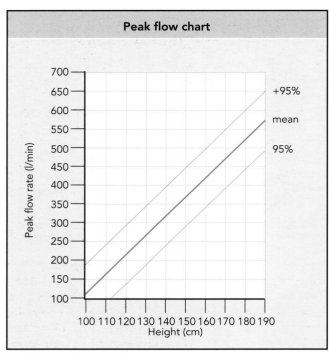

Fig. 12.43 Peak flow chart according to height. These data are valuable in predicting an expected range for peak expiratory flow rate in girls and boys according to their height. Most 5-year-olds can be taught to do reproducible peak flows, which can help in the diagnosis and monitoring of asthma.

plaint and sensitive to the patient's need to be seen with (or without) a parent. Adolescents are usually able to give informed consent for examination and treatment if the reasons are explained to them in a way they can understand. They are still their parent's (or carer's) legal responsibility and problems can arise when there is a disagreement. It is good practice to communicate effectively with both the adolescent and parents.

GROWTH

During the first 10 years there is remarkably little difference between the height and weight velocity in the growth of girls and boys. Both have a slowly decelerating growth until puberty, then there is a growth spurt that lasts for 2–3 years. This will complete the child's physical transformation into a young adult (Figs 12.44, 12.45 and see Figs 8.1, 8.3 and 9.4).

The adolescent phase of growth is initiated by sex steroids that are produced by the gonads, stimulated by gonadotrophins from the anterior pituitary. Along with the dramatic increase in size and growth, these sex steroids will promote the development of secondary sexual characteristics and fertility.

PUBERTY

The onset of puberty is less than 1 year apart in girls (mean age 11.4 years) and boys (mean age 12.0 years)

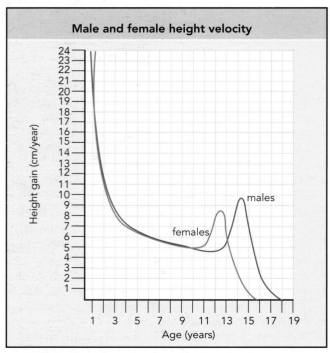

Fig. 12.44 Height velocity in girls and boys. Note how before the pubertal growth spurt there is little difference in girls' and boys' height velocities. Also note that girls' pubertal height velocity peaks are earlier and less tall than those for boys. These are thought to be the main factors determining the difference in adult male and female height.

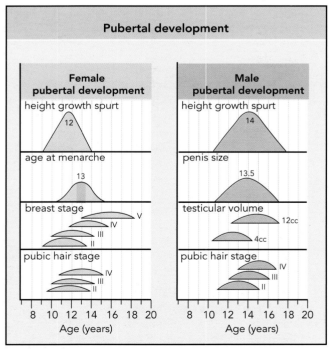

Fig. 12.45 Pubertal staging in males and females. These standard puberty stagings are important to note whenever you plot children's growth in the second decade (see also Figs 8.1, 8.3, 9.4, 12.10 and 12.11).

but the pubertal growth spurt occurs in girls approximately 2 years before boys. The first physical sign of puberty in a girl is the development of breast tissue under the nipples (mean age 11 years); the first physical sign in boys is the enlargement of the testes from their prepubertal volume of less than 2 ml to an endocrinologically active volume of greater than 4 ml (mean age 12 years). However, a boy's growth spurt does not occur until the testicular volume is approximately 10 ml.

A delay in growth and puberty can be a source of great unhappiness for the adolescent who is endocrinologically normal but, because of an inherited tendency, develops and matures more slowly than peers (Fig. 12.46).

A constitutional delay in growth and puberty is more of a problem for boys than girls because boys have their pubertal growth spurt 2 years later than girls and because boys' growth spurts are larger than girls', so its absence is more apparent.

Over the next 2 years in girls, and 3 years in boys, there are changes in body shape and composition (lean mass and distribution of body fat) along with growth of pubic hair (and facial and body hair in boys).

Dx Differential diagnosis
Constitutional delay in growth and puberty

- This condition is most common in boys
- Patients usually have a history of growing in the lower quartile of the normal range but by the middle teenage years are very much shorter than their peers (at this time they present to a specialist clinic)
- Severe psychological stress may result from this genetic and physiological delay in puberty
- Pharmacologically inducing puberty is an effective way of relieving the stress suffered by these patients

In girls, when the growth spurt (height velocity) decelerates to less than 4 cm per year, the menarche can occur; height continues to increase for 1.5–2 years after the menarche. Final adult height is achieved when the bony epiphyses fuse in the vertebrae and along the long bones of the leg. It is impossible to evaluate an adolescent's growth without knowledge of what stage of pubertal development they have reached.

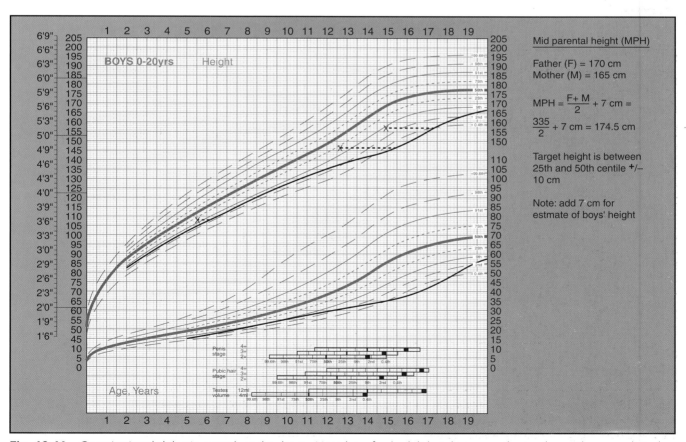

Fig. 12.46 Constitutional delay in growth and puberty. Note how final adult height is near the tenth centile as predicted by the growth velocity observed between age 4 and 10 years. He was most psychologically stressed in his 16th year (see Fig. 12.11 for pubertal stages.) (© Child Growth Foundation, adapted with permission.)

DEVELOPMENT

Development continues long after growth has finished. It is mostly in the spheres of social and behavioural development that adolescents are still progressing. This age group is requesting and gaining more independence from their parents and carers. They have completed their primary education and will be completing their secondary education by the end of this phase. Interests will change and relationships with peers are crucial to the adolescent's self-image.

The gap between the end of growth and the end of development into a fully independent adult is apparently widening. The mean age for pubertal milestones appears to have come down from that of a century ago. In the developed world, there is a decreased need for unskilled workers and an increased need for skills and higher education to be a successful provider. Thus the end of 'development' is often only complete after the age of 20 years.

HISTORY

Depending on the presenting problem, it may be necessary to agree who remains in the consulting room. This is one area in which confidentiality and consent may become a point of conflict. When taking the history, it is important to direct your questions primarily to the patient, and only when necessary to the parent or carer.

Details about the family and relationships between members of the household are important. Details about school, progress with school work, hobbies, sports, pastimes and friendships can all help give an indication of how the adolescent is coping with the increasing stresses of the real world. Again, it is easier to take a quick trip through this part of the history at the beginning because, if problems of psychosocial issues arise later, it can seem awkward to 'go back' and ask the straightforward questions.

EXAMINATION

Most adolescents are very self-conscious of their appearance, so make sure they have suitable facilities to prevent undue embarrassment (e.g. blankets and screens around the examination couch). The examining doctor will need to decide during the history-taking whether the parent is to be invited alongside the patient. Which side of the screens should the parent stay? This can be difficult to get right every time. When an adolescent is seen alone during the physical examination, it is advisable to include a chaperone in the examination room.

Apart from the assessment of growth and puberty and attention to the adolescent and parent relationship, the rest of the examination will be similar to that for an adult patient.

Review
Normal ranges for adolescents

- Heart rate: 60–100 beats/min (> 160 tachycardia)
- Systolic blood pressure: 100–120 mmHg (depends on age and height)
- Respiratory rate: 15–20 breaths/min (> 25 tachypnoea)

Review
Examination of adolescents

- Adolescents are usually very healthy and do not see their doctors much
- They are generally not well served by their doctors
- Psychological factors are important
- Risk-taking is normal but hazardous (sex, drugs and so on)
- Deliberate self-harm is increasingly common and must be properly assessed by a trained counsellor on a case by case basis

Index

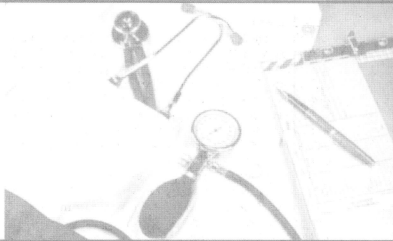